TREATMENT OF SKIN DISEASES
A Manual

Treatment of Skin Diseases

A MANUAL

CHARLES SHEARD, M.D.
F.A.C.P., F.R.C.P. (C), D.A.B.D.S.

Clinical Associate Professor of Medicine (Dermatology),
Cornell Medical College, New York City
Associate Attending Physician, The New York Hospital
Senior Dermatologist, the Stamford Hospital
Senior Dermatologist, St. Joseph's Hospital, Stamford, Connecticut
Visiting Dermatologist to the General Hospital,
St. George's, Grenada, West Indies

YEAR BOOK MEDICAL PUBLISHERS, INC.
Chicago • London

Library of Congress Cataloging in Publication Data

Sheard, Charles, 1914–
Treatment of skin diseases.

Includes index.
1. Skin–Diseases. 2. Therapeutics. I. Title.
[DNLM: 1. Skin diseases–Therapy. WR650 S539t]
RL110.S53 616.5′06 78–53581
ISBN 0–8151–7642–2

Preface

This book deals with the treatment of skin diseases. For diagnosis the reader should turn to the larger and more comprehensive textbooks. The rare and exotic is not dealt with in this manual. The deep mycoses are skipped, and much of the lymphomas are missing. X-ray therapy is condensed, and the section on tumors of the skin is short. More attention is paid to the compounding of lotions, creams and ointments, and to the description of surgical and electrosurgical techniques, as well as sterilization methods *in an office,* since such information is hard to find in standard works. Where applicable, names and addresses of suppliers are given. Thus, one major value of this manual may be analogous to a classified telephone directory. In other words, I have tried to list a variety of useful therapeutic methods and modalities for treating the common skin diseases encountered daily by students and practitioners.

Because dermatology is one specialty where *cure* rather than alleviation *is* possible in many instances (for example, in a drug-induced dermatitis), I have emphasized the management of commonly encountered conditions for which successful treatments are available, although sometimes not well known. Throughout the text, whenever possible, I have keyed descriptions of these conditions to specific illustrations in *Pocket Color Atlas of Dermatology.** As a diagnostic tool this book makes an excellent companion to my own.

The attitude that there is something inherently unscientific in the application of successful empiricism should be abandoned. Gold is still an excellent treatment for arthritis despite the lack of etiologic orientation for the treatment. There are

---

*Joseph Kimmig and Michael Jänner, *Pocket Color Atlas of Dermatology* (Chicago: Year Book Medical Publishers, Inc., 1975).

many equally empiric, yet successful, maneuvers in surgery and medicine. So my feeling is, if it works use it.

Occasionally my personal views may conflict with the reader's cherished concepts, and if this occurs I ask for indulgence. Remember, "Circumstances alter cases."

In an article entitled "Is There a Doctor in The Making?" (*Punch*, January 31, 1970)* John Rowan Wilson writes,

> "The aspect of their teaching which attracts most medical students beyond all else is, naturally enough, clinical medicine—the personal contact with patients. It is doubtful whether any other form of education has such a unique capacity to influence the attitudes of young people subjected to it, and this influence is exerted constantly in favor of individual rather than collective values. Clinical skills are founded on an empirical rather than a theoretical approach. They demand caution and responsibilities. There are incessant reminders of the fallibility of human nature and the limitations of human knowledge.
>
> The medical student is in the position, at once stimulating and harassing, of constantly being asked to do things. Not for him the happy aloofness of the student of political science. . . . He lives in a state of constant apprehension that tomorrow he may be asked to diagnose a difficult case or lance an abscess, or deliver a baby.

Besides the stamina to stand on one's feet for sixteen hours a day, the effective clinician must be able to manage clinically difficult problems; he must have mastered practical, therapeutic skills. The patient must *see* his doctor's concern for his personal problem and sense that something is being done to relieve him.

I write all this to defend the totally clinical orientation of this manual, which is written from the viewpoint of years of practical experience treating patients in a busy office setting. As such it attempts to retain much of the old that is good (that works) and embrace much of the new that shows promise. If it offers the reader one additional way to get his patient better, then it will have been worthwhile.

The author wishes to acknowledge the sometimes pointed but always helpful criticism of the several physicians who offered comments on the early text. Thanks are due to Dorothy Pullman, who typed the manuscript and contributed in many ways to the completion of this book.

CHARLES SHEARD, M.D.
Stamford, Connecticut

Contents

1 / Some General Principles in the Application of All Treatment

It is essential to remember that no matter how little the physician may know about the disease, he always knows more than the patient, that is, if he follows Osler's dictum and listens to the patient. The patient is trying to give the physician the diagnosis. So the physician should listen to the patient and question him systematically and persistently.

Most of the patients coming to the dermatologist's office have had their rashes treated either by the advice of friends or by the most appropriate remedy available in their medicine cabinets at home. Many such patients cure themselves of minor skin problems in this way. However, when the problem persists and they seek help, it is wise to get a list of the previously used medications, including internal medications, and perhaps some pertinent family history and other background data. An atopic family history (eczema, asthma, hay fever or hives) will suggest inherent therapeutic difficulties. Patient histories may also disclose contraindications to systemic steroids, such as in cases of gastrointestinal ulcer, tuberculosis, diabetes and heart disease.

The physician should learn to identify those patients who treat themselves too harshly with home remedies, by too vigorous cleansing (for example, with pHisohex, the one-time panacea), or even with excessively stern application of prescribed treatment. Many patients with bland dermatoses, such as pityriasis rosea, are so emotionally disturbed by the appearance of their inexplicable rash that they scrub themselves harshly and produce irritation.

A difficult problem is the elderly man with winter itch

(xerosis, asteotosis), who wears tweed trousers and takes daily hot showers with antibacterial soaps. He cannot comprehend the advice to stop bathing. It takes at least three interviews to get through to many such patients. They often do much better when given a printed sheet of instructions setting forth in understandable terms the nature of their skin disorder and a means of correcting it.

The printed instruction sheet saves many an after-hours telephone call. It is excellent practice to have such instructions printed, for example, how to make a starch bath, a boric acid compress or Epsom salt soaks, how to care for a hand dermatitis, and how to manage winter itch. In addition, some postoperative instructions for the care of wounds are valuable. In the office, we use Zephiran solution for the face and tincture of Merthiolate elsewhere and have forms printed to tell the patients how to apply these.

The patient's known allergies to medications are important and, if possible, should be noted on the initial visit. We use bright red stickers on the front of the chart for patients who have drug allergies and other essential phenomena; in a busy office this can prevent many an embarrassing incident.

An assessment of the patient's normal skin problems can be made at a glance, with experience, but still should be noted on the chart, such as "redhead," "fair," "thin, sensitive skin," "finds all soaps drying on the face," or "lips chap in winter." A patient with such traits would have to be carefully forewarned of the irritative powers of such acne treatments as sulphur or benzoyl peroxide lotions. The patient should begin with extremely mild local treatment, and as the tolerance to the medication increases, strong medications or higher concentrations of the starting medication can be gradually introduced. One thing to watch for in *all* patients with acne is overenthusiasm.

In general, patients who suffer from skin disorders will have widely varying individual reactions to medication, and this should constantly be borne in mind. Irritation or aggravation, as distinct from true allergic reaction, will have to be watched for until the patient is stabilized. It is essential to set up return visits for every patient. A patient should never be allowed to leave the office without a fixed return appointment. The well-followed patient will be cured and grateful. The patient who is told to "let me know if it doesn't clear up in a week or two" won't let you know and won't be grateful, and will complain that you couldn't cure him! Occasionally we give patients a return appointment but tell them if their skin clears up they can call and cancel.

Occasionally physicians encounter the type of patient who cannot remember to take pills or put on an ointment, and who by masterful inattention has "gone through" four or five other physicians and perhaps seven or eight other ointments and is no better. The patient should bring in his jars and check the amount used. Often about one sixteenth of an inch will be used from each jar. The patient should demonstrate his method of application if possible. This often is an education in itself. Very often the lack of cure in patients is due, *not* to the incorrect choice of medicine, but to the inability of the patient to apply it properly, or to the failure on the part of the physician to carefully instruct his patient on how to do it. With some of these patients, the treatment should be done *in the office.* Either paint it on, rub it in, inject it, or shine a lamp on, but do it in the office even if the patient is charged for only every fourth visit. This may be the only way to cure some of these patients.

"Ut aliquid fieri videatur" (let it be apparent that something is being done) is a good maxim. The physician must get up and do something for the patient besides talk to him even if it is only to take a scraping or look at the skin with magnification. The "laying on of hands," of which much therapy is merely an extension, still has healing power—mystical and perhaps a little ridiculous in our age of debunk, but nevertheless real.

As Sutton says, "A doctor must impose his will on his patient, and this can be done best with graciousness, diplomacy and reason."[1] In these days of moderately sensationalized medical news items, a misinformed intelligent patient can be a trial, and a misinformed unintelligent patient can be a monster. With the constant application of the techniques of persuasion, an attitude of confidence, courage and sympathy, and I might add humor, a physician can bring even "hardened cases" through to a successful conclusion. A good throw-away line that always gets a smile from a serious pessimist is "Cheer up, you'll never get out of this world alive!" Another is Stokes' "What difference will it make 100 years from now?" The physician must not be flip, but certainly the light touch with a cheery smile dispels gloom.

Many patients with continuing skin problems fear they have cancer and are not being told. Most patients will ask about this when a good rapport has been established, but sometimes the physician hears from a relative that the patient is afraid to ask if he has cancer. The patient should be informed whenever possible that what he has is not catching and not cancer. Much of the time if a patient is told that he has his own private allergy, he will like that.

On follow-up visits, changes in medication may have to be made because the patient may have improved greatly up to a certain point and then cannot seem to get beyond that despite very accurate application. This "getting used to it" may be partly due to actually becoming acclimatized to the medication and partly due to a change in the stage of the dermatitis, from acute to subacute or from vesicular to squamous peeling. Early in the management of a dermatosis, it is wise for the physician to see the patient at moderately frequent intervals, say from three to seven days. Later, visits can be spaced at two-week intervals or even longer. Often, when it is a matter of assessing the final result of a compensation dermatitis venenata, several months may elapse between visits.

Principles of Dermatologic Treatment

Vehicles are used to distribute active medication over the skin and hold it on the surface, to absorb water or prevent evaporation, or to assist in cooling the skin surface, depending upon the particular situation. Variability in the type of vehicle is therefore a necessity in the external management of skin disorders, as is an accurate assessment of the type of medication required. In general, if the skin is dry, lubricate it; if it is wet and oozy, dry it. If the skin is acutely inflamed, soothe it; and if it is chronically thickened and indolently unresponsive to mild treatment, stimulate it. Theoretically, it would seem that a drug should be most active if it is less soluble in the base than in the water or oil of the skin, that is, if there were a gradient of solubility that would transfer the drug from the base to the skin. This has not been demonstrated except perhaps in the case of phenol, which is rarely caustic in an oily or alcoholic vehicle in which it is readily soluble, but is more caustic in water in which it is less soluble. The transfer of a drug from the vehicle to a cutaneous base is accomplished by mechanical means, e.g., by rubbing or sometimes by selective solution (dimethyl sulfoxide 30% penetration in 3 hours). In general, transfer is good when the vehicle is miscible and compatible with the cutaneous phase and when the drug is soluble in both the vehicle and the mixture, as, for example, boric acid in water on oozing skin, or salicylic acid in castor oil on oily skin.

Drugs cross the epidermal cell membrane by a process of diffusion, and the concentration of the drug is important. A pH gradient will help penetration, as will a concentration gradient. Other factors of concern are (1) dermal circulation; (2) thickness of the stratum corneum, e.g., palms and soles vs. eyelids and foreskin; (3) temperature, with heat-facilitating transport; (4) maceration or hydration by moisture, which facilitates transport; and (5) disruption of the stratum corneum by excoriation, which also facilitates penetration. The barrier is in *all* layers of the epidermis, not in any special layer.

Compounds with a water partition coefficient close to 1 are the best penetrators. Dr. Richard B. Stoughton says that 5% thiobendazole used on the sole of foot epidermis by a technique of punch biopsy of tissue from corneum after 20 hours resulted in inhibition of known fungus inoculum on Sabouraud's agar in 11 of 26 cases.[2]

If the drug is more soluble in the mixture than in the vehicle, transfer is also good, as for example boric acid in polyethylene glycol on an oozing sore. However, when the vehicle is immiscible with the cutaneous base (e.g., phenol in petrolatum on oozing sores), even though the drug is soluble in both the vehicle and the cutaneous base, transfer is only fair; and if the drug is insoluble in either the vehicle or the cutaneous base, transfer is poor.

The question of chemical compatibility must be borne in mind; for example, sulfur and mercury in the same prescription lead to mercury sulfide (which is highly irritating and dark colored). But it is important that the drug be evenly distributed through the base and stay that way. Accordingly, water-soluble drugs should be dispersed in oil-in-water emulsions and other water-miscible bases, and not in oils such as greases, waxes, fats or petrolatum. Oil-soluble drugs should be dispensed in greases, waxes or water-in-oil emulsions, and not in water-miscible bases. Insoluble drugs such as sulfur may be dispensed in any base in which they form an even, stable mixture.

The vehicle may be important. For example, when strychnine in oil of orange is applied to the skin of the white mouse, the mouse dies, but with strychnine in castor oil, nothing happens—not only because of the physical rate of release from the emulsion or suspension of the active ingredient, but also because of its capacity to aid in penetrating the skin. Possibly this is an effect of strychnine entering the hair follicle or sebaceous gland, because in general nothing penetrates the stratum corneum, although lard (oleic acid) and peanut oil (linoleic acid) get part way through.

The compounding of a lotion or emulsion is of some importance to the ultimate result of its application. A pharmacist who knows how to use an electric homogenizer and makes well-compounded smooth lotions will produce treatments that achieve superior results for the dermatologist's patients. An example of this is lotio alba, which must be made *fresh* with the best zinc sulfate which has not effloresced or lost water. The patient should be instructed to use it up quickly over a six-week, or at the most an 8-week period, as its effectiveness in the compounded lotion rapidly decreases. Lotio alba is very useful in the treatment of acne and rosacea, but it must be borne in mind that all sulfur can produce a chapping dermatitis, often at a slight distance from the area where it is applied. Very often, patients, in applying this lotion immediately before bedtime, will rest their head on the pillow and in turning their head smear the lotion so that the sides of the neck and other areas such as the eyelids will contact the sulfur; this will produce irritation which causes the patient sometimes to be afraid to use the medication. All patients should be warned about the possibility of chapping, irritation and excessive redness and be advised to search in the mirror to see if there are examples of this beginning. If so, the patient should stop using the lotion for a few nights and then resume it. Gradual acclimatization can occur, and the patient can become used to the sulfur and tolerate it so that the ill effects do not occur. The strength of the lotio alba may be gradually increased, starting with perhaps 4 gm zinc sulfate and sulfurated potash (each) in 60 gm rose water (each) and then 8 gm and 12 gm and even 16 gm later on, gradually increasing the strength as the patient requires it or becomes used to it. (See Formulary, no. 1.)

Shake Lotions

Shake lotions are the most commonly prescribed lotions, for example, calamine. (See Formulary, no. 2.) They are suspensions of powders in a watery vehicle, suspended by shaking or in some cases by the addition of a suspending agent, e.g., tragacanth. When the suspensions are applied to the skin, usually with the fingers, the water evaporates, imparting a cooling sensation and leaving the powders drying on the skin in a protective film. Some powders are easily wetted by water, for example, calamine and Neocalamine, calcium carbonate, kaolin, magnesium carbonate, starch, zinc oxide, zinc carbonate and titanium dioxide. Other powders not readily dispersed in water, such as cinnabar, talc, sulfur precipitate and zinc stearate, require the addition of a wetting agent to the lotion.

Aromatic substances usually are only slightly soluble in water though soluble in oils, for example, camphor, menthol, phenol and thymol.

Fixed oils, such as crude coal tar, balsam of Peru and benzyl benzoate, require emulsification. When a lotion is made without a suspending agent, the powders are usually triturated together in a mortar, adding *just enough* of the vehicle to make a thick paste; when smooth, the balance of the vehicle is added, triturating all the while. If hydrophobic powders are included, the addition of a little glycerin will usually correct the problem. This is especially true in the case of sulfur. High concentrations of glycerin should be avoided, however, since glycerin is an irritant on occasion. Another emulsifying agent such as bentonite magma (a paste that contains about 5% bentonite) is often very helpful. Excellent suspension can be obtained when at least 40% of the total volume of the lotion is bentonite magma. Bentonite is a native hydrated colloidal aluminum silicate. Note that it takes 24 hours to make bentonite magma. Burow's solution and other acids coagulate bentonite magma, and cannot therefore be used in combination with it. Bentonite magma is also incompatible with resorcin monoacetate, but not with resorcin. (See Formulary, no. 3.)

In the manufacture of lotio alba, the active ingredients, chief of which is probably hydrogen sulfide, are formed by chemical reaction. The use of sulfurated potash of excellent quality and fully hydrated zinc sulfate is an absolute necessity for obtaining a satisfactory therapeutically active lotion. If the pharmacist has zinc sulfate in a cardboard container so that it loses water, the sulfate lotion will produce an excess of zinc sulfate and it will be irritating. The same holds true if the pharmacist uses a poor-quality sulfurated potash. The ordinary white lotion prescription is usually zinc sulfate 4%, sulfurated potash 4%, and rose water q.s. to 100%, which might be termed a starting lotion, since often the patient with acne has used this for a month or so before he finds that it is becoming ineffective. Then he can have the strength of the lotion increased by doubling the quantity or later tripling or quadrupling the quantity. Irritation, which is usually manifested by chapping erythema and excessive desquamation, has to be watched for, as mentioned.

In making shake lotions in general, it is advisable to keep the powders to about 40% of the total and use no more than 15% glycerin, since glycerin can irritate tender skin in higher concentrations and tends to make the lotion too sticky. The following is a suitable drying shake lotion:

Zinc oxide	20
Talc	20
Glycerin	15
Alcohol 70%	
Water $\overline{aa}$ q.s. ad	100

If to this basic lotion you add active drugs in the form of powder, you decrease the other powders to keep the total amount of 40%:

Sulfur precipitate	20
Zinc oxide	10
Talc	10
Glycerin	15
Alcohol 70%	
Water $\overline{aa}$ q.s. ad	100

Some drugs will change the consistency of the lotion. Salicylic acid will make the lotion stiffer. Resorcin and Ichthyol will make it thinner, so in the case of the former, the percentage of liquids should be higher, and in the latter, the percentage of powders should be higher. (See Formulary, no. 4.)

Tars and oils (except liquor carbonis detergens or coal tar solution) do not go into lotions well unless an emulsifier, e.g., tragacanth, is used.

It takes 6 oz of shake lotion to cover the average adult body. Lotions are best for treating superficial dermatoses, especially if there is slight oozing, and should not be applied to hairy areas where they tend to get crumbly or to a markedly oozing dermatitis where they tend to cake and form hard, cement-like plaques under which infection often supervenes.

Lotions should not be removed more than once a day, although they can be applied four to six times a day, applying fresh over old as long as possible. The dermatitic skin can be cleansed by warm boric compresses, warm water or mineral oil (olive oil plain or 30% olive oil in benzine), gently swabbing with dabs of cotton soaked in the cleansing ingredient and blotting with tissue afterward to soak up the oil.

Emulsions

Oil-in-water emulsions, e.g., milk or hydrophylic ointment, and water-in-oil emulsions, e.g., butter or cold cream, are discussed here.

Oil-in water emulsions can be made with tragacanth (around 1/30), bentonite magma (between 40% and 50%) or triethanolamine oleate or stearate. When an oil-in-water emulsion is applied to the skin, the aqueous phase is in direct contact with the skin and hence is more cooling and compatible with serum. Such an emulsion is less occlusive than a water-in-oil emulsion. Bentonite magma is probably the best emulsifying agent to use. A hand homogenizer or blender, such as is used in soda fountains, speeds up the work and gives superior results. Emulsions containing more than 30% oil are very thick and should be dispensed in wide-mouthed jars. They are also less stable.

An example of an oil-in-water emulsion is as follows:

Cade oil	4
Zinc oxide	15
Glycerin	8
Olive oil	24
Bentonite magma	50
Lime water q.s. ad	120

Another oil-in-water emulsion is Pusey's calamine emulsion (oil in water):

Phenol	0.2	
Bergamot oil	0.3	(may be omitted)
Tragacanth	1.0	
Zinc oxide	6.0	
Calamine	6.0	
Olive oil	33.3	
Water q.s. ad	100.0	

(Also see Formulary, no. 5)

Carron oil is a water-in-oil emulsion containing about 50% oil, with a divalent or calcium soap as the emulsifying agent.

Solution of calcium hydroxide
Linseed oil $\overline{aa}$ q.s. ad 120

The linseed oil must be at least 50%, and the emulsion is mixed with lime water (solution of calcium hydroxide). If the oil is rancid, the free fatty acids present are saponified by the alkali to form calcium soaps (calcium oleate). However, if the oil is of good quality, it may separate out. The addition of 0.5% oleic acid to each 50 cc linseed oil before mixing with the lime

TABLE 1-1.—EMULSIONS

WATER IN OIL	OIL IN WATER
Hydrous lanolin	Acid mantle cream
Eucerine (Duke) aquaphor and water	Almay emulsion base
Lubriderm	Cetaphil
Nivea cream (scented eucerine)	Dermabase (Marcelle)
Velvachol (Texas Pharmacol)	Neobase (Burroughs and Wellcome)
Polysorb (Fougera)	Hydrophilic ointment USP
Qualatum (Almay)	Unibase (Parke-Davis)
Aquaphor (Duke)	Multibase
Hydrosorb (Abbott)	Dermovan (Texas Pharmacal)
Hydrophilic petrolatum USP	Keri
	Vanibase

water helps considerably. This is Carron oil, so called because it was used at the Carron Iron Works in Scotland for burns. A thicker emulsion can be achieved by adding zinc oxide and calamine.

A good watery emulsion that is very useful for treating atopic patients utilizes ready-made lotion emulsion, e.g., Cetaphil lotion (Texas Pharmacal), which contains no true fats:

Kenalog suspension for intralesional use 50 mg
Cetaphil lotion q.s. ad 240

Another proprietary lotion emulsion is acid mantle lotion, oil in water (Dome Company), which contains aluminum acetate and has a pH of 4.5. Lubriderm, water in oil (Texas Pharmacal), contains lanolin.

Table 1-1 lists several emulsions and their manufacturers.

A formula that Dr. Sulzberger has suggested for cold cream is:

White wax	4.5
Light mineral oil	18.0
Sodium borate	0.92
Distilled water q.s. ad	30.0

Ointments

Ointments are salves, greases or grease-resembling substances with a butter-like consistency at room temperature.

Ointments can be mixed by using a slab and spatula for less

than 2 oz or mortar and pestle for more than 2 oz. The principle of having just enough of the vehicle to make a thick paste with the previously triturated solids still holds true. A smooth ointment can be made in this manner, whereas some substances, such as ammoniated mercury, have to be levigated (ground to a fine powder in the presence of a liquid in which it is insoluble) with a little mineral oil. In washable bases, a little water may be used. When the insoluble substance is finally dispersed, then it should be gradually incorporated into the ointment base.

Once crystalline solids are dissolved in a little water, the solution can be incorporated into the ointment base. Balsam of Peru should be mixed with castor oil, chloroform or soft soap before incorporating it into an ointment base to make it a smooth, permanent, nonseparating ointment.

Ointments serve to relieve dryness, brittleness and the fissures occurring in erythematous skin. Their most important role is as vehicles for chemically active agents. The solubility of a drug varies with the base used, and the drug's clinical effect on the skin may vary from one ointment base to another. Chrysarobin has a much stronger effect in petrolatum than in lanolin. Salicylic acid dissolves in oils better than in petrolatum, but is more active in aquaphor.

Greasy ointments should not be used for treating acutely inflamed oozing dermatoses as a rule. They are much better adapted for treatment of chronic scaling or deep processes.

Ointments can be applied by rubbing them in, with the patient wearing thin cotton material next to the affected skin (e.g., Surgitube), or covering them with a dressing, preferably linen or old cotton, and bandaging them in place. Except for use on extremities, this technique is not too practical for ambulatory patients; squares of dressing (e.g., linen or Telfa gauze) can be held in place more easily with plastic or adhesive tape. For the scrotum, jockey shorts are an excellent, comfortable dressing. They should not be washed with bleach and detergent to get the ointment stain out; mild laundering is enough.

Oils

Oils are used in the softening and removal of crusts, especially where there are thick masses of scale from the hairy scalp. They are also used to decrease the drying effect of the alcohol scalp lotions and to soften ointment bases. *Olive oil* is comparatively nonirritating, although it readily becomes rancid. *Sesame oil, rapeseed oil* and *peanut oil* are cheaper than olive oil and just as good as a rule. *Oil of almonds* is odorless and colorless, but expensive. *Castor oil* is wonderful for dissolving salicylic acid and imparting sheen to the hair in scalp lotions. *Linseed oil* has an unpleasant odor and is slightly drying, and *cod liver oil*, of course, smells.

Oils are used on the scalp if ammoniated mercury or sulfur precipitate (or something relatively insoluble) has to be applied to the scalp and kept on overnight prior to a shampoo. A mixture of castor oil and olive oil is a very effective base, although slightly unpleasant.

Other seldom-used preparations such as *benzoinated lard* NF (hog fat), the 10% powdered benzoin added to prevent rancidity, is an excellent base for oil-miscible medicaments. It has a pleasant odor but tends to liquefy in warm weather. A mixture of equal parts of benzoinated lard and hydrophilic petrolatum makes a base for mercury or sulfur scalp ointments which can be washed out without great difficulty. *Cocoa butter* (oltheobromatis), not to be confused with coconut oil (which is sometimes called "coconut" butter), has a high melting point of 30–35 C because its acids are 31–33% stearic. It is a good lubricant and is often used in massage, lip salves and cosmetic preparations. It probably deserves wider use as an ointment base.

Ceresin (ozocerite or mineral wax) is a naturally occurring mixture of hydrocarbons found chiefly in Galicia; there are also deposits in Utah. It is used in some creams and is said to have a blending effect, keeping solutions of waxes in oils from separating.

White ointment USP consists of 5 gm white wax and 95 gm white petrolatum. Waxes usually give an additional amount of smoothness to an ointment or a cream.

Petrolatum is the most common ointment base. It should have no petroleum odor, although it is derived from residual products in the refining of petroleum. It keeps well and never turns rancid. It keeps the skin supple and has a melting point close to skin temperature, so that it is sometimes absorbed by the clothing. It is often mixed with other greasy bases.

Pure anhydrous *lanolin* is very thick and does not apply easily to the skin, but it takes up water readily and then lubricates more easily. Anhydrous lanolin (in many respects similar to human sebum) can absorb between two and three times its own weight in water but is smelly and very thick, whereas hydrous lanolin (USP), which is 27% water, is a much more suitable ointment base.

Aquaphor, a cooling ointment consisting of petrolatum with the addition of lanolin derivatives, or *hydrophilic petrolatum USP* is as water miscible as pure lanolin and is an excellent base for extemporaneous compounding. It has the disadvantage of being greasy, of course, and the water droplets are sealed in grease (water in oil). But by mixing it with other bases, e.g., unguentum aquae rosae USP, a very suitable base can be obtained which is chemically effective and esthetically acceptable.

Cerates are mixtures of wax with oil or grease, fused while melted. There is no sharp distinction between ointments as to properties and uses. The main difference is that the cerate leaves a smooth, somewhat hard and less greasy surface when spread thin and is more difficult to wash off.

Ceratum has been dropped from the pharmacopeia but is retained as ceratin NF and is 30 gm white wax in 70 gm benzoinated lard. It is a fairly hard mixture, which needs warming before it can be spread well. With 2–5% salicylic acid, it makes an excellent treatment for rough xerotic skin in old people, and for pruritus hiemalis and ichthyosis.

Creams

Some ointments have a great capacity to absorb water, hence they can absorb oozing serum and produce a soothing, cooling effect, probably because of the evaporation of the absorbed water. They can therefore be called *cold creams.* (See Formulary, no. 6.)

Vanishing creams are oil-in-water emulsions made by rather complicated procedures with the aid of emulsifying agents. Many commercial bases of this type are available in pharmacies throughout the world, and since their preparation is complex, it is better to become familiar with a few bases of this type and their incompatibilities rather than try to have the compounding pharmacist make his own. Neobase (Burroughs & Wellcome) is an excellent vanishing cream with very few incompatibilities (but is currently hard to find). USP hydrophilic ointment is another standard one. Velvachol and Topisol (Texas Pharmacal) are also examples of creams with wide ranges of compatibilities. Almay's Qualatum is another elegant base that is compatible with most drugs used by dermatologists.

Since the water content is high, drugs that are not stable in aqueous media (e.g., antibiotics) should be used within a week or so, and refrigeration will help prolong their life.

The lack of occlusiveness of vanishing bases often lessens the therapeutic effect of the incorporated drugs, so that the patient has to be instructed to "rub in well until it vanishes" many times a day. It is often unfortunate to learn from a referred patient that the instruction was once or twice daily, which is hardly enough to have any real effect on the dermatosis. Vanishing creams are best suited for use on nonirritable dry dermatoses, but they must be rubbed in.

In general, ointment bases that are cosmetically elegant are not therapeutically effective. Most cold creams are essentially soap with a little oil added.

A washable nongreasy base recommended by Downing a few years ago consists of the following:

Sodium lauryl sulfate	0.8
Cetyl alcohol	15.0
Glycerol	5.0
White petrolatum	14.0
Water	35.0

Carbowaxes (see polyethylene glycol ointment USP)

By polymerization of ethylene glycol, a series of compounds has been produced, of which those with higher molecular weight have the consistency of fats or waxes, although they are soluble in water. This combination of properties has obvious advantages for pharmacies, especially for preparations used on the scalp. The compounds are good vehicles for water-soluble drugs, and they can be washed from the skin and hair with warm water with or without soap.

Carbowaxes are sold under the trade name of *carbowax compound* with a number that indicates the molecular weight of the predominating glycol; the one most commonly used is Carbowax 4000, which resembles beeswax in consistency and melts at 50–55 C. Carbowax 1500, which is about the consistency of petrolatum, melts at 35–40 C. Carbowax 1500 may be used alone as a vehicle, but is somewhat sticky when applied to the skin. If a considerable quantity of an aqueous or alcoholic solution is added, it liquefies. These disadvantages may be overcome by mixing Carbowax 1500 with Carbowax 4000 to make it harder and less sticky, or with propylene glycol to make it softer. By mixing these three ingredients in varying proportions, bases of almost any consistency can be prepared. Propylene glycol is used as the liquid ingredient, because ethylene glycol is toxic.

The following formulas are representative:

Propylene glycol	35 cc	Water	25 cc
Carbowax 1500	25 gm	Carbowax 1500	35 gm
Carbowax 4000	40 gm	Carbowax 4000	40 gm

Carbowaxes are very useful for treatment of the scalp. They make satisfactory pastes with sulfur or ammoniated mercury and are the best bases for zinc peroxide (which has not been used recently). They are unsatisfactory bases for oils, tars or oil-soluble substances, although Zetar makes a good mixture with carbowax, with or without zinc oxide.

Pastes

Pastes are 50% powders in a greasy base, basically zinc and talc as in the shake lotion, for example:

Zinc oxide	25
Talc	25
Petrolatum q.s. ad	100

Starch can be used, but it decomposes and tends to mat in the presence of moisture, although Lassar's paste (without salicylic acid) is still very popular. By reducing the content of powder to 40%, a softer zinc oxide paste (pasta zincie mollis) is made, which is less drying, less stiff and perhaps easier to apply although occasionally more "heating" to some patients.

Zinc oxide	20
Talc	20
Petrolatum q.s. ad	100

Adding small percentages of active ingredients requires no change in the basic paste formula. However, if larger amounts of liquid, for example, *tars,* are added, the weight has to be subtracted from the grease component. Powder ingredients similarly reduce the amount of powders in the base, for example:

Sulfur precipitate	20
Zinc oxide	15
Talc	15
Petrolatum q.s. ad	100

Pastes in general absorb moisture from the oozing surfaces and tend to "splint" the skin and put it at rest. They tend to be drying while keeping the skin somewhat supple and soft. Pastes stick better than ointments, have a more superficial effect than ointments and in general are soothing and rarely irritating. They should not be removed too often unless caked, although they should be cleaned off at least once every 24 hours with either mineral or olive oil as with lotions. A thick coating of paste is usually applied with the fingers and rubbed in well and then covered with tissue and wrapped with Kling or Surgitube to hold it in place.

Suspending Agents

Glycerin is miscible with practically all water-miscible bases and emulsions. It is a solvent for most water-soluble compounds and also for phenol, salicylic acid and iodine. It is used also for its emollient effects and for its hygroscopic properties, which keep aqueous preparations from evaporating to complete dryness, it is useful. It also serves as a pharmaceutical aid in dispersing hydrophobic powders and lessens drying, although in high concentrations it is very dehydrating and irritating especially to exposed tissue, usually in concentrations of more than 15%.

Acacia tends to be sticky and is not used much since it requires large quantities for suspension or emulsification of solids. It often imparts a sensation of tautness to the skin on drying.

Methylcellulose is a water-soluble, white, fibrous substance, which is stable, colorless and effective as a thickening or suspending agent when used in 2–4% concentrations. It can be obtained in various viscosities, of which the 1,500 and 4,000 centipoise viscosity types are the most useful. Pouring ability can be enhanced by the addition of 0.1% polysorbate 80 and 0.1% sorbitan mono-oleate (span 80) without disturbing the suspending properties.

Tragacanth is an effective suspending agent in concentration of 1% or so. Variability in quality occasionally lessens its effectiveness and #1 grade should be specified. Tragacanth is readily attacked by molds in solution, hence should be preserved by the addition of phenol, resorcin or one of the parabens. In oil-in-water emulsions, it should be about one thirtieth of the amount of fixed oil to be emulsified; if a volatile oil is used, approximately twice as much is needed.

Bentonite magma is the suspending agent of choice except in formulas containing Burow's solution, resorcin monoacetate, acids and acid salts. Excellent suspensions are obtained when 40–50% of the total volume of the lotion is bentonite magma. It takes between 12 and 24 hours to make bentonite magma.

Triethanolamine oleate and stearate are excellent emulsifying agents for some oil-in-water emulsions. However, they are incompatible with all acids, acid salts, divalent (Ca, Mg, Zn, Hg) and trivalent (Al) metal salts, but they are compatible with starch, titanium dioxide, phenol, camphor, menthol, liquor picis carbonis and sulfur. The triethanolamine soaps are formed during the preparation of the emulsion; the required proportions are one part of triethanolamine and 2.2 parts of the appropriate fatty acid. If oleic acid is used, the mixing can be carried out at room temperature, but with stearic acid or other waxes and fats with high melting points, heat is needed.

Solvents

Propylene glycol resembles glycerin chemically and in appearance. It is a remarkable solvent for many substances, including most sulfonamides, vitamins A and D, stilbestrol, thymol, menthol, 5-fluorouracil and some essential oils. It is, however, *not* miscible with fixed oils, fats and waxes. It is hygroscopic and emollient. When added to a vehicle, it assists in the penetration of these drugs, especially steroids.

Alcohol is the standard solvent for alkaloids, many dyes and most essential oils and frequently used skin applications with phenol, menthol, camphor, salicylic acid, resorcin and iodine. It is immiscible with most fixed oils, fats and waxes, but does dissolve castor oil and coconut oil. It may be thought of as an intermediate between water and true fat solvents.

In practical application alcohol is more irritating, especially if concentrated, than glycerin or propylene glycol. Because of its volatility, its preparations are cooling but also drying and slightly defatting.

Acetone, also an intermediate solvent, is closer to the true fat solvents than alcohol. It is miscible with water and disolves most fixed oils and fats freely. It does not dissolve phosphatides, lanolin, petrolatum or waxes. It dissolves most of coal tar, but not the black asphalt-like portion. It is inflammable.

Ether, chloroform, carbon tetrachloride and *benzol* are true fat solvents. They are immiscible with water and glycerin but freely miscible with alcohol and acetone. Chloroform and propylene glycol mix.

Spans, Tweens and Arlacels

Nonionic surface active agents (Atlas Powder, Wilmington, Delaware) are largely supplanting the older emulsifying agents. (Tween 80 is the compound with which Dubos obtained diffuse growth of the tubercle bacillus.) Their activity is not disturbed by many conditions that inactivate the ionized types. *Spans* are formed by the union of fatty acid radicles with cyclic anhydrides of sorbitol or mannitol. *Arlacels* are purified spans prepared for pharmaceutical use. *Tweens* are more water-soluble, modified spans.

In preparing emulsions, a span is sometimes dissolved in the oil phase and the corresponding tween in the aqueous phase before emulsifying. (The Atlas Powder Company publishes numerous formulas.) The Texas Pharmacal Company manufactures an excellent vehicle for scalp medication incorporating this principle, called Topisol. Hydrophobic powders, such as sulfur and ammoniated mercury, are readily accepted by Topisol, and cade oil is easily dispersed with agitation.

Tween 80 = Polysorbate 80, or polyoxyethylene sorbitan mono-oleate
Span 80 = Sorbitan mono-oleate

Externally Active Drugs

Salicylic acid, one of the "reducing agents," reduces epithelial proliferation and normalizes faulty keratinization. In weak concentrations (1–2%) it has a keratoplastic effect; i.e., it exerts favorable influence on the formation of new keratin. It is therefore suitable for treating acute dermatoses. It also is antipruritic in low concentration. It is soluble in alcohol and ether and relatively insoluble in water, although it goes into ointment bases, especially petrolatum, very well. It is antiseptic and antifermentative.

In high concentrations (5–20%), salicylic acid is a keratolytic and is therefore the most important additive in treatments for heavy scales or severely keratotic dermatoses. It is useful where a caustic effect is intended. It is considered to be antieczematous, probably because strong salicylic acid ointments have beneficial effects on some squamous eczemas. Salicylic acid reinforces the action of sulfur, forming an excellent skin softener in combination with an ointment base. The 40% salicylic acid plaster is useful in the treatment of corns, calluses and plantar warts.

Boric acid is believed to be antieczematous, although probably its greatest value is in its mild acidity, thereby reducing the pH of a compress of, say, cool wet cloths, to that of the skin. (Water has a pH of around 7.2, and skin has a pH of around 5.0.)

Boric acid in an ointment prevents spoiling. It also has mild astringent disinfectant properties on the skin. It is poisonous if ingested; cases of it being mistaken for saline and given intravenously have occurred, resulting in death, so that it is often barred from hospital use. Boric acid should not be used on extensive burns because it can be absorbed percutaneously.

Resorcinol, one of the "reducing agents," is used in low concentrations (0.1–2%) in compresses, lotions and pastes and is often used at the start of eczema treatment in Europe, probably because of its astringent effects. It is soluble in water, alcohol and ether. It is antipruritic in concentrations of 0.5–3% and in ointments in concentrations of less than 5%. It is keratoplastic in concentrations of 10–30% and in lotions in concentrations of 3–8%.

Resorcinol stains skin and hair and fairly often induces an irritative dermatitis by its overuse in fair-skinned teenagers; but it has markedly beneficial effects in treating patients with seborrheic disorders such as acne, seborrheic dermatitis, rosacea and seborrhea capitis, especially when used in combination with sulfur. Its keratolytic properties can be of help in prickly heat lotions. If used in the scalp, resorcinol monoacetate stains less.

Sulfur, one of the "reducing agents," is also an oxygen accepter. It is insoluble and used principally in the treatment of scabies, tinea, acne, rosacea and seborrheic dermatitis with comedones. It is keratoplastic in low concentration (1–2%) and keratolytic in high concentration. It can be stimulating. Sulfur's effect on the skin is probably oxidative through assisting cornification by the formation of the disulfide groups from SH groups present in cysteine. Some of the sulfide combines with oxygen from the air to form polythionic acids, which have hygroscopic properties and may dehydrate the epidermis. They may also reduce parakeratosis, e.g., that seen in actinic keratoses.

The keratolytic effect of salicylic acid with sulfur is better than that of either substance alone, and petrolatum is probably the best base for this purpose, although the base is not important.

Sulfur is usually used as a sulfur precipitate; the sublime sulfur is used in Vleminckx solution, and colloidal sulfur, having a finer particle size, is probably the most active form.

In alkaline solution, the disulfide bands in keratin are broken, converting it to protein digestible by trypsin and pepsin, which may explain the keratolytic effect of high percentages of sulfur in ointments. If large amounts of hydrogen sulfides are being formed, more than the oxygen present can convert to polythionic acids; then the reducing action leads to keratolysis.

Sulfur has antibacterial properties against gram-positive bacteria, through blocking an enzyme system, by direct toxicity or by making some nutrient unavailable. Its antiscabetic effect is probably because of the direct effect of the sulfides produced. Its effect on cases of seborrhea and acne is harder to explain and probably is because the process of keratinization of follicle openings is "normalized."

Sulfur dermatitis, which is a typical "crackilee" irritation of the skin, can be seen in overtreated patients with acne or in children treated too long for scabies. One of the factors in its production is the temporary relief of itching achieved by the use of 10% sulfur ointments, and when the itching returns, the unsuspecting patient, believing his scabies not yet cured, reapplies the ointment, leading to eventual sulfur dermatitis.

Danish ointment is 10% sulfur, with 2% balsam of Peru and 1% phenol.

Paradoxically, a thick sulfur paste containing between 30 and 50% sulfur in petrolatum often irritates less than paste with lower concentrations and has antiphlogistic, antipruritic and antiparasitic effects that are useful in treating rosacea, seborrheic dermatitis, psoriatic erythroderma and other diseases.

Colloidal sulfur was preferred by Combes[4] in his article on sulfur and it is noteworthy that sulfur and mercury are incompatible on the skin in any vehicle, except cinnabar (hydrargyrum sulfurate rubri 0.1–2%).

A good sulfur resorcin lotion that is extremely effective in treating prickly heat is as follows:

Sulfur precipitate	5
Resorcin	2
Zinc oxide	20
Talc	20
Glycerine	10
Alcohol 70%	35
Lime water q.s. ad	120

Make a lotion and apply as needed.

An ointment that is very useful in treating athlete's foot is 3% sulfur and 3% salicylic acid in petrolatum, to be used at night. Vleminckx solution is excellent for compressing cystic acne and rosacea. (See Formulary, nos. 7, 8 and 9.)

Ichthyol is soluble in water. It is a sort of transition phase between sulfur and tar, and it is a distillation product of a bituminous shale, the remains of fossilized fish from the Austrian Tyrol. It is soluble in water, alcohol and ether. It is generally bland in its effect on the skin, having its greatest use in concentrations of 2–10% in ointments. Its antiseptic action is slight, but it is a mild reducing and exfoliating agent. In high concentration, i.e., between 30% and 50%, it produces a drying effect on outer layers of the epidermis. It is useful for rosacea and occasionally for acne in pastes for night use. It colors zinc paste a light beige in 2–3% concentration, and its stains, if any, are washable. It is mildly keratoplastic, antipruritic, astringent and vasoconstrictive. It is sometimes useful in treating chronic eczematous conditions when moving toward more stimulating treatment.

Tars are not soluble in water. They have a complex composition and their usefulness cannot be denied. They consist mainly of phenols and aromatic hydrocarbons. Mostly they are derived from wood or coal by dry distillation. Wood tars come from birch (oleum rusci) or juniper (pix juniperi or cade oil) or pine (pix pini or pix liquida NF). Siemens[5] mentions beech tar (oleum fagi) though it is not in the NF or USP. Coal tar is the most useful tar (pix carbonis USP), and coal tar solution (liquor picis carbonis NF or LCD), a solution of coal tar in tincture of Quillaja, is suitable, milder and less apt to photosensitize. Naftalan (Lascoff's Pharmacy, New York City) and Tumenol are tars derived from bituminous earths from the Caucasus and they do not photosensitize.

Discussions about the virtues of various tars often appear to be like those on "how many angels can dance on the head of a pin." In general, learning how to manage one or two tar preparations in various concentrations and becoming familiar with them is the best way to acquire skill in the use of tars.

Juniper tar (cade oil) is black or brown and has a very objectionable odor. All tars stain, and the stains may be difficult to remove. In moderate strength, tar is soothing and antipruritic, and if stronger applications are used, tar is stimulating and even irritating.

White's coal tar paste (which is black) is a favorite prescription:

Crude coal tar	5
Zinc oxide	5
Cornstarch	40
Petrolatum	40

A modification that is sometimes useful is Sutton's modification, which is as follows:

Crude coal tar	1
Lanolin q.s. to mix	
Zinc oxide	10
Cornstarch	10
Liquid petrolatum	10
Petrolatum q.s. ad	100

This makes a 1% coal tar ointment.

Tarpaste (Doak Company, New York City) is a good proprietary ready-made tar.

In general, tars are highly variable substances containing naphthalene, oils, pitch, cresol, phenol and anthracene. Depending upon the manufacturer and raw material source, tars may have a higher or a lower concentration of any of these substances. The antiseptic and antipruritic qualities of the tars appear to be related to their phenol content. Irritant qualities relate to the naphthalene content.

Coal tar is a photosensitizer, and this fact should be recognized, especially in summer. Therefore, tar is useful in the Goeckerman treatment of psoriasis. Tar is a potent carcinogen; the benzopyrene in it probably being the worst offender. It should never be used in combination with x-ray and grenz-ray therapy.

Coal tar will not go into petrolatum directly, but the addition of lanolin or Aquaphor will enable it to be absorbed. Many proprietary bases, e.g., Neobase, absorb crude coal tar nicely. Zetar is a commercial preparation that is water soluble and makes nice tar ointments. Many prefer liquor carbonis detergens (LCD) and usually start off with 5%, gradually increasing the strength. However, for treating a stubborn nummular eczema there is nothing like a 1% crude coal tar paste.

Tar is the chief antieczematic and is very useful in treating atopic eczema, infantile eczema, lichen simplex chronicus, psoriasis and any other chronic eczema. Occasionally a tar folliculitis will be produced, and it should be watched for. (See Formulary, no. 10).

Mercury is classified as one of the weaker antieczematics. It is still often quite useful in treating seborrheic dermatitis, tinea and bacterial infections.

Ammoniated mercury (hydrargyrum ammoniatum USP) is the most common form in use, usually in 2–20% strength. It is used in treating seborrheic dermatitis. It can be effective in combination with salicylic acid and in a concentration of 2–4%, whereas it may be used in combination in 10–20% concentration for treating psoriasis. The Carbowax bases are useful in treating scalp psoriasis. The use of mercury in impetigo and other superficial pyodermas has largely been supplanted by the antibiotic ointments, but there is a 3% ammoniated mercury ophthalmic ointment that sometimes is useful for blepharitis. The USP 5% ammoniated mercury ointment is useful for psoriasis, too. (See Formulary, nos. 11 and 12).

Mercury bichloride (corrosive sublimate-mercuric chloride), usually in dilutions of 1 : 1,000 aqueous, can be useful in treating scalp and other hair follicle infections and is often almost specific for acne necroticans miliaris when applied frequently. (There is 0.03% USP mercury bichloride ophthalmic ointment.) (See Formulary, no. 14.)

Yellow oxide of mercury, usually 1%, is used in eye salves and seborrheic blepharitis; in stronger concentrations it is used for treating pediculosis when nits are on the eyelids (see the 3% ammoniated mercury ophthalmic ointment above). (See Formulary, no. 14.)

Tincture of Merthiolate (1:1,000 or 1:750) is useful, like Metaphen, as an antiseptic.

Mercury cannot be used with sulfur, except cinnabar. Mercury can sensitize, and frequently does.

Anthralin and *chrysarobin*, reducing substances, are very useful in the treatment of nonirritable psoriasis. (See Formulary, nos. 15 and 16.) They must be *rubbed in* and used with full awareness of their almost invariable ability to produce eventual reaction. Contact with the eyes should be avoided, since a rather severe conjunctivitis can result. However, repeated washes of 1:5,000 potassium permanganate and hydrocortisone eyedrops will clear this quickly.

In general, patients can learn to use these substances, at least anthralin, safely in the scalp. Chrysarobin can be used from 1% to 20% strength in pastes, ointments or paints. Anthralin is generally used in an ointment form 0.1–1% strength.

Anthralin is preferable, used in gradually increasing strengths and rubbed in using a clothespin covered with cloth as a rubbing stick. It can irritate the kidneys if it is used extensively, and it stains skin and clothing although not as badly as chrysarobin. It is supplied as 0.1%, 0.25%, 0.5% and 1% strength by manufacturers (Dermik—"Anthraderm").

Vioform (iodochlorhydroxyquin USP—Ciba), a potent bactericidal and fungicidal agent containing iodine, comes in ointment or cream in 3% concentration and also in lotion form in combination with 1% hydrocortisone. This drug can also be incorporated in any desired concentration in extemporaneous compounding by prescribing for the Vioform powder, for example:

Vioform powder	0.3
Ammoniated mercury	0.6
Zinc oxide	2.0
Aquaphor	
Cold cream USP $\overline{aa}$ q.s. ad	30.0

Vioform stains the skin yellow; this is more marked with ointment than with cream. It has a wide range of uses in dermatology, being antipruritic (very useful in treating pruritus ani) and antieczematous, and is especially valuable in treating vesicular finger dermatitis and splits on the heels and hands. It is also useful in treating intertriginous sebopsoriasis fissures. (See Formulary, no. 17.)

Anti-inflammatory, antibacterial and antifungal agents for local application come as ointments, creams, lotions and powders, as well as eyedrops, eardrops and suppositories.

Anti-inflammatory agents are chiefly corticosteroids and are useful in treating all allergic dermatoses and many granulomatous and infiltrative disorders, as well as many metabolic and other disorders where the cause is obscure, e.g., psoriasis and necrobiosis lipoidica. The fluorinated steroid creams penetrate best, but have a higher incidence of striae, telangiectasia and even atrophy, which may be permanent; hence there should be limited refills on the prescription. (For a list of available formulas, see Formulary, no. 22.)

Occlusion with plastic coverings hydrates the keratin layer to make it more permeable, and the resultant "bank" of soaked-up steroid is subsequently released over 7–10 days. Occlusion does enhance sequelae and may predispose to miliaria and undesirable organisms overgrowing to produce odor. Hypopigmentation may occur.

Intralesional steroid injection may be the method of choice for treating a number of conditions, e.g., acne cysts, stubborn psoriasis, lichen simplex, keloids, granulomas from insect bites, swimming pool abrasions, granuloma annulare. Even Dupuytren's contracture and ganglions have succumbed to this method of treatment. Dilution lessens the risk of atrophy. Kenalog (triamcinolone acetonide) and Aristocort (triamcinolone diacetate) appear to be most effective.

Most *antibacterial agents* (See Formulary, no. 23) used locally are too toxic for systemic use, e.g., bacitracin, neomycin, polymyxin B, Chloromycetin, tyrothricin (gramicidin and tyrocidine). Erythromycin has additional strength against the organisms causing erythrasma, while bacitracin, the most commonly used, is effective against tetanus, diphtheria, and anaerobic and gram-positive cocci (Table 1–2). (For available preparations, see Formulary, no. 23. For skin disinfectants, see Formulary, no. 24.)

Antifungal agents—commonly 3% sulfur–3% salicyclic acid in either greasy or hydrophilic base; and one-half strength Whitfield's ointment, e.g., 6% benzoic and 3% salicyclic acid in USP hydrophilic ointment, are the classic reme-

TABLE 1-2.—ANTIBACTERIAL AGENTS AND THEIR EFFECTIVENESS

ANTIBACTERIAL AGENTS	EFFECTIVE AGAINST GRAM POSITIVE	EFFECTIVE AGAINST GRAM NEGATIVE
Bacitracin	+	0
Gentamicin	Some	+, including pseudomonas, Proteus and *Escherichia coli*
Neomycin	0	+
Polymyxin B	0	+, except *Proteus Serratio*
Tyrothricin	+	0

dies for athlete's foot. The development of griseofulvin has made the management of the scaly *Trichophyton rubrum* infection (one palm–two soles) easier and even occasionally curative. The blistering and fissuring toe web *T. mentagrophytes*, however, does not respond as well, and *Candida* and tinea versicolor do not respond at all. Local treatment still is needed here. Usually a combination of soaks, powders, salves and creams will clear the average case. (See Formulary, no. 25.)

Paints or tinctures are a convenient medication, using a dye or caustic which can be applied directly to the lesion or affected area with a swab, glass rod or even a paint brush, usually one to three times daily.

Castellani's paint is a rather complicated formula which essentially is basic fuchsin with 1% resorcin, 5% acetone and 1% boric acid in a phenol solution. It is probably the best single remedy for tinea cruris, monilial or otherwise. (See Formulary, no. 18.) It must be compounded by a skilled pharmacist, and it is messy. Lotrimin lotion (Delbay) is a pleasant and very effective, though more costly, substitute. Castellani's paint should be applied daily for 3 weeks, extending 1 in. beyond the visible margin of the lesion. The patient should be reexamined in the fourth week. Since the physician cannot see through the scarlet paint, the patient should discontinue use for a week before the examination. Castellani's paint is used in combination with Caldesene powder (Calcium Desenex—Maltbie). It also can be used on toenails and other fungus infections, although it is perhaps less effective there.

Using 1% Aqueous gentian violet is a good way to lose a patient, but it is an excellent treatment against *Monilia*, especially paronychia (also Vincent's angina in the mouth).

Aqueous 20% sodium caprylate is no longer manufactured, but can be made up by a pharmacist on prescription. It is excellent for treating monilial paronychia, too.

Onychophytex (Wynlit Labs.) is a proprietary drug, consisting of tannic acid and boric acid with salicylic acid, for the treatment of onychophytosis. I think it helps.

Verdefam (Texas Pharmacal) is sometimes a useful fungus paint.

The following is a prescription for a paint for fungus nails:

Salicylic acid	5%	
Sodium propionate	2%	in water and
Sodium caprylate	2%	isopropyl alcohol
Propionic acid	3%	to make 100%
Undecylenic acid	5%	
Copper undecylanate	0.5%	
Sodium dioctyl sulfosuccinate	0.1%	

A solution of 3% chrysarobin in chloroform is used in the treatment of monilial paronychia and occasionally psoriasis. It is dark brown to black, however, and should be painted on daily. A solution of 3% thymol iodide in chloroform has similar uses and is lighter in color.

Ten percent ichthyol in collodion is an occlusive paint, which for some reason, perhaps because it keeps the air out, seems to help in splinting and protecting the tender skin in acute herpes zoster.

Quatrasol (Dome Co., New York), a mixture of 5% salicylanilide in 1% trimethyloctadecyl ammonium pentachlorophenate (iamine 3258) and 94% isopropyl alcohol, is unbelievably effective, but is no longer available. When painted between the toes religiously twice a day, it would often clear soft corns in 4 to 6 weeks. (See Formulary, no. 19.)

A mixture of equal parts of 25% podophyllin in acetone and tincture of benzoin is excellent for treating soft warts in the genital region. It can set up an extremely severe reaction in some people, so the first trial should be in a small area only. Instructions to the patient should be to wash off in 6 hours. Weekly follow-up is imperative. It can be used in concentrations up to 50% if the pharmacist allows the mixture to stand overnight and sort of "sink in" while mixing. It can be used for the treatment of hairy brown tongue in lower concentrations. (See Formulary, no. 20.)

Wart paints, such as 10% each of salicylic acid, lactic acid and glacial acetic acid in collodion, are effective treatment. (See Formulary, no. 21.) Patients or parents have to be instructed in shaving, rasping or sandpapering the wart surface and then making a "dimple" in the center of the wart with a toothpick, almost tattooing the paint in when applying it daily. Every few days, the paint can be either cleaned off or removed with nail polish remover and pared. If the skin becomes irritated, perhaps a resting period should be ordered.

Various other paints can be improvised for special purposes, such as 3% salicylic acid and 2% thymol iodide in tincture of Merthiolate used on toenail fungus infections.

Aerosol sprays that form a coating on wounds when dry are useful in the scalp after sutures have been placed, e.g., Aeroplast dressing in spray can (Aeroplast Corporation, Dayton, Ohio).

Wet Dressings

The closed (plastic-wrapped) wet dressing has almost no place in dermatology, although surgeons use it in treating severe infections of the extremities. It is very "heating" and macerates the epidermis. The wet soak or bath is preferable to the closed wet dressing, using a basin to soak an infected hand, or in the hospital, in arm bath or foot bath.

Open wet dressings soothe and cool inflamed skin, dry oozing secretions, soften crusts, aid in cleansing and assist in draining purulent lesions. If ice cold, they help to stop itching. Plain tap water can be used for wet dressings. I prefer 1 teaspoon boric acid per pint, while others prefer saline and still others Burow's solution or aluminum acetate (which I find very astringent). Boric acid must be labeled if it is in solution because there have been occasions when used intravenously, it has resulted in death.

Bur-Veen powders (Fougera) are a mixture of Burow's solution with oatmeal, which seems to lessen the sometimes biting astringency of the solution. Dome-Boro powders (Dome) come in packets which, when opened into a pint of water, make a 1:20 solution for wet compresses. Burow's solution USP (5% aluminum acetate solution), if used 1:20, 1 oz of stock solution is added to 1.25 pints of water to make a suitable strength for soaks.

Silver nitrate is very useful in treating monilial intertrigo, under pendulous breasts, in groins and under uncircumcised foreskins. It can be used in dilutions from 1:400 to 1:1,000. One-quarter percent strength is preferred, which in some communities is best made up with distilled water, depending upon the mineral content of the water. If the mineral content is high, distilled water should be used. The solution stains. Patients should be cautioned to avoid overuse.

Acetic acid in 5% aqueous solution (e.g., vinegar) is helpful occasionally in combating pseudomonas.

Magnesium sulfate or epsom salts is useful in trying to localize infection, e.g., a furuncle. One tablespoon per quart of water is about right.

For a saline dressing, one teaspoon of sodium chloride or table salt to one pint of water makes an isotonic solution that is compatible with tissue fluids. It is inactive though soothing.

Potassium permanganate ($KMnO_4$)—five grains to 3 qt make a 1:9,000 solution. Stained, brownish red toenails were formerly the mark of intensively treated athlete's foot. Potassium permanganate is seldom used now because it stains the skin and clothing and makes it difficult to see what is going on. Stains in tubs and bowls can be removed by dilute oxalic acid, which usually takes off some of the finish as well.

D'Alibour solution is prepared as follows:

Zinc sulfate	1.4
Copper sulfate	0.4
Camphor water saturated q.s. ad	240.0

This is an excellent soothing and germicidal solution which is sometimes useful in treating impetigo and occasionally for flat warts. Dali-Sol packets (Dome), when placed in a quart of water, make a 1:16 solution.

ANTIBIOTIC DRESSINGS.—These are expensive and very little used. *Bacitracin* (Upjohn) comes in 3,000, 10,000 50,000-unit vials and uses 100 units per 1 cc saline. It is useful against *Staphylococcus aureus, Streptococcus, Corynebacterium diphtheriae, Bacillus welchii* and *tetanus* organisms, as well as *Entamoeba histolytica. Polymyxin B sulfate* (Burroughs Wellcome) comes in 20-mg vials, which are useful in a dilution of 1 mg/cc saline against *Pseudomonas aeruginosa, Escherichia coli* and *Staphylococcus aureus.* For *neomycin sulfate* (Upjohn—5,000-mg vial), use 2 mg/cc saline, effective against *Staphylococcus, diphtheria, tuberculosis, Bacillus welchii, P. aeruginosa* and *E. coli. Terramycin* or *Aureomycin* in 50-mg tablets (Pfizer and Lederle), 1 mg/cc saline, is effective against *Staphylococcus, Streptococcus, diphtheria, welchii, tetanii* and *coli,* but not against *P. aeruginosa.*

Powders

Dusting powders have a very superficial effect on the skin, mainly acting to decrease friction in areas of mechanical irritation, in intertrigo, chafing, jock-strap itch, or in reducing inflammation with little exudation. Occasionally they are applied on top of ointments to prevent clothing from absorbing the ointment.

In general, powders are drying and cooling and absorb moisture, exposing more surface for quicker evaporation. These effects are mainly the result of the physical properties of the powder. Their medicinal components are therefore usually inert or almost so.

Plain talc, or a mixture of equal parts of zinc oxide and purified talcum, is the powder most frequently used. Several commercially available standard powders are excellent, e.g., Johnson & Johnson Baby Powder, Ammen's Powder and Zeasorb Powder (Stiefel).

Antiseptic powders such as bismuth formic iodide (BFI—Merck, Sharp & Dohme) or Aristol powder have value in the care of small wounds, e.g., after the removal of skin tags from the side of the neck. *Antibiotic powders*, e.g., Terramycin powder or Neosporin powder (Burroughs Wellcome), are helpful in healing wounds in intertriginous areas. *Astringent powders*, such as equal parts tannic acid and zinc oxide, are helpful in treating balanitis and hyperhidrosis.

Powders can be applied with a cotton puff or shaker. They should not be used in the presence of marked oozing and exudation, since they tend to cake into hard granules, especially with purulent exudate.

In chronically ill patients, the liberal use of powder can assist in the prevention of bed sores or pressure sores. For treating diaper rashes and some adult fungus infections, e.g., monilial intertrigo, Caldesene powder (Maltbie Labs.) is helpful. Desenex powder is very useful in treating moist dermatophytosis, as are several other commercially available powders, e.g., Enzactin (Ayerst).

Baths

Soaking in a tub is a relaxing and soothing pastime, even in the absence of any medication. In cases of extensive eruptions, bathing can be a convenient way of achieving widespread exposure to a medication, soothing or otherwise, with a minimum of trouble to the patient and therapist.

Starch baths are made from one-half box of Linit or cornstarch per tub, but to make them properly, the starch should be mixed with a little water to make a thin paste, then add boiling water while stirring. This will burst the starch granules to make a gelatinous mixture, which is then dumped into the bathtub with about 6 inches of water in it. The patient soaks for about 10 minutes. It is useful as a soothing and antipruritic measure in treating widespread eruptions, such as lichen planus, pityriasis rosea, urticaria and other oozing eczemas where there is crusting.

The indications for *Aveeno* baths are much the same as those for starch baths, although the precooked and packaged oatmeal is more convenient to use. There is also oilated Aveeno.

Epsom salts baths—3 cups of the bulk magnesium sulfate

per 6-inch tub—are useful in treating pyodermas, furuncles and necrotic acne, especially of the back, shoulders and buttocks.

Several excellent commercial *tar* bath products are available, e.g., Balnetar (Westwood Labs.) and Zetar, which are soothing and helpful therapy for itching eczemas and often psoriasis before sunlamp. Occasionally the patient can smear the tar bath solution directly on the lesions just before taking ultraviolet lamp exposure. The USP coal tar solution, or liquor carbonis detergens, can be used for this purpose (3 oz per tub).

Potassium permanganate baths may be needed on some occasions. They are useful in treating smelly bullous or ulcerating generalized conditions, such as pemphigus or mycosis fungoides. For the average bath, 2 teaspoons of the crystals or 25 of the 0.3-gm (grain V) tablets, finely ground and stirred up in 5 qt of warm water and then dumped into the bath, make about a 1:10,000 solution. The patient should get in directly when the bath is mixed; otherwise its oxidative effect may be lost.

Bath oils are useful in treating severe xerosis or dry ichthyotic skin (e.g., winter itch) and are available as Alpha-Keri, Domol, Lubath, Kauma and Syntex. You can make your own with 2 oz olive oil in a cup of milk. Stir and then dump into the tub. Nivea skin oil can be used in a similar manner.

Antipruritics

All cooling measures, e.g., open wet dressings, alcohol daubing, dusting with powder and others, will reduce the sensation of itching. Folk remedies include holding the itching part under very hot water from the tap and applying household ammonia, or soaking in a dilute solution of Clorox—all effective, I might add, and probably no more injurious than Surfacaine or Nupercaine obtained from the drugstore. On occasion an ice bag may be helpful.

Camphor, 0.125–2%; menthol, 0.25–2%; Thymol, 0.25–2%; phenol, 1–2%; and resorcinol, 1–2% are useful as antipruritics. Occasionally chloral hydrate, 1–1.5%, is helpful. Salicylic acid, 0.5–1%, is also mildly antipruritic.

In general, use twice the concentration in a paste as you would an ointment, and half that percent in a cream or lotion emulsion.

Principles of Prescription Writing

The prescription is a written order for the pharmacist to dispense medication for a patient. It includes directions for the pharmacist as well as for the patient. It may become a legal document someday, so it has to be preserved and should be written in ink. With ball-point pens available, carbon copies can be kept in the patient's file for later review, or an accurate note may be written in the record for every prescription given to the patient. It is extremely embarrassing when a miraculously effective "remedy" cannot be identified and there is no pharmacist's number to look up! The physician's aura of expertness suffers! Therefore it is an excellent principle to note the prescription on the patient's record *at the time* it is written, not later in the day when there is more time—for some or all of it may be forgotten.

The prescription should be written in the presence of the patient if possible. It should be written without hesitation, with confident efficiency and in a manner conveying to the patient that the writer knows what he is doing and *is* writing this prescription specifically for this patient. This little scrap of paper represents the culmination of the physician's skill, experience and diagnostic and therapeutic acumen as applied to the patient, and it extends relief.

In general, it is better to write all directions in English and all measurements in the metric system. The metric system is a decimal system, and grams and cubic centimeters are usually interchangeable; Arabic numbers are written. In the apothecary system, grains and minims, drams and ounces are used; this is a rather inexact measurement at best although convenient, since one teaspoon equals one dram, which is 4 or 5 cc, and bottles and jars are usually measured in ounces. That is to say, if you prescribe a face lotion in a 4-oz bottle and you write the prescription for 100 cc, there will be 20 cc (1 oz = 30 cc, so 4 oz = 120 cc) of empty space in the bottle, which may lead the patient to suspect that the pharmacist has "shortchanged" him by not filling the bottle. So one should remember to make the prescription up to the multiples of 30 that correspond to the common sizes of bottles and jars: 120cc, 180 cc, 240 cc, and so on. In recent years the use of bottles that contain 100 cc and 200 cc are becoming popular, so this may not be so necessary in the future.

Many physicians substitute a line instead of using decimal points. This decimal line may be printed on the prescription pad, giving the prescription this appearance:

Salicylic acid	0	9
Sulfur precipitate	0	9
USP hydrophilic ointment		
q.s. ad	30	0

The apothecary system is also official in the USP, and one should become familiar with it and be able to interchange from metric to apothecary. For instance, the over-the-counter aspirin tablets are always "5 grains," which is written gr v with the Roman numeral following the symbol. When the number is *one*, a dot is placed over it as added insurance to emphasize the *exact* number, e.g., mi̇.

In the case of fractions, one-half (1/2) is written s̅s̅ so that 2 1/2 minims becomes mi̇i̇s̅s̅. The s̅s̅ is the abbreviation of the Latin "semis." Other fractions are expressed as fractions (not decimals) using the arabic numerals, e.g., atropine gr 1/150. Grams are always written with the capital G, as Gm, whereas grains always with a small g, as gr.

In general, gr v to the ounce equals 1% when compounding a prescription.

1 mg = gr 1/60	1 cc	= 15 minims (actually 16.23)
1 Gm = gr xv	1 L	= 1 qt ± 3–4 oz
1 dram = 4 cc	1 pt	= 500 cc
	1 gr	= 60 mg
	1 qt	= 1,000 cc
	1 oz	= 30 Gm or 30 cc

Drops vary with the size of the dropper and the liquidity of the fluid being dropped, so when medication is being pre-

TABLE 1-3.—HOUSEHOLD MEASURES

MEASURE	METRIC	APOTHECARY
1 drop	0.05 cc	1 minim
1 teaspoon	5 cc	1+ dram
1 dessert spoon	8 cc	2 dram
1 tablespoon	15 cc	0.5 oz
1 wine glass	60 cc	2 oz
1 glass	250 cc	8 oz

scribed in dropper form, it is wise to use the USP standardized dropper and request the pharmacist to calibrate and mark a spot on the dropper that gives the exact dose desired. When eyedrops and scalp lotion are applied with the dropper, this does not apply.

Household measures are almost always used to measure medications (Table 1-3). Teaspoons more often are 5 cc than 4 cc, which should be borne in mind when estimating how many doses are in 30-cc or 60-cc bottles of expensive medication. There will more often be 6 teaspoons than the customarily expected 8 teaspoons in an ounce of syrup of Periactin (Merck), for example.

Construction of the Prescription

Traditionally there are four parts of a prescription.

SUPERSCRIPTION.—This includes the patient's exact name, address (if for a narcotic), age (if minor) and date. The symbol Rx is an abbreviation for the Latin recipe "take thou." Some consider the stroke through the tail of the Rx an ancient invocation to Jupiter, whose symbol is ♃.

INSCRIPTION.—This part contains the names and amounts of the ingredients, which are best written in full. Classically these consist of the *basis,* or principal drug, the modifying drugs (*adjuvant* and *corrective*), which assist the action of the principal drug and perhaps reduce some of the undesirable effects, and the *vehicle,* which carries the drug to its point of action. In the case of ointments, this is usually the ointment base.

SUBSCRIPTION.—This contains the directions to the pharmacist, usually a somewhat curt *misce fiat unguentum* (mix and make an ointment) or even merely the abbreviation M. for mix.

SIGNATURE.—This is actually derived from the Latin *signa*, meaning write, mark or label, which can be written "label" in English, or "sig." Then the directions to the patient follow, either in English or in the customary abbreviated Latin form, as in "one teaspoon three times a day after meals," or ʒi t.i.d.p.c." or even "rub in well t.i.d. and h.s.," a combination of both languages which, while not correct, suffices. The use of "as directed" should be avoided. If directions are complicated, they should be separately written and given to the patient and then the signa can be "as per written directions."

If a narcotic is dispensed, the directions should specify "for pain," "for itching" or "for cough"; and if the directions would embarrass the patient, they should be given to the patient privately and not displayed on the label of the medication.

If no refills are desired, as in the case of arsenic, the use of "non rep." (*non repetatur*—do not repeat) conveys the message to the pharmacist. This is not necessary with narcotics. If an unusually large dose is prescribed, the letters "Q.R." (*quantitum rectum*—correct amount) will save an unnecessary phone call, since it notifies the pharmacist that this is not a mistake. If the patient is an impoverished individual and the physician is receiving little or no compensation for his services, the initials "Pp" (*pauperisimus*—pauper) will indicate this to the pharmacist, who may do likewise.

Then the physician signs his name with the traditional M.D. following it. It is not in good taste to add other degrees, desirable and honorable though they may be, e.g., M.R.C.P. (London), F.A.C.P. or D.A.B.D.S.

In writing prescriptions for ointments, much can be left to the discretion of the pharmacist, as in the following:

Salicylic acid	1.8
Benzoic acid	3.6
Lanolin	
White petrolatum to make	60.0

Here the exact proportions of lanolin and white petrolatum are not given, and the pharmacist can use his own judgment.

The percentage form may be used, as in the following:

Salicylic acid	3%
Benzoic acid	6%
Lanolin	
White petrolatum to make	60.0

M. Label: Apply a thin film to the affected parts night and morning.

Familiarity with the official preparations, that is, those that are in the USP or NF, may save the writing of sometimes lengthy prescriptions and, since many of the more common official preparations are manufactured by drug houses and kept in stock in pharmacies, may save time and money.

A prescription for Whitfield's ointment, which is 6% salicylic acid and 12% benzoic acid in wool fat (5%) and petrolatum, and is referred to as the compound ointment of benzoic acid NF, can be written as follows:

Rx. Compound ointment of benzoic acid (NF) 30.0

Label: Apply a thin film to affected parts night and morning.

Since these percentages are just double those of the 3–6% previously written, a modified prescription would be:

Rx. Compound ointment of benzoic acid (NF)
White Petrolatum $\overline{aa}$ q.s. ad 30.0
diluting the official preparation to make it milder

It is wise to bear in mind the story about the man who ate the suppositories, silver paper and all, and who then complained to the doctor that for all the good it did him, "he might as well have shoved them up his rectum." All preparations that are to be used externally should have this stated somewhere in the directions. The part to which the application is to be made should be identified and the frequency and mode of application clearly given; for example, "sop on freely four times daily to forearms," or "rub in gently t.i.d. and h.s.

hands," or "paint on daily for three weeks–inguinal area."

The amount prescribed wil! vary, depending upon the area to be covered. In general, when prescribing ointments, we use:

For the face, groin or anus	1 oz
For the hands or scalp	2 oz
For a patchy eruption on the body or on both arms and legs	4 oz
For a generalized eruption	8–16 oz
For three generous applications of an ointment well rubbed in all over	4–6 oz

When prescribing lotions, we usually use:

For the face	4 oz
For the face and back	8 oz
For scattered patches on the trunk and extremities	6–8 oz
For the hands, frequent use	6 oz
For face, body and extremities, as in a bath lotion	16 oz
For the scalp	8–16 oz
Powders	Mostly 2 oz
Paints	Mostly 1 oz

A Few Phrases and Abbreviations

Ad libitum (ad lib.)–freely
Ana (aa)–of each
Ante (a)–before
Ante cibum (a.c.)–before meals
Bis in die (b.i.d.)–twice daily
Chartula–powder
Cum (c)–with
Fiat–let it be made
Gutta–guttae (gt.)–a drop, drops
Hora somni (h.s.) hour of sleep (at bedtime)
Lotio–lotion
Misce (M.)–mix
Pigmentum–paint

Post (p) — after
Post cibum (p.c.) — after meals
Quantum satis (q.s.) — sufficient amount
Quaque hora (q.h.) — every hour
q.s. ad — a sufficient amount to make
Secundum artem (s.a.) — according to the practice
Sine (s) — without
Si opus sit (s.o.s.) — if necessary
Ter in die (t.i.d.) — three times a day
Unguentum — ointment

Incompatibilities and Disadvantages of Some Medications

Tincture of iodine and mercurial lotions and ointments are incompatible because mercurous iodide is violently irritating and leads to an acute contact dermatitis. Mercurials are also incompatible with sulfur, which turns the skin black. Mercury ointments, if rubbed in with the fingers unprotected by finger cots or gloves, may color the nails slate gray by the formation of mercury sulfide from the sulfhydril groups in the keratin. Cold waves can cause mercury-treated hair to turn greenish black also.

Resorcin colors blonde or gray hair; and while resorcin monoacetate is not reported to do so, it does eventually discolor light hair.

Anthralin can produce a conjunctivitis, and all ointments containing this should be labeled "keep away from the eyes." Patients should also be warned of this. Anthralin can be used on the scalp, however, by a sophisticated patient. Excessive use can produce kidney damage by absorption. Anthralin stains linen quite often, although not as badly as does chrysarobin.

Occasionally a strangely irritating compound is formed when salicylic acid is mixed with ammoniated mercury in a vanishing base. Sometimes when salicylic acid and mercury bichloride in high concentrations are mixed in any kind of base, a marked irritation of the skin or scalp can occur, although just how this occurs is rather obscure.

Phenol, when applied to the scalp, has a more clinging odor of carbolic acid than when used in ointments applied to the skin. Sulfur has a rotten-egg odor when the skin gets warm, e.g., in intertriginous areas. Birch tar has a strong odor, as does cade oil. Mercury, if absorbed, can cause quite a stomatitis. Tars can photosensitize and lead to folliculitis. Vioform stains linen and *can* act as an "etcher," making keratin peel. Selenium sulfide shampoos occasionally seem to cause cold wave failures, so that this should not be attempted until several regular shampoos have intervened. Occasionally the use of mercurials in the scalp preceding a cold wave will cause the formation of mercury sulfide and cause the hair to turn greenish black later.

Sulfur may produce a red pruritic peeling irritation of the neck, particularly in patients with acne who of course have not applied lotio alba to the neck, but can pick up some by turning on their pillow. The same thing can happen from the use of strong sulfur soaps.

Ichthyol is black, and if used in 10% ointment, everything gets soiled, but if it is used in a paste, then it stains only a dark brown. In 3% concentration with 10% zinc oxide in an ointment, one gets a light skin-colored tan shade. With pyrogallic acid, on the other hand, the addition of zinc oxide makes everything stain black. Chrysarobin becomes black when exposed to soap (or alkali).

Salicylic acid in higher concentrations combined with ammoniated mercury causes severe irritations because the two agents together produce mercury sublimate.

"The larger the number of combinations in an ointment, the closer one gets to quackery, i.e., treatment with therapeutic measures the effect of which is difficult or impossible to predict." Avoid package prescriptions.

REFERENCES

1. Sutton, R. C.: *Diseases of the Skin* (St. Louis: C. V. Mosby Co., 1956), p. 65
2. Stoughton, R. B.: Symposium on the Pharmacology of Drugs, New York University, October 1969.
3. Polano, M. K., and Ponec, M.: Dependence of corticosteroid penetration on the vehicle, Arch. Dermatol. 112:675, 1976.

4. Combes, F. C.: Colloidal sulfur, N.Y. State J. Med. 46:401, 1946.
5. Siemens, H. W.: *General Diagnosis and Therapy of Skin Diseases* (Chicago: The University of Chicago Press, 1958), p. 263.

SUGGESTED READING

Domonkos, A. N.: *Andrews' Diseases of the Skin* (6th ed.; Philadelphia: W. B. Saunders Co., 1971).

2 / Viral Diseases

The observations by Jenner that milkmaids had lovely complexions though their hands were covered with cowpox lesions led to the development of vaccination for smallpox. The milkmaids' beautiful complexions were a by-product of their not getting smallpox, not a result of drinking milk, which is sometimes a point of confusion to this day.

Perhaps our knowledge of virus disease has advanced since that time, but we still have no truly specific treatment for viral disease. Viruses contain either RNA or DNA.

Antiviral Drugs

Iododeoxyuridine (IDU herplex) prevents certain aspects of DNA synthesis and is an effective antiviral drug, with its chief use in treating herpes keratitis. It has to be used early and very often and has apparently been effective in treating herpes simplex of the skin, too.

Thiosemicarbazone (Marboran) was apparently useful in preventing a smallpox epidemic in India in 1963 and in preventing the spread of alastrim in 1965. Recently doubt has been cast on its effectiveness.

Interferon is produced by cells that have harbored viruses; it exerts an antiviral action. Perhaps this will lead the way to further advances.

Immune globulin, when taken from adults who were vaccinated with a primary take 4–6 weeks earlier, contains virus-inactivating antibodies against vaccinia and variola.

Specific Viral Diseases

Herpes simplex (DNA – 100 – 200 mμ) (see p. 81, PCAD)* can infect infants with no cutaneous symptoms and may be

*PCAD refers to: Joseph Kimmig and Michael Jänner, *Pocket Color Atlas of Dermatology* (Chicago: Year Book Medical Publishers, Inc., 1975).

fatal in newborns. It can lead to gingivostomatitis in very young children, and in others it tends to produce clusters of vesicles around mucosal orifices of the face or genitals. (In atopic persons, it can lead to widespread explosive dissemination—Kaposi's varicelliform eruption.) The Tzanck smear from blister fluid shows eosinophilic intranuclear inclusions in giant cells. It is often recurrent at or near the site of the original infection, indicating that local tissue immunity must be lacking. Treatment rests largely in uncovering the trigger that sets off each attack, suspecting such things as a menstrual period, sun, wind, chocolate, nuts, constipation, smoking, drinking, and a visit to the dentist (stretching of the lips), which can be guarded against when discovered.

Weekly vaccinations with smallpox vaccine for 8–10 weeks suppress attacks at least for a while, and the Lilly experimental herpes simplex vaccine, which was given subcutaneously weekly for 10 weeks and then a booster every 2–4 weeks, offered promise. Changing the internal environment by large doses of acidophilus milk (or Bacid or Lactinex tablets) occasionally works, as does the use of sun-screening ointments.

Herplex Liquifilm (Allergan Labs.) applied locally to the suspected herpes *at the first sign* (usually burning and stinging) every 5 minutes for the first hour, then hourly thereafter for the first 2 days, then every 3 hours, occasionally aborts the herpes. Ether applied for 5 minutes every 6 hours is occasionally effective. The use of proflavin 0.1% or neutral red tattooed in, followed by 2 minutes of "black light" (Wood's lamp ultraviolet) at 6 in. distance, is another method, which is currently controversial.

Full-blown herpes can be treated with steroid antibiotic cream or ointment depending upon how much crusting there is. Burow's solution or boric acid soaks and peroxide dabbing help the lesions dry up and accelerate resolution. Vioform hydrocortisone lotion 1% is excellent for herpes progenitalis, and 1% gentian violet and occasionally Neosporin powder superimposed on this help also. Burow's compresses seem to accelerate recovery.

For more intensive and expensive therapy of recurrent debilitating herpes, several suggestions have been made by Dr.

Lewis B. Pipkin of San Antonio, whose extensive experience is sparked by his own lifelong infection with the virus. He suggests the use of Lupidon H (type 1) or G (type 2), a vaccine available from Germany. He advises weekly injections for the first 12 weeks, then a gradual decrease in frequency with continued boosters for several years. In addition, he believes that Symmetrol (amantadine HCl—Endo), 100 mg three times a day after meals and tapering to smaller doses as indicated, is helpful in suppressing the viral activity. He favors four daily doses for a month and then decreasing the treatment over a period of 4 months or so. Using the syrup at 50 mg/teaspoon provides easier dose control during the tapering-off period. For local use, Doctor Pipkin prefers Vira-A ophthalmic ointment 3% (adenosine arabinoside—Parke-Davis) applied to vulvar lesions eight to ten times a day; the area should be covered with Telfa and snugged up with panties. In men with a foreskin, a similar application should be used sparingly. This drug used in treating herpes encephalitis has reduced the mortality from 70% to 25% and possibly is helpful in local application.[1] Women can have the virus in the cervix and reinfect the male without clinical evidence; cervical cultures will assist in the diagnosis. (Media are available from Microbiologic Associates, Walkersville, Maryland.)

Ice cubes applied for 15 minutes followed by the Vira-A rubbed in gently is the most effective method of treatment.

Herpes zoster is characterized by painful blisters following the distribution of a sensory nerve. (Figs 2–1 and 2–2 show the arrangement of nerves in the body.) In the head, watch for facial nerve palsy (Ramsay Hunt syndrome, a geniculate ganglion involvement) and corneal ulceration if the side and tip of the nose are involved (nasociliary branch of the trigeminal). Generalization can occur without lymphoma being present, but the physician should be suspicious. (See pp. 83–84, PCAD.)

If pain is severe, treatment should include rest at home with sedation; Empirin, codeine and Darvon are helpful. Local hyperesthesia of the involved region can be treated with a snug padded dressing to keep the temperature even and protect from friction from clothing. Occasionally an electric heat-

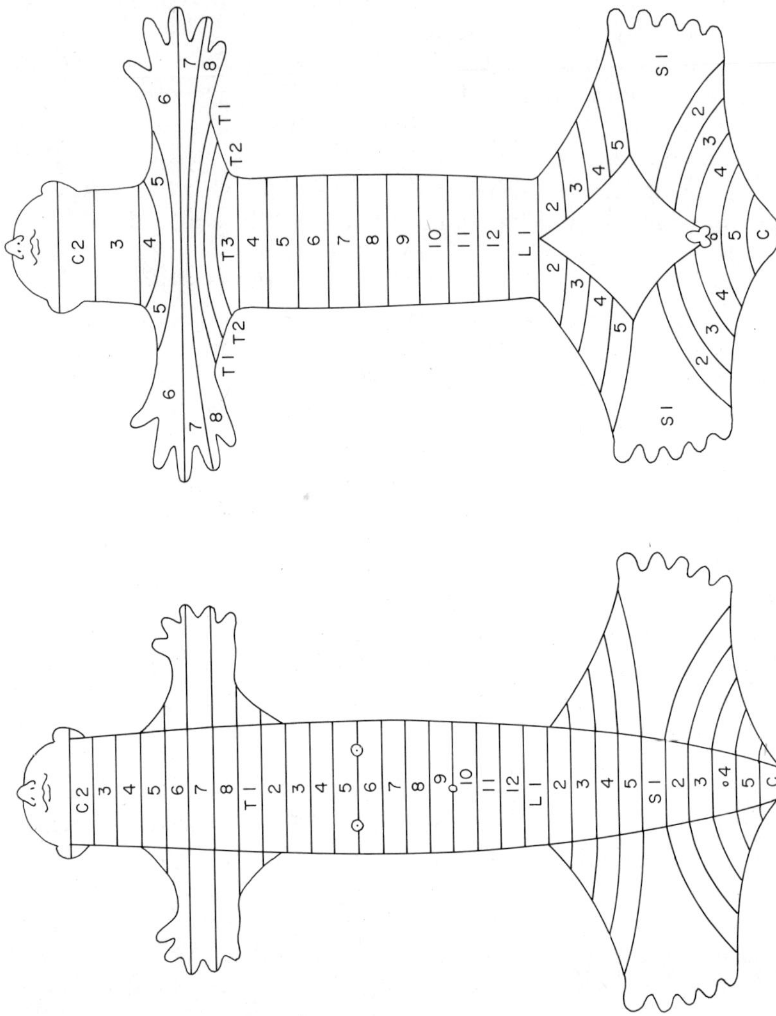

Fig 2–1.—Arrangement of the spinal nerves, anterior division. (From McGregor, L.: *Synopsis of Surgical Anatomy* [Bristol: John Wright & Sons, Ltd., 1943], after Purves-Stewart.)

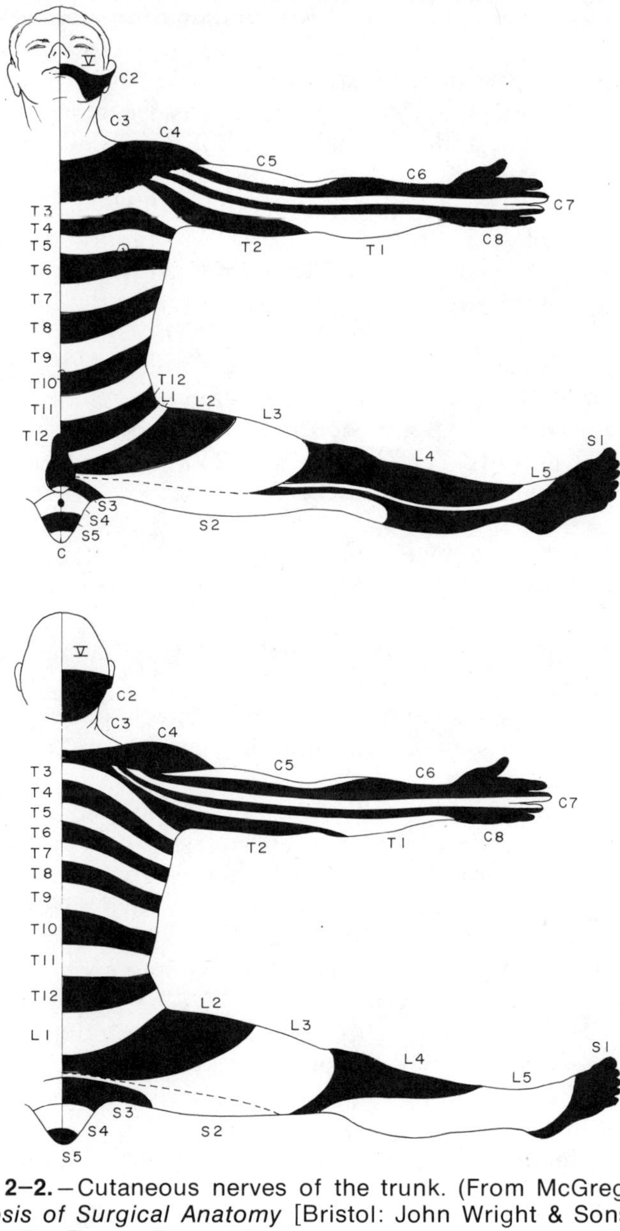

Fig 2–2.—Cutaneous nerves of the trunk. (From McGregor, L.: *Synopsis of Surgical Anatomy* [Bristol: John Wright & Sons, Ltd., 1943], after Purves-Stewart.)

ing pad assists this. A well-known Buffalo dermatologist used to prescribe 10% Ichthyol in collodion painted on daily to form a protective film. This splinted and protected the skin.

A dusting powder, warm compresses twice a day, steroid-antibiotic cream and even calamine lotion are all useful on occasion. To prevent postherpetic neuralgia, which in elderly patients is to be feared most, treatment should be aimed at the prevention of scarring in the dorsal root ganglion. For this purpose, adrenocorticotropic hormone (ACTH) or steroids (e.g., 80 mg Kenalog given intramuscularly) are the best. If the disease has been present for 4 days prior to the institution of such treatment, the risk of dissemination is practically zero. Determining that the patient is free from tuberculosis, diabetes, peptic ulcer, hypertension (and pregnancy?) is wise before using steroids. Taractan (Roche), 25 mg three times daily, is helpful (bearing in mind the frequent side effects of this drug).

Prior to the age of steroid usage, pituitary extract given 14 times daily by injection had a reputation of preventing neuralgia, as did occasional protamide injections, perhaps daily for a week. X-ray treatment over the spinal dorsal root ganglia was sometimes advocated, as was sodium iodide given intravenously. However, once the neuralgia is firmly ensconced, little helps. Neurosurgical intervention has to be considered sometimes.

A form of counterirritation to block the pain sensation (gateway theory)—a sort of do-it-yourself occupation—has recently demonstrated merit. The affected region is sprayed with fluoroethyl and then rubbed briskly with a towel repeatedly. This will stop the neuralgia. Also, diluted intralesional steroid injected into the course of the cutaneous nerve occasionally relieves zoster neuralgia.

Eczema vaccinatum results when an atopic individual gets near someone recently vaccinated. (See p. 86, PCAD.)

Kaposi's varicelliform eruption occurs when atopic individuals get herpes simplex infection. They are very sick and require systemic antibiotics and steroids plus soothing baths and local antibiotic creams. (See p. 82, PCAD.)

Rubeola (measles) is best treated by pediatricians. (See p. 8, PCAD.)

Rubella (German measles) produces deafness in children of women who catch it in the first trimester of pregnancy. The rash is very transient, usually on the face first, and disappears in 72 hours.

Enteroviruses (coxsackie and echo) can produce a variety of rashes, e.g., hand-foot-mouth syndrome.

Varicella (chicken pox), though usually a childhood disease, presents vesicopapules in all stages, with the trunk, face and scalp being the chief sites. The lesion has been described as a "dewdrop on a rose petal"—tiny vesicles at the tip of an erythematous papule. Soothing lotions, baths, antihistamines and antibiotics offer comfort.

Cytomegalic inclusion disease is detectable by the immune globulin test. It usually occurs in infants and has been thought to be rare and fatal, producing necrotic liver and spleen with large inclusion bodies in the lungs, skin and intestines. The autopsy findings are similar to those in a disseminated herpes simplex infection.

For *cat scratch disease*, the Foshay antigen skin test is diagnostic. An insignificant bite, scratch or puncture is followed in 3 weeks by regional lymph gland enlargement. This may subside or suppurate. Continued antibiotics seem to be the treatment of choice, either tetracycline or chlortetracycline. This disease is probably more common than is realized.

Lymphogranuloma venereum (LGV) usually occurs after an insignificant initial lesion; inguinal nodes (often unilateral) become matted and drain to produce sinuses in men and rectal stricture in women. There is an albumin globulin reversal; the Frei test shows positive results in 72 hours (nodule larger than 7 mm). Watch for the anorectal syndrome (stricture of 4–6 cm). (See p. 203, PCAD.)

Tetracycline, 500 mg, should be given four times a day; or you can use Aureomycin, sulfa, Chloromycetin or streptomycin, in decreasing order of effectiveness. The treatment should be prolonged.

Molluscum contagiosum has an incubation period of about

2–6 weeks, producing small pearly tumors. It is found in swimmers, Turkish-bath devotees and locker-room habitues. The tumors are usually in the axilla and groin. (See p. 79, PCAD.)

Treatment involves removal with a curette with ethyl chloride spray, or by application of phenol on a toothpick, by electrocautery using very low current, or by liquid nitrogen cryotherapy. Some authors claim that sulfadiazine, 4 gm/day, is curative in several weeks.[2] Others claim that Terramycin will do the same thing,[3] with which I disagree. Lately, griseofulvin has been reported to favorably affect molluscum warts in children.[4]

Warts may have an incubation period of up to 3 years. (See p. 80, PCAD.) *Verrucae vulgaris,* including filiform and periungual warts, are best treated with electrosurgery, although occasionally the application of phenol or trichloracetic acid on a toothpick suffices. If this is done at all, it should be done with a sharp round "World's Fair" toothpick and tattooed into the wart a little. Sometimes shaving the hard outer keratin layer permits better absorption. The application of the cantharides paint covered with plastic adhesive and held in place with Elastoplast for 72 hours, which produces blistering, will often destroy periungual warts. It is somewhat disconcerting, however, when the patient returns with a new ring of warts around the former site, the so-called doughnut effect.

Other local cauterants can be used, e.g., Freezone (zinc chloride, salicyclic acid, castor oil, alcohol, ether) or a prescription for wart paint (10% salicylic acid, 10% lactic acid, 10% glacial acetic acid in collodion), Ver Acid (Depelle) or Duofilm (Stiefel), all of which the patient can be taught to apply at home. For large warts, a rim of vaseline can be built up around the wart to enable the cauterant to be applied to the wart only, wiping the vaseline off after the medication dries to a film. The patient should be instructed to desist and resume later if excessive irritation occurs. (See Formulary, no. 21.)

"Strangulation" of the warts by occlusively wrapping them with elastic adhesive, leaving it on for weeks and replacing it if too messy works occasionally and is useful in very small frightened children.

Intralesional injections of various substances from vitamin A to Novocain itself, if done at the dermal-epidermal junction, involute a wart, but if you are going to go this far, you might as well remove the wart with electrosurgery.

Vitamin A in oral doses of 100,000 units daily for 3–6 months may help to clear warts, as might bismuth (Barclay Pharmacy, Philadelphia) given intramuscularly weekly. This method of treatment is out of favor currently.

Suggestion therapy, if accompanied by a convincing display of belief in its efficacy, can and does clear warts, though the mechanism may have more to do with the fallacy of the positive instance than with changes in the blood or nerve supply to the wart. Hypnosis often is efficacious, though probably expensive.

Refrigeration techniques using liquid nitrogen applied to the wart for 15–40 seconds (depending on wart size) on a cotton-tipped (loosely wrapped) applicator often produce a scarless result, which is especially useful around the elbows and knees. It is painful, though most children tolerate it well. The object is to produce a blister, which is left alone to dry up and drop off, taking the wart with it. For storing the liquid nitrogen, we use a pint thermos with a little fiber glass *inside*, using a cork with a hole in it and then a screw-on top. This usually lasts 48 hours and is refilled from a local vacuum tube manufacturer. Local welding supply companies will provide liquid nitrogen in large containers. I have found the cotton-tipped applicator satisfactory and free of breakdown problems. The "Foster Froster" is faster. (See the chapter on cryotherapy.)

CO_2 snow pencils, such as can be made with the Kidde apparatus, can also be used to treat warts. They can be applied with moderate pressure for 30–120 seconds, depending upon the size and depth of the wart. It is important to observe patients 4 weeks after receiving such treatment and re-treat if not clear.

The application of monochloracetic acid (saturated solution), tattooing it in after paring and then covering with 40% salicylic acid plaster and wrapping with Elastoplast, is another treatment for stubborn periungual warts. The dressing should be left on 5 days or so and the resultant maceration removed. Retreatment in another week should be done if needed.

Whereas many dermatologists no longer have x-ray machines in their offices, and in fact the proper use of the x-ray machine is being taught less and less in many dermatologic training centers, it is a therapy of great value. Its *proper* use must be emphasized. The x-ray machine can be a dangerous weapon, and accidental overdose can produce late sequelae of considerable severity. X-ray therapy of benign lesions, such as warts, should be done only by those with proper training in radiotherapeutics. The machine must be calibrated annually by a physicist, and have an automatic timing device.

X-ray treatments occasionally are helpful when a profuse explosion of warts suddenly occurs after a thermal burn. Here the number of warts makes individual treatment almost impossible. Seventy-five rad of superficial therapy administered to the area once a week at 30 cm tube–skin distance will often cause involution.

X-ray treatment to individual warts, especially to periungual or subungual warts, is often extremely efficacious. This must be done skillfully and can be administered in one dose of about 1,200 rad, shielding to within 1–2 mm of the margin with lead and using a cone.[5] I prefer 100 kv at 20 cm tube–skin distance, although Andrews recommends 60 kv with a half-value layer of 0.7 mm aluminum, which unless the wart is very thin, might not penetrate deeply enough.[6] The warty thick keratin should be shaved off as much as possible. Fractionating the periungual wart treatment to 200 rad, 100 kv, unfiltered at 20 cm tube–skin distance every 2 weeks for four treatments is a little safer and has been curative. Shielding must be done carefully and the finger must be strapped to a sandbag with tape. If the single-dose technique is used, the patient should be brought back 40 days later to have the warty remnant removed.[7] This can be easily peeled off and usually reduces the reseeding risk considerably. X-ray treatment of warts should be reserved for the most difficult therapeutic problems; it should not be used routinely.

Verruca plana juvenilis.—Often Vleminckx solution applied

straight out of the jar every night will cause these to involute. Since many of these patients are small children, other mild peeling lotions can be used, for example, "freckle peeler" (see Formulary, no. 13) or D'Alibour solution two or three times a day. Sometimes a strong 20% lotio alba will effect a cure. Painting with 2% podophyllin in alcohol, or 20–50% trichloracetic acid or light electrodesiccation, leaving the crusts to drop off and following with BFI powder, are other suitable methods. Liquid nitrogen can be used very lightly, or CO_2 slush applied at intervals. Hot Vleminckx compresses occasionally are successful, too. Digitate warts of the beard in men are best treated by electrodesiccation, either with low current without Novocain, or with procaine anesthesia in the case of the larger lesions. This should be done in a very bright light using a strong magnifying loupe, and the whole bearded region should be inspected carefully to get every last wart. Monthly reinspection should be scheduled, and shaving articles should be thoroughly cleansed and on occasion even sterilized after use. Disposable razors are useful here. Ten percent benzoyl peroxide in a cream at night occasionally is also helpful. Retin-A, 0.1% cream every night to beard warts, is occasionally curative.

Plantar warts must be differentiated from clavi or plantar corns, which characteristically occur over the heads of metatarsal bones and have a hard central translucency that is pearly and very sensitive to lateral pressure. A wart has small loops of capillaries which become traumatized, leaving small black dots in it which often bleed when shaved, and is soft after shaving.

Electrodesiccation is an effective and, with good technique, a comparatively painless way of dealing with these problems. After cleansing the area thoroughly and wiping with alcohol, ethyl chloride (Gebauer) is sprayed on until the area is hard and white, after which 2% procaine (or Carbocaine, Xylocaine or Cyclaine) is injected. Using a Luer-Lok 3-cc. syringe with dental grips and a 30 needle, one has good control. The spark is applied to the surface of the wart using a medium strong setting, and then inserted into the wart so that the tissue fluids boil. When the wart puffs up and becomes luminescent, the steam has lifted the wart off the underlying tissue, and after clipping with small scissors, it can be lifted off and the pulp curetted out. The edges should be trimmed clean, and the base lightly desiccated to control bleeding. Tincture of merthiolate is applied, and an Elastoplast dressing over a gauze pad wrapped around the foot several times to provide effective hemostasis is the dressing. This can be left on for 12 hours, and then the patient applies tincture of merthiolate and a bandage in the daytime and tincture of merthiolate without the bandage at night. A "ball-o-foot" cushion (Dr. Scholl) will assist postoperative walking comfort. Generally the wound heals with a scab forming in 10 days and dropping off in 4–6 weeks, leaving a soft pliable white flat scar. It is good practice to ensure that the patient understands something of the natural history of warts, since development of satellite warts around a solitary wart, if it occurs following removal of the solitary wart, is often blamed on the physician. Therefore the patient should understand the relation between the duration of plantar warts and the chance of new ones developing, regardless of what method of removal is used.

Liquid nitrogen and carbon dioxide snow are not used on plantar warts very much in my office because of the severity of the pain for the patient. However, liquid nitrogen has a very definite place in the treatment of such plantar warts (using Xylocaine first).

Another effective method after paring is the application of a saturated solution of monochloracetic acid using a cotton-tipped *sharp* World's Fair round, hard toothpick, tattooing the solution into the wart quite thoroughly with multiple punctures and using finger cots or rubber gloves so that the monochloracetic acid will not creep up on the toothpick and produce annoying splits on the fingers of the operator a few days later. Covering this treated area with 40% salicylic acid plaster (Beiersdorf) over which a much larger piece of moleskin is applied and then the whole wrapped on with 2-inch Elastoplast to hold it in place is very effective treatment. It should remain fixed in position for one week, and it should be wound around the foot two or three times and not get wet. On the patient's return visit, after cleaning off the adhesive with ether or acetone, the resultant sterile abscess is easily deroofed with a Schick injector razor blade or a sharp 15 scalpel blade; often that cures the wart. Dressings for one day are all that is necessary, and healing is remarkably prompt.

For elderly, debililated or other problem patients, or as a last resort, x-ray treatment of plantar warts may be a "lifesaver." X-ray treatment of plantar warts should be done only after extensive paring, since the thick keratin can effectively filter out most of the rays. The lead shield should be 1 or 2 mm wider than the wart to be treated. If the patient lies on his stomach and a cushion is placed on a wastebasket or stool for a foot rest, the position is satisfactory for treatment. If the single-dose technique is used, the smaller the wart, the larger the dose, e.g., a 5 mm or smaller wart should get 2,000 rad, whereas 1,500 rad is the dose for a 5–10 mm wart; 1,200 rad for a 10–15 mm wart; 1000 rad for a 15–20 mm wart. Sixty kilovolts unfiltered (0.7 mm Al) is recommended by Andrews, although I prefer 100 kv unfiltered (0.9 mm Al) at 20 cm tube–skin distance, with a spot cone and a lead shield. Another method of treatment is 600–750 rad every 2 weeks for three visits depending upon the size of the wart. This last method seems to have a slightly higher rate of success. Careful diagrams should be kept of the location of radiation-treated warts and the patient should be advised that *no more should be given there—ever!*[5]

Another method of treatment that offers promise is 5% 5-FU in Neobase under occlusion. Successful treatment of plantar warts by injection of bleomycin using the Dermajet has been described by Hudson.[8]

Mosaic plantar warts are generally considered to be resistant to radiation therapy. Repeated paring and application of monochloracetic acid or 100% silver nitrate, liquid nitrogen or carbon dioxide snow, after which the area is covered with 40% salicylic acid plaster over which moleskin is placed, is a moderately successful method of treatment; but many patients tire too soon. If continued long enough, it *will* cure very stubborn mosaic warts, but the patient should be encouraged to be conscientious and continue for about a year. Twenty-five percent formaldehyde ointment, e.g., formalin 4.0 in aquaphor q.s. to

15, under occlusion at night, or soaking in a dilute solution of formalin 1:5 in a saucer or ashtray or small watch glass for 20–30 minutes at night, protecting the surrounding skin with vaseline, is also effective though slow. One patient became allergic to formaldehyde as a result of this treatment, with ensuing shoe-leather problems, so this method of treatment is not without hazard. Also, glutaraldehyde paint is very often helpful. (See Formulary, no. 21.)

Verrucae acuminata almost always occur in sweaty moist people, so recurrences are very common. Twenty-five percent podophyllin in acetone and tincture of benzoin is very effective, but patients with many lesions, or in whom reaction to the podophyllin is to be feared, should be instructed to wash off the paint in 6 hours. Phisohex washing and Neosporin dusting powder with or without daubing with peroxide will lessen recurrences. In anal condylomas, a proctoscope will often disclose unsuspected rectal verrucae, which otherwise will reinfect the anal skin and may have to be removed under general anesthesia. Similarly, condylomas in the vagina and even on the cervix can lead to reinfection and recurrences. With scattered, few or solitary condylomas, electrodesiccation using procaine is an effective "cure." Occasionally 50% podophyllin in acetone and tincture of benzoin are more effective; and Dr. W. B. Swarts of Greenwich says that if this is allowed to sit overnight, it goes into suspension fairly well.[9] Occasionally trichloracetic acid will help in those who cannot tolerate podophyllin, and 3% podophyllin in polyethylene glycol once a day by the patient often suffices in modest involvement. Cryotherapy with liquid nitrogen (20–60 seconds) is another modality. (See p. 80, PCAD.)

Other useful treatments for condylomas are the application of thiotepa locally three times a day and, for intraurethral soft warts, 5-FU applied carefully and repeatedly with a swab. Extensive condylomas may be softened with potassium iodide solution soaks, after which the podophyllin dry resin powder may be carefully daubed with a swab.

Complications of electrosurgery in wart removal include keloidal scarring, especially in patients in the 11–18 age group, where warts tend to occur. Follow-ups therefore should be complete, and the patient and the patient's parents should be warned that in this age group scarring can be a cosmetic problem; the patient should be carefully observed for several months. Keloidal scarring is fortunately rarely seen in periungual warts. However, occasionally in an extensive old periungual or subungual wart, some distortion of the nail may result from removal of the wart. This is more apt to happen when there is a need for hemostasis with much electrodesiccation. Trichloracetic acid used for hemostasis often is less destructive.

Liquid nitrogen is less scarring but less reliable for cure. Keloids can be either flattened with liquid nitrogen or injected with diluted Kenalog intralesionally. The technique for injecting intralesional Kenalog into keloids is discussed more thoroughly later in this book.

There has been an instructive discussion of wart regression with wart antigen, when complement-fixation antibodies developed.[10] Lewis has developed a technique of sensitizing the patient with recalcitrant warts to dinitrochlorobenzene (DNCB – Aldrich Chemical), then applying it daily in a reactive concentration under Telfa (usually 0.01%) for 5 – 10 days. Warts usually disappear in 3 – 6 weeks.[11]

In a Portuguese fowl slaughterhouse, where there was an epidemic of warts, Goncalves cured 50% of the cases using 5-FU with 4% salicylic acid.[12]

REFERENCES

1. Whitley, R. J., et al.: Adenine arabinoside therapy of biopsy-proved herpes simplex encephalitis, N. Engl. J. Med. 297:289, 1977.
2. Sommerville, J.: Molluscum contagiosum and M & B 693, Br. J. Dermatol. 53:255, 1941.
3. Mopper, C.: Terramycin therapy of molluscum contagiosum, Am. Arch. Dermatol. Syphilol. 65:613, 1952.
4. Singh, O. P., and Kanwar, A. J.: Griseofulvin therapy in molluscum contagiosum, Arch. Dermatol. 113:1615, 1977.
5. Pipkin, J. L., et al.: The treatment of plantar warts by single dose roentgen ray, South. Med. J. 42:193, 1949.
6. Domonkos, A. N.: *Andrews' Diseases of the Skin* (6th ed.; Philadelphia: W. B. Saunders Co., 1971), p. 553.
7. Sutton, R. L.: *Diseases of the Skin* (St. Louis: C. V. Mosby Co., 1956).

8. Hudson, A. L.: Treatment of plantar warts with bleomycin, Arch. Dermatol. 112:1179, 1976.
9. Swarts, W. B.: Personal communication.
10. Pyrhönen, S., and Johansson, E.: Regression of warts: An immunological study, Lancet 1:592, 1975.
11. Lewis, H. M.: Topical immunotherapy of refractory warts, Cutis 12:863, 1973.
12. Goncalves, J. C. A.: 5-fluorouracil in the treatment of common warts of the hands, Br. J. Dermatol. 92:89, 1975.

3 / Atopic Dermatitis

Atopic dermatitis includes eczema, infantile allergic eczema and disseminated neurodermatitis. (See p. 36, PCAD.)

In infancy atopic dermatitis starts on the face, usually when the infant is 2 or 3 months old. There is usually a family history of eczema, asthma, hay fever or hives. It may commence in childhood after age 2, with papules on the extensor areas (excoriated usually) and lichenification in the flexures, particularly in the antecubitals or popliteal areas, sides of the neck and eyelid areas. These patients are usually better in summer, although not all are worse in winter. Occasionally they outgrow their condition at the ages of 8 to 12, *or* it may persist into adolescence and early adult life, with much the same localization. There is intense pruritus, which despite much scratching, seems to become infected surprisingly seldom. Intraepidermic vesicles occur only in infants and are not seen in children or adults, the pathology being mostly in the dermis, and the epidermal changes being entirely secondary to rubbing and scratching. The skin is often dry, and atopic persons are intolerant of rough materials, e.g., wool and often soap. The areas of involvement are those where sweat glands are concentrated, and indoor exercise when there is no breeze to assist in the evaporation of sweat from the skin surface, often produces severe itching, e.g., in a basketball game in a gymnasium. Atopic persons tolerate hot, humid weather poorly and often flare with emotional stress or simple fatigue. They tend to develop cataracts, exhibit white dermagraphism and react unpredictably and unreliably to all intradermal skin tests. Response to elimination diets is disappointing in adults, although helpful in infants, where allergies to milk, wheat, eggs, orange juice, spinach, tomatoes, fish oils and vitamins containing fish oils are often significant.

Hospitalization always improves the condition of atopic

persons, probably by getting them away from their families. Treatment is not very satisfactory, although an understanding of the above factors is essential to the management of such patients. Often greasy occlusive applications will aggravate rather than help them, and dusty atmospheres and hot spicy food will aggravate itching. Commonly there is eosinophilia. Eczema is seldom difficult to diagnose although it has to be differentiated from a chronic contact dermatitis with lichenification due to a continuous undisclosed cause. Seborrheic dermatitis occasionally is difficult to differentiate; nummular eczema can confuse the physician, too. Persons having prurigo (mitis and ferox) should be managed as are atopic patients.

Infantile Eczema

The first step in treating infantile eczema is to reassure the anxious parents that the chances are greatly in favor of eventual spontaneous clearing of the eruption after around age 2. They should be assured that there will be no scars or other sequelae. Atopic children are often go-getters who become successful adults, and this, of course, is of value for the parents to know. Atopic children usually look worse than they feel. No one can catch the condition; and the patients seldom get blood poisoning or other infections as a result of their constant lesions.

The parents should be told not to overdress the baby. They should use light loose clothing and keep the house at an even temperature, around 70 F. In other words, sweat should evaporate from the skin surface easily. Rough material next to the skin is forbidden, especially wool. Strong detergents with strong bleaches or whiteners are also offenders. If drooling is a problem, a waterproof mattress cover under the sheet keeps the baby's face bathed in saliva with or without detergent; a pad under the sheet will absorb much of this so that the facial dermatitis will be lessened. Fabric softeners used in washing machines will do much to impart softness to the materials next to the atopic skin. Diapers can be rinsed in Diaparene or boric acid or boiled for 10 minutes to destroy the bacteria that split off the ammonia from the urine, if diaper rash is a problem.

Reduction of environmental allergens, such as dust, blanket fuzz, feathers, mattress ticking, animal danders, and Teddy bears, by common-sense choice of foam rubber or other allergen-proof zippered covers on things, plus using plastic toys is wise, not only to help the eczema condition, but also to forestall future inhalant sensitization.

Elimination Diets

Elimination diets, especially those eliminating wheat, milk and eggs, orange juice, tomatoes, spinach, fish and fish oils, often cure children. It is difficult to instruct a mother in the avoidance of these foods since so many baby foods contain one or more of these allergenic foods. Often soybean milk, such as Mull-Soy or Sobee, or even goat's milk will have to be resorted to, with the resultant loose stools. Occasionally just the slight denaturing of the manufactured evaporated milk is sufficient; and this can be used instead of cow's milk. Soybean wafers, Ry-Krisp and various other substitutes for bread, which of course contain no wheat or egg, may be used and careful reading of the labels on baby foods can lead to the proper selections. A hospital dietitian can be of great assistance.

Food Allergies

Food hypersensitivity in children should not be confused with food intolerance, such as gluten intolerance. Food additives, such as tetracyclines and penicillin in poultry, cheese and milk, saccharine and soybean products, and gums (acacia, karaya, tragacanth), produce a variety of reactions which often are inadvertently blamed on the food. Some artificial sweeteners have a photosensitizing effect (e.g., cyclamen).

Food allergy is more common in children less than two years of age. Usually allergy to milk is the first to disappear, while fish and nuts allergies persist longer. Cooked or canned foods are often tolerated when raw foods are not. Following an allergic reaction to a food, there occurs a brief refractory period. Then there is a period of increased sensitivity, which fades. Multiple food sensitivities are the rule.

Immediate Reactions

Reactions occur within a few minutes of eating some whole

proteins (e.g., milk, eggs, peanuts, fish, crab, lobster, shrimp, oysters, pork, nuts, tomatoes, strawberries and occasionally buckwheat). Symptoms are either acute gastrointestinal, urticaria, angioedema or allergic rhinitis, asthma *or* a shocklike picture with pallor and syncope.

The treatment should be to give antihistamines, or 0.05–0.2 cc of 1:1,000 epinephrine injected intramuscularly or subcutaneously.

Delayed Reaction

A delayed reaction occurs several hours later, and skin test results are usually negative. The sensitizer is usually a breakdown product of the whole protein, e.g., milk chocolate, cola, eggs, legumes (including peanuts), orange, tomato, corn, wheat, pork or food coloring.

Treatment is essentially identification and avoidance. This is done with elimination diets or provocative diets and food diaries. Avoidance of wheat is especially difficult, since most commercial rye breads contain wheat. Parents must know the "hidden sources" and read *all* labels.

Sources of menus for diets are listed below:

1. American Medical Assoc., 535 N. Dearborn, Chicago, Ill.
2. Gerber Products Co., Fremont, Mich.
3. Hollister-Stier Labs., 550 Industrial Park Drive, Yeadon, Pa.
4. American Dietetic Assoc., 430 N. Michigan Avenue, Chicago, Ill.
5. Sheldon, J. M., Lovell, R. G., and Matthews, K. P.: *The Manual of Clinical Allergy* (2d ed.; Philadelphia: W. B. Saunders Co., 1967)

Cow's milk substitutes are listed below:

1. Soybean formulas
   Sobee (Mead Johnson)–liquid and powder
   Mull-Soy (Borden)–contains no corn products, no vitamins–liquid and powder
   Soyalac (Loma Linda)–liquid or powder
2. Meat base formulas
   Lambase (Gerber)–liquid
   Meatbase (Gerber)–contains no corn

3. Refined soy protein
   Prosobee (Mead Johnson)
   Neo-Mullsoy (Borden) – no corn
   Similac, Isomil (Ross)
4. Protein hydrolysates
   Nutramigen (Mead Johnson)
   Amigen (Baxter)
   Stuart amino acids (Stuart)

The formula should be started at 1:3, gradually increasing to the standard 20 calories per oz. If soybean formulas are not tolerated, then lambase formulas should be used, 1 – 2 oz water (and one teaspoon sugar or Karo), and gradually increased to a 1:1 dilution. Meatbase formulas may be tolerated better by some children.

The casein in cow's milk and goat's milk appears to be identical, and there is some cross antigenicity in their albumins, so avoid goat's milk in suspected cow's milk allergy.

If the infant's allergic symptoms subside in 7 – 14 days (after a cow's milk substitute or with plain cooked tapioca, flour and sugar), then add other foods at 5- to 7-day intervals, starting with the following: applesauce or apple juice, strained pears, carrots, beets, squash (severe reactions have been reported), rice cereal, banana flakes, lamb or veal.

A strict elimination diet includes a cow's milk substitute (Soyalac), apple juice, pear nectar, apricot nectar, apple cider, applesauce, cooked apples, canned pears, peaches, apricots, tapioca or gelatin flavored with vanilla or honey, Ry-Krisp, Rice Krispies, rice cereal, rice, puffed rice, rice wafers (Celler Co., Chicago), boiled carrots, and milk-free margarine (e.g., Willow Run margarine or Marv-Parv.), beets, string beans, squash, sweet potato, lamb (boiled ham is also often allowed), soy oil for cooking, sugar, salt, honey, rock candy, blueberries, cranberries (canned), lettuce, okra, and artichoke for older children. Vitamins and calcium supplements should be given.

Local Treatment

In extremely generalized eruptions, oilated Aveeno, starch or tar baths are always soothing and antipruritic when used with care not to overdry the patient's skin. They are helpful in removing accumulated scale, crust and old ointment as well. In less widespread cases, mineral oil soaks, or washing with Phisoderm or a bath oil, or boric acid or Burow's compresses will soothe and cleanse effectively.

Scalp

If there are caked scale and crusts and they are a problem, the following prescription is very useful:

Salicylic acid	2.5
Castor oil	12.0
Peanut oil q.s. ad	120.0

This will cleanse the scalp very well when rubbed into the scalp two or three times daily and shampooed out every three days.

In babies, use Johnson & Johnson Baby Shampoo or Phisoderm for normal skin, or even Phisohex on occasion. For older people, tar shampoos, such as Tersa-Tar (Doak), Polytar (Stiefel), Zetar (Dermik) and Sebutone (Westwood) are good commercially available shampoos. (See Formulary, no. 31) Plain Dara shampoo, or 5% sodium lauryl sulfate in distilled water is an effective shampoo.

Steroid lotions, such as hydrocortisone scalp lotion (Texas Pharmacal) or Synalar 0.01% solution in propylene glycol (Syntex), are effective, as is a compounded prescription as follows:

Hydrocortisone-free alcohol powder	0.3
Cade oil (or 5–10% coal tar solution USP)	0.9
Topisol cream (Texas Pharmacal) ad	30.0

Directions: Make an ointment and rub in the scalp at night.

Ze-Tar-Quin Creme, 0.5% (Dermik), is occasionally helpful here also.

Generally speaking, the best treatment for atopic eczema in the adult scalp is to keep it clean.

Face

Sometimes the following is an effective treatment for very crusty oozing eczemas in infants:

Cade oil	1.5
Zinc oxide ointment q.s. ad	30.0

More often, the following is preferable and cleaner: 1% hydrocortisone cream or lotion form, e.g.

Hydrocortisone	0.3
Allercreme skin lotion (Texas Pharmacal) q.s. ad	30.0

or

Hydrocortisone	0.3
USP hydrophilic ointment q.s. ad	30.0

Other bases, such as Cetaphil lotion, can be used since many atopic persons seem to tolerate a lipid-free lotion better than a greasy base. Lubriderm creme (Texas Pharmacal) or Shepard cream lotion can be used as the base. Some atopic patients respond extremely well when Cetaphil lotion is rubbed in and then, immediately afterward, Synalar lotion is rubbed on top.

Tar intolerance can develop and worsening of the eruption or increased itching or pustulation indicates that it should be discontinued. The triamcinolone preparations, e.g., Cordran-Aristocort-Kenalog or Synalar creams, are always very effective, too, although they are proprietary drugs and the therapist does not have complete control.

One can use:

Aristocort 0.5%	5 gm
Acid mantle base (Dome)	
or	
mixture of aquaphor and water	
q.s. ad	30.0

or other variations in these extemporaneous prescriptions, so that you can have triamcinolone in combination with other drugs.

Trunk

Over large body areas, the cost of the commercially available steroid preparations, e.g., $5 for a 2-oz tube of 0.025%

Kenalog or 0.01% Synalar, makes extemporaneous compounds much preferable. For instance, a vial of Kenalog suspension used for intralesional injections, which is 5 cc and contains 50 mg Kenalog, may be dumped into 8 oz of Cetaphil lotion. This makes approximately the same percentage as the commercially available preparations. The same thing can be done with hydrocortisone powder, of course, and other bases such as Lubriderm, Allercreme and Cetaphil. A commercially available lotion that is relatively inexpensive is the 0.25% Cort-Dome lotion, which comes in the acid mantle base and has the disadvantage of the Burow's solution present.

Lidex ointment (Syntex), while greasy, seems to be extremely well tolerated and also extremely effective in treating atopic patients almost anywhere. Care must be taken to avoid excessive use in intertrigenous areas or too prolonged use under occlusion in order to avoid the atrophy occasionally seen with the use of strong fluorinated steroids. It does not sting as does Lidex cream (which is also very effective). (See Formulary, no. 22.)

One can throw a few capsules of Chloromycetin into the lotion to control follicular infection, e.g., eight capsules of Chloromycetin in 8 oz Cetaphil lotion gives about a 1% concentration, which is adequate.

Limbs

When the skin is oozy, crusty and dry, the following prescription is helpful and also useful in treating infected eczemas on the face:

Hydrocortisone	0.3
Bacitracin q.s. ad	30.0

This should be rubbed in three times a day after meals.

Occasionally the following prescription is used to make an effective ointment:

Hydrocortisone	0.3
Coal tar solution USP	1.5
USP hydrophilic ointment q.s. ad	30.0

Systemic Treatment

Antihistamines, particularly Chlor-Trimeton, 4 mg in either a syrup or tablet, Pyribenzamine elixir, 10 mg per teaspoon, or

Benadryl elixir, 10 mg per teaspoon, 4 to 5 teaspoons a day, perhaps 2 at bedtime, can be very helpful. Syrup of Periactin is my favorite, which is approximately 2 mg per teaspoon. It is excellent at bedtime because it seems to keep children from scratching through the night. It can be given in the daytime, although it does make the patient quite drowsy, at which time the dose can be reduced to one-half teaspoon. Temaril syrup, one-half teaspoon at bedtime, or three or four times a day unless too soporific, occasionally helps, too. Syrup of Atarax, one teaspoon three times a day, helps hyperkinetic atopic patients.

Systemic steroids should be resorted to only rarely because of the cessation of growth which may occur in growing children. (It is regained later.) The danger of a person contracting varicella while taking steroids is a real one, with an increased risk of death. However, if steroids are used, local treatment should be pushed to minimize the withdrawal flare-up when discontinued. Sometimes if all else fails, a complete change of environment, perhaps to a desert clime or a beach where the breezes are offshore, will clear the condition of the stubborn patient.

It cannot be emphasized too strongly that in atopic children, a home atmosphere of love and affection with plenty of physical contact between the child and the parents often does more than any other single factor to prevent exacerbation of eczema. An attitude of rejection, withdrawal of affection, or even hostility can occasionally be observed in the parents of such children; and the value of tender loving care should be emphasized to them.

Excessive bathing should be interdicted, and the parent should be cautioned not to be "too clean," neither constantly having the child in freshly and strongly laundered linen, nor spending too many minutes in the shower or bath. Baths must *not be daily,* but perhaps only twice a week—with bath oil and superfatted soap and short and cool (no bubble bath).

In older children and adults, the management is essentially the same, although antihistamines have to be given with great care since the side effects may be risky in certain occupations and interfere with cerebration. Grenz rays or x-rays used to be very helpful in the treatment of stubborn areas; they are seldom used today. The various steroid creams and ointments applied are often extremely effective, and occasionally a change from hydrocortisone to triamcinolone, or back again, seems to enable the patient to switch around so that he doesn't get too used to one particular steroid and have its effectiveness reduced. In rare cases, help from a psychiatrist may clear a patient, although this is always a long and tiring proposition for the patient and not always one that he can be persuaded to accept.

The administration of systemic steroids by injection in patients who do not have diabetes, hypertension, peptic ulcer, tuberculosis, thrombotic or psychotic phenomena seems to be the safest, cheapest and most effective management technique for the adult with severe atopy. The dose reduction coupled with the long-acting effect (often 3 months or more of remission from a single intramuscular injection of 60–80 mg Kenalog suspension) minimizes the side effects when the steroids are injected intramuscularly. Present evidence indicates that all circulating steroid is gone after 21 days, although it would be perhaps safer to estimate 30 to 40 days. ACTH occasionally and intermittently can do the same thing, as can other steroids injected intramuscularly (e.g., Celestone, Soluspan, Depo-Medrol and Aristocort). However, the favorite of the moment seems to be triamcinolone acetonide (Kenalog). Side effects to watch out for are hirsutism, weight gain, acne, peptic ulcer, ankle edema, osteoporosis, hypertension, diabetes, disseminating infection, thromboses, uremia, adrenal insufficiency, and potassium depletion leading to muscle weakness and pain. All of these side effects can be dealt with. However, it is a wise physician who realizes the power of many of our present medicines and discusses the possible dangers with his patient thoroughly. A mention that atopic persons tend to develop cataracts without steroids may forestall later blame. The surgeons who do things at prearranged times in front of expert witnesses are now much safer than physicians who can, with a stroke of a pen, add a really potent force to the life of an individual patient.

The effects of the powerful medicines we now have at our command can alter the thinking of a patient, can make him more courageous and expansive and even produce personality changes that may lead to poor judgment in a business or political situation. I have had patients start terrific building projects while under the influence of steroids, only to cancel everything when they were tapered off the medication. Drugs can affect people in very strange ways, and caution must be used. This is known to all but neophyte physicians, and is stated here mainly to reinforce the fact that caution is essential at all times.

4 / Urticaria

Urticaria results from dilation of the superficial blood vessels with extravasation of fluid subcutaneously to produce whealing. (See p. 118, PCAD.) The surrounding erythema, called the "flare," is the result of an axone reflex. There is pronounced itching, which is not relieved easily by scratching. Dilation of the deeper vessels produces giant hives, or angioneurotic edema, with predilection for the mucocutaneous junctions and the palms and soles. The cause is commonly a large protein allergy; histamine is released (probably along with other substances) at the site of the antigen-antibody union to cause the leakage and itching. Acute attacks usually follow the ingestion of certain foods or drugs and are quickly relieved by steroids administered intravenously or adrenalin subcutaneously, but chronic or recurrent attacks respond better to antihistamines or ataractics, e.g., Pyribenzamine, Benadryl, Chlor-Trimeton, Atarax and Vistaril. (See Formulary, no. 26.) Careful investigation and removal of the cause, of course, also are essential.

Cholinergic Urticaria

Cholinergic urticaria (widespread 2–3 mm urticarial papules) responds to Pro-Banthine (15 mg) or atropine sulfate (See p. 118, PCAD.) and may result from physical allergy (light, heat, cold) or emotion. It is rather rare. A large flare response is obtained to intracutaneous injection of 1/5,000 Mecholyl. Atarax is the drug of choice here.

Angioneurotic Edema

Angioneurotic edema may involve the larynx and lead to death from choking, so the patient should be warned to seek help at once if talking, swallowing or breathing seems difficult.

In an attack, patient history may elicit the cause since events are fresh in the patient's mind. Questioning and requestioning about food, drugs, infection, parasites, nerves, sneezing attacks (inhalants), newly dyed clothes, suppositories, dental packs and injections sometimes turn up some pertinent information. Often, however, "cross-fixes" are required after repeated attacks over many months. For this purpose, a food diary is helpful.

Acute Urticaria

In acute urticaria or giant hives, adrenalin or epinephrine hydrochloride, 1:1,000, 0.2–0.4 cc subcutaneously, or Susphrine (long-acting), 0.1–0.2 cc, or adrenalin in oil intramuscularly, usually is the quickest and most reliable method of controlling an acute attack, although it may make the patient quite shaky at times. The administration of Chlor-Trimeton intramuscularly, Benadryl intravenously in a dose of 2 cc, and lastly Solumedrol intravenously can occasionally be very helpful. The steroids take a little longer to be effective, however.

Once the immediate threat is controlled, depot steroids, e.g., Kenalog intramuscularly 60 mg, are effective in suppressing the attack for a few weeks while the patient recovers to normality. Meanwhile he should avoid the cause, if known or strongly suspected; and if not, he should be given a list of the most common offenders and told to avoid them. Among the foods to be strictly avoided are: shellfish, fish, nuts, berries, tomatoes, oranges, cheese, pork, chocolate, eggs and food tenderizers. The drugs that commonly incriminate are: penicillin (this includes milk and certain moldy cheeses, as well as "achronized" poultry, or any kind of meat that has been preserved with antibiotics), sulfonamides, quinine, phenolphthalein, bromides and iodides, barbiturates and ipecac.

Urticaria is not commonly caused by inhalants, but in cases where the cause is in doubt, avoidance of the common inhalant allergens is wise. This list includes feathers, down, Orris and Lycopodium powders found in makeup, animal dander, house dust, gums and oils and sprays used on the hair, pollens, insecticides, and dyed material which can by percutaneous absorption lead to urticaria.

The local application of 1% phenol in calamine lotion, mild menthol-camphor lotion or steroid cream lotion is helpful in relieving the itching, as are soothing baths, especially starch baths. Calcium gluconate, injected intravenously very slowly, often seems to be helpful when all else fails to give relief. It was popular in the presteroid era and still has value.

Chronic Urticaria

The cause here is usually more difficult to identify and the longer I deal with such cases, the more skeptical I become that staple foods, such as milk, wheat and eggs, are ever to blame. Certain somewhat more exotic foods, such as mustard, chocolate, lobster, and even pork, are easier to uncover as the cause, but many cases are caused by the repeated taking of a drug of which the therapist is unaware, despite repeated questioning. The patient should be made to understand that *all* medications have to be eliminated for a trial period, including vitamins, hormones, oral contraceptives, laxatives, tonics, cold tablets, nose sprays, hair dyes, eardrops, eyedrops, toothpastes and mouth washes, douches and suppositories, especially water pills and diet pills, nerve pills, as well as visits to the dentist involving packs in the teeth. Food preservatives, e.g., sodium benzoate, can occasionally be responsible for repeated acute attacks. A *stool examination* for ova and parasites is wise in persistent cases, especially if there has been a visit to a tropical climate or any recent change in bowel habit. A search for *foci of infection* in teeth, tonsils, sinuses, gall bladder and prostate occasionally leads to clearing of the urticaria. Patients should avoid inhalant allergens in bedding and overstuffed furniture, wear synthetic fabrics, and avoid animals and perfume. Hypoallergenic cosmetics should be used. Tartrazine cross-reacts with aspirin, and occasionally is a factor to consider in chronic urticaria. The 25–50 mg Atarax tablets are colored with tartrazine, but the 10 and 100 mg tablets are not.

Careful history, good observation and physical examination will uncover occasional uncommon, unsuspected, underlying diseases such as hyperthyroidism, malignant tumors, lymphoma, diabetes, malaria, brucellosis and other subclinical diseases. Occasionally dermatophytosis will underlie chronic urticaria, as will incipient uremia and liver damage. Menstrual and climacteric hormone changes can produce urticaria, although the wise therapist will never underestimate his capacity to credit the cure to the "wrong" etiology in chronic urticaria. Other conditions such as dermatitis herpetiformis, Loeffler's syndrome and mastocytosis, plus the onset of an acute exanthem in a child very often will be ushered in with urticaria. Subacute lupus, at least systemic lupus erythematosus, occasionally manifests itself initially as urticaria, too.

Nervous strain and emotion probably play the greatest part in prolonging chronic urticaria. There may be a coincidental food or drug allergy manifested only when, due to emotional influence or alcohol, penetration of the raw protein through the gut into the bloodstream occurs more readily. An example of this is lobster with champagne producing hives, when either one alone does not.

Vasomotor urticaria is seen in xanthine abusers, those whose intake of coffee, chocolate, nuts and junk food is excessive. There is a good deal of caffeine in most soft drinks, and beer also can be part of this spectrum.

Antihistamine therapy using Periactin (Merck), with its antiseritonin effect, at night since it is very soporific, and Atarax, 10 mg or 25 mg (Roerig) three times a day, or Vistaril (Pfizer), 25 mg or 50 mg twice a day, as suppressive maintenance therapy is of distinct value. For occasional attacks, Pyribenzamine or Chlor-Trimeton, Dimetane or Benadryl, every 3 hours as required, will enable the chronic sufferer to bear his illness while being investigated.

Physical Urticaria

Passive transfer of antibodies has been demonstrated in *light urticaria* due to wavelengths of less than 3,700 Å. Some patients with this condition have to work at night and sleep in the daytime. Many such situations appear to be precipitated by intense overexposure to sun, e.g., building swimming pools. Sunscreens can be very effective here if chosen carefully and applied well. Atabrine occasionally seems to be effective, too.

For treating *cold urticaria,* rule out cryoglobulins and cold agglutinins as well as syphilitic paroxysmal cold hemoglobinuria. The traditional treatment is with large doses of vitamin C. Desensitization by daily baths, or applied wet cloths, of gradually cooler temperatures can be effective, but should be carefully and cautiously done – *not* by the patient when alone since too abrupt a change can produce shock. One investigator reports that benanserin hydrochloride (Merck) improved cold urticaria (this is a specific antimetabolite for serotonin).

In *heat urticaria,* knowledge of the refractory period that follows an attack, with the consequent depletion of antibody for a few hours, has led more than one dancing daughter to stand in front of the fire or take a hot shower to precipitate her hives before an expected dance.

Dermographism

In dermographism, production of wheals in the morning shower by scrubbing with a brush often leads to a more quiescent day. While these measures have a certain practical value, antihistamines or anticholinergics have generally marked effects in physical allergies, and if the individual's variable response to any *one* kind of antihistamine is taken into account and trials on different antihistamines are made, satisfactory control can generally be achieved.

Aquagenic Urticaria

Water contact produces fine hives in people with this disease. Protection by a film of oil before immersion often helps, and antihistamines of course help, too. Atarax can be very helpful.

Quincke's Edema

Quincke's edema (hereditary angioneurotic edema) is transmitted as a Mendelian dominant trait with irregular penetrance. Twenty-five percent of these patients die of laryngeal edema. There is a deficiency of inhibitor, C′ esterase inhibitor (neuramino glycoprotein), for serum globulin permeability factor. Antihistamines are of no help. Trauma has to be avoided here, and treatment is fresh frozen plasma in an attack. In hereditary angioedema, methyltestosterone is reputed to be very effective treatment.[1]

Persons who are susceptible to the stings of insects should have Isuprel linguets and Isuprel spray available and should carry a small epinephrine injection kit as well.

In general, skin test results are unreliable in patients with urticaria and very often an exhaustive history, occasionally a change in environment and careful observation over a period of time are necessary to elucidate the important factors and eliminate them. I am impressed with the importance of emotional factors in chronic urticaria, less so in acute urticaria.

TABLE 4-1.—ANAPHYLAXIS EMERGENCY STEPS

Supine posture—Patent airway
Proximal tourniquet—Constant attendance

Anaphylaxis (protein)	Corticosteroid intravenously Epinephrine 0.4 ml subcutaneously
Allergy (drug)	Corticosteroid intravenously Epinephrine 0.2 ml subcutaneously
Local anesthetic (toxic absorption)	Nembutal 2 ml intravenously
Epileptic seizure	Nembutal 2 ml intravenously

In all cases of emergency, place the patient in a supine posture with constant attendance, cease or block administration or absorption of medicament if possible, and maintain a patent airway.

An intravenous corticosteroid solution, epinephrine (1:1,000) solution, a barbiturate solution, and a syringe with needle should be available in every treatment room at all times.

Table 4–1 shows a very useful reference that should be posted in a key spot in the treatment room.

REFERENCE

1. Shaffer, A. L., et al.: Methyl testosterone therapy in hereditary angioedema, Ann. Intern. Med. 86:306, 1977.

5 / Drug Reactions

At a time when excessive publicity is given to side effects, with the implication that the physician neither knows nor cares about them, it behooves every practitioner to be extremely familiar with the toxic and allergic effects of drugs of all kinds. These may be *cumulative,* as is the case of argyria, where continued use of silver compounds leads to a slate gray skin color, or the yellow color of the Atabrine taker, the retinopathy in patients who continue taking chloroquin, and the mercurial pigmentation of the nails in ammoniated mercury ointment users. Hypervitaminosis A, leading to pseudo-tumor-cerebri, thinning hair or localized periosteal swelling in small children, is also an example. (See pp. 42–44, PCAD.)

Overdosage effects, such as too much anticoagulant producing bleeding into the skin, or a mixture of too much aspirin with Coumadin, leading to a dose-related purpura (usually more than six aspirins per day leads to the rash), are seen. Hair loss as a result of heparin or Coumadin is also seen.

Trigger effects (biotropism) of certain drugs or foods activating a latent herpes simplex infection are seen.

Ecologic effects are seen in the destruction of friendly intestinal organisms leading to monilial overgrowth after antibiotic therapy.

Pharmacologic effects include a reaction against Triparenal (MER/29), which produced ichthyotic skin changes with alopecia while reducing serum cholesterol and had to be withdrawn.

The *Jarisch-Herxheimer* reaction is the sudden destruction of spirochetes by penicillin in early syphilis, which releases allergenic products to which the tissue reacts with fever and rash within 24 hours.

The *Schwartzman* reaction leads to a hemorrhagic type of reaction to a drug to which the patient has, in an interim, developed antibodies, usually purpura from a barbiturate sleeping pill taken intermittently.

In *hepatotoxic* effects, phenothiazine derivatives (e.g., thorazine) can produce jaundice imitating biliary obstruction, as can methyltestosterone, triacetyloleandomycin (TAO) and erythromycin estolate, and can produce alteration in the serum glutamic oxaloacetic transaminase (SGOT), indicating allergic reaction in the liver in a small percentage of the healthy population. Other drugs can do this also, for example, carbarsone, norethandrolone, para-amino-salicylic acid, chlorothiazide, novobiocin, dinitrophenol and isoniazid.

Bone marrow depression notably occurs from Chloromycetin, though sulfapyridine, methotrexate, sulfones, antihistamines, Butazolidin, gold, arsphenamines, griseofulvin, novobiocin, Orinase and Tridione also produce it.

Eighth nerve damage can result from streptomycin, kanamycin and colimycin.

Hemolysis can be expected to result from long continued sulfone treatment of dermatitis herpetiformis, although it responds to iron orally. Primaquine, pamaquine, sulfonamides, acetophenetidin, acetanilid, para-amino-salicylic acid, probenecid, aspirin and nitrofurantoin are prone to produce this in some individuals with an inherited susceptibility.[1]

Special Reactions

FIXED DRUG ERUPTION.—This is usually a persistent purplish erythema that lasts a long time and recurs at the same spot on taking the drug again. Many drugs can cause this, perhaps the most common being phenolphthalein and amidopyrine.

TOXIC EPIDERMAL NECROSIS.—The sudden onset of a widespread severe involvement of the whole skin in an eruption is at first bullous, and later desquamating in sheets and also fatal. Butazolidin, sulfonamides, hydantoin and antipyrine have reportedly been involved. There may be a greater staphylococcal or viral role in the cause than has been acknowledged up to now.

TUMOR-LIKE REACTIONS.—Bromides and iodides produce large granulomatous nodules often of frightening appearance. Arsenic can lead to warty growths on the palms and soles, around the sweat ducts, and even to epitheliomas.

POLYNEUROPATHY.—Large amounts of mercury, usually from overuse of ointments, can produce enzyme changes causing neuropathy, e.g., the salivations of old syphilitics years ago, "mad as a hatter" mercury poisoning seen in hatters, and acrodynia in children. British anti-Lewisite (BAL) helps this.

PSEUDOTUMOR CEREBRI.—This is found classically in vitamin A overdoses, but usually headache and diplopia are the earliest signs. Sudden changes in the type of steroid maintenance therapy occasionally result in hypertensive encephalopathy.

PSEUDOLYMPHOMA.—Dilantin can cause enlargement of the spleen, liver and lymph nodes, as well as hypertrophy of the gums; hydralazine leads to lupus erythematosus cells in blood and enlarged lymph nodes, liver and spleen.

PARA-AMINOSALICYLIC ACID (PAS) ISONIAZID.—This can cause a mononucleosis-like syndrome.

LONG-ACTING SULFONAMIDES.—These drugs, particularly Madribon, can cause Stevens-Johnson syndrome, although in one case the patient's disease appeared to be a virus infection from the start, ending with a virus pneumonia from which we were able to extract a change in titer.

TEETH CHANGES.—Changes resulting from tetracyclines taken by pregnant women or infants lead to hypoplasia of tooth enamel and staining with yellow fluorescence and a mottled appearance. The permanent teeth can be affected in children, with fibrocystic disease of the pancreas.

METHOTREXATE.—Methotrexate can lead to abortion in pregnant women or presumably monstrous offspring if administered to either father or mother at the time of conception.

DECLOMYCIN.—Declomycin can produce onycholysis, and

old tetracycline can produce Fanconi's syndrome (failure of the tubules to reabsorb, with frequent thirst and urination).

MUCOUS MEMBRANE LESIONS.—Dilantin can produce hypertrophy of the gums (Tridione can be substituted) and bismuth produces the blue line along the gum margins (like the lead line). Various antibiotics and on occasion vitamin B complex can produce hairy black tongue, and stomatitis can occur from mercury, phenolphthalein and streptomycin. Cheilitis can come from fluoridated toothpastes, as can an ulcerative stomatitis. Diodoquin and codeine produce pruritus ani with regularity, and chloroquin can bleach hair. Lipoiodine can lead to recurrent painful folliculitis of the nostrils.

DRUG FEVER.—Drug fever is caused by some drugs, particularly Potaba, sulfonamides, PAS, iodides and thiouracil.

Allergic Reactions

Characteristically drugs tolerated for days or years *suddenly* cause a reaction, and once this happens, it will invariably happen again. As a general rule, the eruption is not characteristic of either the drug or the patient. Some drugs, however, do seem to favor one type of eruption, e.g., penicillin will produce urticarial eruptions usually, and this can later be reproduced by the person ingesting a small amount of penicillin in blue cheese or contaminated milk or poultry. Barbiturates produce morbilliform eruptions; atropine, scarlatiniform eruptions; bromides, acneform; and quinine, bullous eruptions. The eruptions produced by Valium seem characteristic also—bright swaths of irregular erythema blotched haphazardly over the body.

In the main, drug eruptions are bright red, pruritic, widespread, symmetrical and of sudden onset. They do not fit any distributive pattern for atopy or contact, and there is little systemic disturbance to the patient despite the widespread eruption.

The simple chemical in the drug probably combines with part of the serum protein to form the hapten eliciting the allergic reaction, and configurations of the causative chemical being sufficiently changed so that the situation cannot be duplicated in either scratch or patch tests. There is therefore no easy way to test for drug sensitivity except by provocative ingestion. This may be so risky as to make it unwise. Skin testing for penicillin can be done by using a freshly made solution of crystalline penicillin (10,000 units per cc) and a scratch test observed for 20 minutes (with a tourniquet handy) for the appearance of wheal flare and pseudopods. If the results are negative, this can be followed by an intracutaneous injection of 0.02 cc of the same material; and if again negative, then penicillin is presumed safe. This is not 100% reliable. If the patient has an allergic background, he is more likely to become allergic to penicillin.

Anaphylactic Reactions

Oxygen in a simple tank with a turnbuckle and mask plus an airway should be on hand in any office where penicillin is given by injection. A routine procedure typed out in red and pasted inside the door or drawer of the instrument cabinet detailing steps to take in case a severe reaction occurs is good insurance. Most of us may never have an anaphylactic reaction in the office, but we should be prepared for one. The treatment involves the use of either *epinephrine,* 0.3–0.5 cc intramuscularly at once (1:1,000), a *tourniquet* above the injection site and intravenous *Benadryl,* 50 mg, or 500 mg aminophylline with or without Solu-Cortef intravenously at once. Sometimes ephedrine given intravenously is lifesaving.

General Management of Drug Reactions

The first order of the day is the identification and removal of the causative drug. A knowledge of the basic products underlying many of the trade-name drugs is very helpful. The AMA book on new drugs usually classifies drugs in chemically related groups, in such a way that common allergenic reactions to them can be quickly understood. Excerpta Medica also publishes several volumes on the side effects of drugs, which are fairly current. Doriden and Noludar are both piperazine derivatives and hypnotics. Allergy to one is invariably accompanied by allergy to the other.

Tacaryl and Temaril, Phenergan and Compazine are all

phenothiazine drugs, and while the first three are effective antihistamines used in the treatment of allergic reactions, they would not do at all for the treatment of an eruption from Compazine or Thorazine. On occasion a hidden ingredient in a household remedy may be the cause of a drug rash, and the inciting agent cannot be identified. Phenolphthalein in Hailey's M.O. (mineral oil) is an example. When questioning the patient about his drug intake, never make the mistake of asking about "drugs." This implies narcotics, and the patient will deny everything, thereby quite unintentionally misleading the physician. Specific inquiry about laxatives, headache remedies, sedatives, tonics, stomach or water pills, vitamins, appetite and weight pills, kidney pills, gallbladder pills and cold or digestion medicines may elicit a barrage of information. Acid in the system, purification of the blood, clearing the sinuses and bringing down the blood pressure all should be solicitously inquired about.

In homes for the chronically ill, convalescent nursing homes and the like, patients may be taking so many drugs that an effort to correlate the onset of a reaction to one particular drug may be impossible. Good records and accurate observations by the nursing attendants will assist this objective. In cases where pinpointing is doubtful, it is best to stop all but the essential drugs, for example, Digitalis, and substitute for the others. This usually means discontinuing barbiturates and sleeping medication and substituting either a soporific antihistamine, such as Benadryl or Periactin, or chloral hydrate, which infrequently gives an extremely characteristic drug reaction which can be recognized (erythroderma). Similar substitution of mercurial diuretics for thiazides (or ammonium chloride) and Darvon for aspirin can be used to "wipe the slate."

On occasion, an eruption caused by the linen, incontinence, or from a rubber sheet next to the mattress, especially in very hot weather, in a heavy paraplegic patient can be difficult to differentiate from a drug rash. In such cases, limitation of drugs and vigorous local treatment with neutral linens, good nursing, and Cort-Dome lotion, for example, will usually clear the eruption.

Specific Management

This treatment is usually not possible beyond elimination of the offending drug. However, in bromide or iodide eruptions (iodides are found in the kidney, gallbladder and lung x-ray opacifiers, as well as in vitamins with minerals and table salt), substitution of chlorides by intravenous saline will eliminate the offending drug quickly. A temporary nephritis can occur from excessive bromide in the urine if this is done too quickly. Salt is effective as well.

In severe urticarias or exfoliative erythema multiforme drug eruptions, steroids are the treatment of choice. Initial large doses, e.g., six to eight Aristocort tablets, tapering quickly for two or three weeks, are usually effective. Itching can be relieved by local treatment with baths, lotions, steroid emulsions and creams; and itching around the eyes can be treated by cold boric acid compresses. Antihistamines given orally or calcium gluconate injected intravenously can be additionally helpful. The aid of family or attendants must be enlisted to prevent accidental recurrence. I will never forget one drug rash that escaped me for several months. An elderly patient's housekeeper, kept awake by her employer's noisy late-late television shows (he couldn't sleep because he was itching), fed him a hypnotic every night. She kept it in *her* medicine cabinet where it was not discovered, of course. Several trips to the hospital later, it was finally unearthed.

Occasionally the patient will continue to scratch his skin long after the eruption has faded. Continuing symptomatic local and antihistamine therapy, with reassurance and support, usually will promote normal recovery.

In barbiturate eruptions, Dr. George Andrews recommended 1 gm of vitamin C given intramuscularly daily.[2]

REFERENCES

1. Meyer, K., and Ley, A. B.: Hemolysis of red cells due to sulfones, Ann. Intern. Med. 72:711, 1970.
2. Andrews, G.: Personal communication.

6 / Bullous Diseases

The major disease group of dermatitis herpetiformis, pemphigus and erythema multiforme has been enlarged to include generalized bullous pemphigoid, benign mucous membrane pemphigus, pemphigus foliaceus, subcorneal pustular dermatosis of Sneddon-Wilkinson, Stevens-Johnson syndrome, herpes gestationis and epidermolysis bullosa. Bullae are seen on the hands of elderly porphyric patients on occasion also. Bullous drug rashes from sulfonamides, quinine, arsenic, Mesantoin, phenobarb and phenophthalein, as well as bromides, can also confuse the diagnosis, even in the newborn baby. Bullae may be seen with poison ivy and insect bites.

Pemphigus Vulgaris

A formerly fatal bullous disease shows acantholysis as a constant feature. (See p. 113, PCAD.) The separation is chiefly above the basal layer in the epidermis. Nikolsky's sign, or the ability to extend the margin of the bulla peripherally by pressure, is a diagnostic feature. The etiology is obscure, although a degeneration of the epidermal cell with loss of the intercellular bridges is an early feature.

Lesion skin shows direct and indirect immunofluorescent studies with intraepidermal intercellular deposition of IgG and C3 (complement) consistently. Titers on indirect serum immunofluorescence (IF) reflect the activity of the disease.

Oral lesions are almost always present, sometimes extensively, and the disease may start in the oropharynx. Bullous lesions occur in crops on normal skin with no itching, no erythema surrounding (as with erythema multiforme) and *no grouping,* and circinate forms on the shoulders, buttocks and axilla (Fig 6-1), as with dermatitis herpetiformis (which itches). The bullae are flaccid and rupture easily, leaving a raw surface.

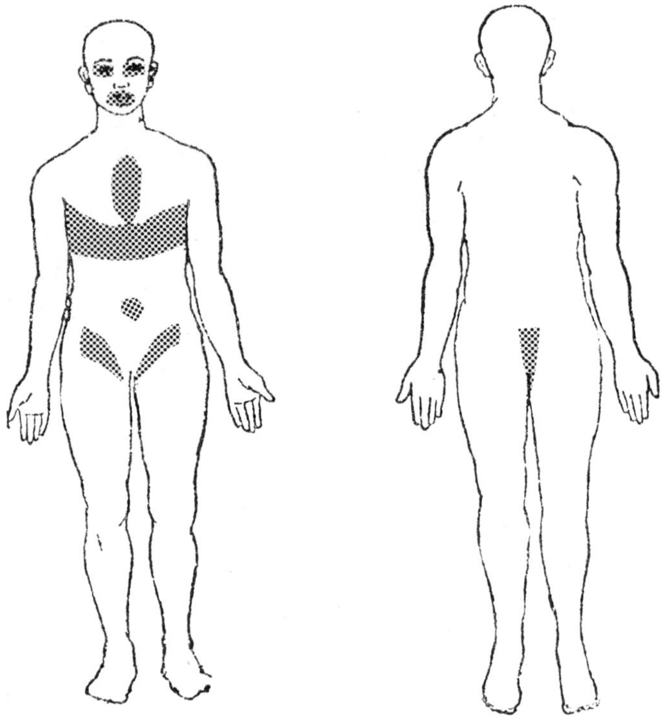

Fig 6–1.—Locations of lesions in patients with pemphigus vulgaris.

Systemic steroids are the method of choice for treatment, using ACTH, prednisolone or triamcinolone. The dose must usually be high at first, then gradually stepping down (start with 60–150 mg per day). If the process is not controlled in a week, the dose should be doubled and *then* stepped down gradually. Antibiotic support with tetracyclines and great care to ensure adequate nutrition and care of the oral lesions are important. Walter Lever advocates methotrexate as an adjunct and sometimes as sole treatment in mild cutaneous pemphigus vulgaris.[1]

Penneys, Eaglestein and Frost at the University of Miami have sucessfully treated 14 of 15 patients with pemphigus using gold sodium thiomalate weekly, given intramuscularly, usually 5 mg per dose.[2] Total doses are around 1,000 mg per patient, and most patients were able to get along without steroids at the end of 3 years. The side effects might be preferable to those noted in the report by Nelson et al.[3] Certainly osteoporosis, diabetes, thromboses (five deaths in 107 patients), perforated gut (three deaths), myopathy and heart failure are unpleasant problems encountered with steroid treatment. One patient was given ACTH alone for 8 years with no side effects—certainly a fortunate outcome. Alternate-day therapy has definite value in reducing side effects and does not seem to lead to less control. Each patient must be treated individually.

Mouthwashes, such as Cepacol, diluted 1:4, and viscous Xylocaine or antibiotic solutions, are of great assistance. Tetracycline syrup occasionally is of value, as is the Water Pik. If the patient is young or survives 3 years, the prognosis is good. Local treatment with Kenalog spray, special baths, starch, Aveeno, potassium permanganate, Phisohex, heat cradles and white vaseline has its place in treatment. Phenergan, 2 drams/oz water, is helpful as a mouthwash before meals.

Pemphigus Vegetans

This occurs when inguinal or axillary folds produce warty, hyperkeratotic, thickened crusted areas. Microscopically they are usually intraepidermal abscesses filled with eosinophiles. The treatment is the same as for pemphigus vulgaris.

Pemphigus Foliaceus

Oral lesions are rare, and while the conditions may start off with bullae, these tend to change to form greasy flakes detached on all sides but one. They are extensive and usually generalized. (See p. 114, PCAD.)

Here, as above, the treatment is antibiotics with systemic steroids, plus antimalarials, one daily on occasion. In treating Brazilian pemphigus (fogo salvagem), quinine and quinacrine have been helpful. Jamarsan is also helpful, although rugged. Prognosis is good. Topical steroids are quite effective. Antihistamines control occasional urticaria.

Benign Mucous Membrane Pemphigoid (Essential Shrinkage of the Mucous Membrane)

This occurs in the conjunctiva chronically and progressively and can lead to blindness ultimately. It may begin in the genital region or mouth and has been described in association with Stevens-Johnson syndrome, dystrophic epidermolysis bullosa and even pemphigus vulgaris. There is no acantholysis in the epidermis. It is usually chronic, but general health is unimpaired.

Immunofluorescence (IF) studies on lesional skin show *direct* linear deposition of mainly IgG at the basement membrane. *Indirect* IF studies show IgG and IgA in low titers against basement membrane.

Treatment here also involves systemic steroids, antibiotics and antimalarials, which may allay progression, while repeated local injections of Kenalog suspension, 5 mg/cc, help if carried out over a long period of time.

Generalized Bullous Pemphigoid

Large tense bullae are mostly in the groin, axilla and flexor surface of the forearms. When the bullae become denuded, they tend to heal and not enlarge, as in pemphigus vulgaris. In addition to bullae, there frequently are areas of erythema with an irregular outline and central clearing. The oral cavity is usually not involved. Though the bulla is subepidermal, as it gets older the roof may degenerate, leaving only a cover of horny layer. There is no acantholysis. Hidden malignancy is the fear here, especially if the onset is sudden in a young patient recently treated for a localized cancer. Direct and indirect immunofluorescence tests show linear deposition of IgG at the basement membrane. Titers on indirect IF do *not* reflect disease activity.

The disease does not respond to sulfapyridine as a rule. In some elderly patients, it may be eventually self-limiting, and it *may* respond to sulfapyridines or Fowler's solution, which should not be used for any *but* older patients. The usual eventual treatment is systemic steroids or antibiotics. Drugs should be carefully ruled out, as should malignancy.

Dermatitis Herpetiformis

This is a chronic recurrent pruritic disease showing papulovesicles or bullae on an erythematous or hyperpigmented base. (See p. 115, PCAD.) Microscopically the bullae form as subepidermal pressure bullae, and the cellular infiltrate often contains many eosinophiles. Biopsy diagnosis is by no means certain. The lesions are usually symmetrical, crusted, grouped or circinate, over the shoulders, buttocks, elbows and posterior axillary line with burning, itching and usually no mucous membrane involvement. (Fig. 6–2). Perhaps some cases of erythema annulare perstans are a form of dermatitis herpetiformis. It can also occur as a sign of hidden malignancy and may be severe. One case of lung abscess cured by lobectomy (which cured the dermatitis herpetiformis) was encountered. Dermatitis herpetiformis in children may not itch and may not respond to sulfapyridine.[4] Direct IF IgA deposition is usually in a granular pattern either in the basement membrane zone or just below it (less often in a linear pattern). Indirect IF test results are negative.

Harold Perry says if the patient is over 60, Fowler's solution is an effective treatment,[5] which has been found to be true. The dose is usually 3 drops three times a day, gradually increasing to 7 drops, then decreasing again to 3 drops. This may be useful when a glucose 6-phosphate-dehydrogenase deficiency makes it impossible to use sulfones. The late sequelae usually will not be a major factor. The historically effective treatment is sulfapyradine, which some patients have difficulty tolerating. Sometimes, Madribon works, and antihistamines such as Benadryl or Chlor-Trimeton assist in controlling the pruritus. The sulfones are very effective and do not depress the bone marrow level quite as much as does sulfapyridine; dapsone 100 mg, Diasone 0.165 gm, Promacetin 0.5 gm, and Roniacol 50–200 mg can be used. The sulfones make the patients look blue and occasionally feel blue, but sulfones seem to be as effective and perhaps safer than sulfapyridine. Once the disease is controlled, the dose to maintain a patient may be very small. Drug rashes are

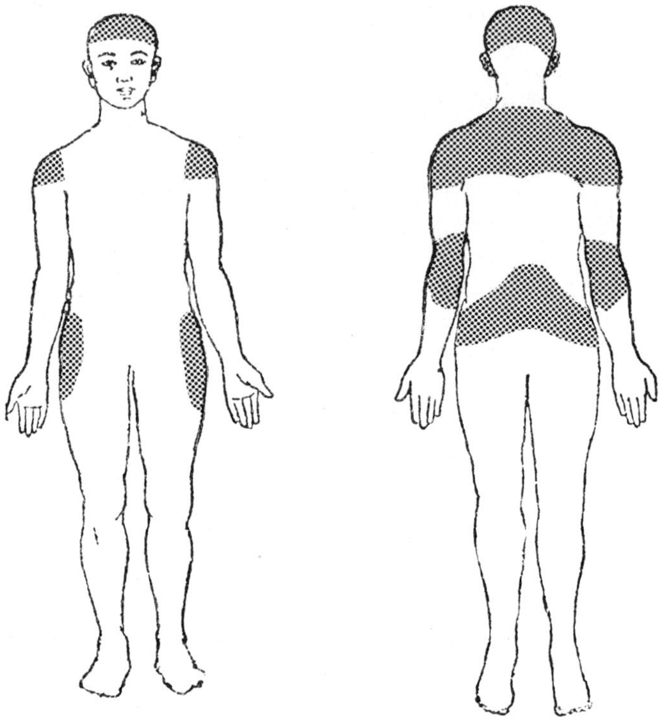

Fig 6–2.—Locations of lesions in patients with dermatitis herpetiformis.

by no means the least of the side effects and must be watched for. Generally, nausea, hematuria and red blood cell suppression are the main side effects. The mild anemia, which is hemolytic, seems to be controlled by iron administration. Focal infections should be eradicated, and iodides and bromides should be forbidden. Locally, steroid sprays and 3–5% sulfur lotion and even sulfur baths help allay the itching. (Physicians should watch for glucose 6-phosphate dehydrogenase deficiency.) For more on the sulfones see p. 150.

Herpes Gestationis

Symptoms of this disease look like those of dermatitis herpetiformis in pregnant women and usually clear after delivery, but can last a few months. In the three patients I have treated, two were treated successfully through their entire pregnancy with dapsone, though one baby was blue at birth (methemoglobinema), which quickly cleared. The third woman was not controlled with anything and simply suffered until the end of her pregnancy. Domonkos says the treatment is varied, which is a mild understatement.[6] Pyridoxine did not help any of my patients and it is expensive.[7] There is little in the literature to guide us, although I believe herpes gestationis is a variant of dermatitis herpetiformis. Immunofluorescent studies, which are not always completely reliable, place it in the bullous pemphigoid group[8] or in its *own* group.[9] Steroids occasionally act dramatically. One patient had her disease reproduced after taking oral contraceptive therapy.[10] There may be a specific circulating complement binding factor found in serum (IgG).[9] Be sure to avoid the tetracyclines in treating these patients.

Prurigo Gestationis

The onset of prurigo gestationis in the 3rd or 4th week of gestation with lichenified papules and excoriations over the buttocks and abdomen requires urgent control (See p. 116, PCAD.)

Treatment with 50–100 mg progesterone daily until controlled, then 25–50 mg daily (Keaty) usually suffices,[11] although if not, Costello recommended steroids, e.g., 10–30 mg prednisolone daily.[12] He thought they were better than sulfapyridine or Promacetin. Another suggested treatment by Fosnaugh et al. was pyridoxine, 50–300 mg daily.[13] After pregnancy, the disease can continue because of a retained placenta. Topical steroids usually help.

Impetigo Herpetiformis

This disease is more serious and rare, occurring late in the last trimester with pustules in the groin and mucous membranes with septic fever. Lever regards it as a variety of pustular psoriasis of Zumbusch.[14]

Erythema Multiforme Bullosum

This includes Stevens-Johnson syndrome and is usually characterized by an acute self-limited dermatitis. (See p. 10, PCAD.) It can on occasion be very recurrent, e.g., spring and fall attacks. When the onset is very acute, with fever, prostration and mucous membrane bullae, this is generally considered the Stevens-Johnson syndrome. Microscopically the bullae are subepidermal and the cellular infiltrate in the dermis is perivascular with lymphocytes, polymorphs and eosinophiles. The etiology here is diverse and any one patient may have food allergy, drug reaction, virus infection, bacterial infection or toxic absorption. It appears as an acute polymorphic bright red target or bullous lesion on hands, feet and face (Fig 6–3);

Fig 6–3. — Locations of lesions in patients with erythema multiforme.

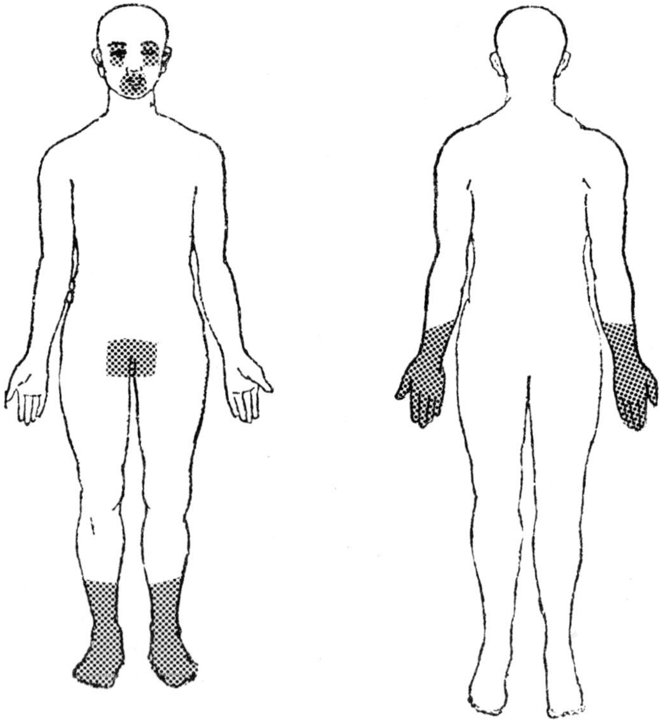

and the mucous membranes are occasionally involved. Involution usually occurs in 3–6 weeks. Direct and indirect immunofluorescent test results are also negative.

Treatment is essentially steroid-antibiotic combined with systemic and symptomatic local treatment. Occasionally sulfapyridine works in an unresponsive patient. Erythema multiforme may usher in another disease such as systemic lupus erythematosus, dermatomyositis, chronic ulcerative colitis, a rheumatic state or lymphoma.

Other Less Important, Less Common Bullous Diseases

Pemphigus Erythematosus, Senear-Usher Syndrome

Early lesions are erythematous with crusting, and clinically resemble lupus erythematosus, usually on the nose, cheek or ears. Occasionally crusted bullae on the chest and extremities occur; and the condition can resemble seborrheic dermatitis. It is a benign form of chronic pemphigus and can possibly switch to pemphigus vulgaris or pemphigus foliaceus, although there is disagreement about this. Pathologic examination of biopsy specimen, especially if taken from the upper back, is usually of great help in making the diagnosis, since a granular dyskeratosis, as well as acantholysis, is seen in pemphigus erythematosus.

Treatment should include steroids, antibiotics, antimalarials, local steroid spray and even estrogens by injection. There is questionable relationship to sun exposure. Maintenance of good health is important here.

Subcorneal Pustular Dermatosis, Sneddon-Wilkinson

This disease consists of vesicles which rapidly change to pustules just under the stratum corneum. Acantholysis is absent. Clinically the disease characteristically occurs in a middle-aged woman with a chronic pustular disease like a chronic impetigo arranged in an annular serpiginous pattern, usually on the abdomen, axilla and groin. Direct and indirect IF test results are negative.

Sulfapyridine is usually an effective treatment. Occasionally steroids are needed. Dapsone induced motor polyneuropathy in a patient who had been controlled for 16 years.[15]

Epidermolysis Bullosa

This starts at birth or soon after, with bullae, vesicles and epidermal cysts. (It should be differentiated from a drug rash via delivery drugs). It is hereditary and involves the extensors. It is worse in hot weather. Microscopically small epidermal cysts occur, and there is an absence of elastic tissue. (See p. 109, PCAD.)

The *benign* (simplex) type (dominant) consists of sparse lesions with no scarring. The condition improves at puberty.

In the *dystrophic* type (dominant or recessive) blisters are followed by scars with cicatricial clawlike hands. Nails and teeth are usually lost.

The *tarda* type appears in adult life.

In the *localized* type (Weber Cockayne), feet and hands are involved. Often other members of the family have it. It is worse in hot weather, and occasionally disappears at puberty.

The treatment is to clip the blisters and rub in steroid cream. Systemic antibiotics are helpful at times. Antimalarials have helped a patient of mine. Protection and genetic counseling and avoidance of trauma are the methods of handling this condition.

Bullous Impetigo

Bullous impetigo can be caused by either staphylococci or streptococci. Streptococcal bullae rupture sooner to produce crusts. (See p. 63, PCAD.)

Pemphigus neonatorum is caused by staphylococci, usually in the newborn, with onset on the 4th to 10th day. It is primarily a skin infection, which may lead to green stools and nephritis.

In *Ritter's disease,* the bullae become larger and rupture, so there is an exfoliative dermatitis.

Penicillin given intramuscularly is the prescribed treatment; isolation is needed.

Syphilitic Pemphigus

Newborn present with bullae on the palms and soles, pea to cherry-sized, which quickly become purulent and break, leaving raw areas. In a biopsy, obliterative vascular changes are present. Bullae are also seen in the eponychium and wrists and ankles. Other stigmata of syphilis may assist in the diagnosis. Penicillin is the treatment of choice. Other antibiotics may be used.

Collodion Baby

This is a bullous variety of ichthyosiform erythroderma, now referred to as *epidermolytic hyperkeratosis*. If the child survives, he may be left with a little or a lot of ichthyosis.

The present thinking is that the treatment of choice is to wash with a soft cloth and hydrate the removal of scale, using emollients to prevent water loss. A 3% salt ointment is helpful, and later 2% salicylic acid ointment and gentle soothing baths can be used.

Familial Benign Chronic Pemphigus (Hailey-Hailey)

This type of pemphigus presents as recurrent bullae and vesicles. It is worse in hot weather and usually appears on the sides of the neck. Pathologically the bullae occur suprabasally. It is usually familial and runs its course in a few weeks only to recur throughout life. (See p. 109, PCAD.)

The condition responds to steroid-antibiotic cream locally and has been reported to be cleared by skin grafting. Intramuscular treatment with estrogens has been recommended by Andrews.[6] One deep-sea diver responded to seasonal intramuscular steroid treatment. Vincent Cippolaro reported control with Cleocin solution (Schoch letter Jan/78.)

Lymphangioma Circumscriptum

These grouped clusters of deep-seated vesicles resemble frog spawn and are localized to one region. Treatment is by proper deep electrodesiccation, but they can be very recurrent. Generalized herpes zoster, chickenpox, variola, Kaposi's varicelliform eruption and vaccinia are described elsewhere.

REFERENCES

1. Lever, W. F.: Methotrexate and prednisone in pemphigus vulgaris, Arch. Dermatol. 106:491, 1972.
2. Penneys, M. S., Eaglestein, W. H., and Frost, P.: Management of pemphigus with gold compounds, Arch. Dermatol. 112:185, 1976.

3. Nelson, C. T., et al.: Pemphigus: 20-year review, Arch. Dermatol. 112:962, 1976.
4. Kim, R., and Winkelman, R. K.: Dermatitis herpetiformis in children, Arch. Dermatol. 83:895, 1961.
5. Perry, H.: Personal communication.
6. Domonkos, A. N.: *Andrews' Diseases of the Skin* (6th ed.; Philadelphia: W. B. Saunders Co., 1971).
7. Osmundsen, P. E.: Herpes gestationis, Dermatologica 131:393, 1966.
8. Person, J. R., and Rogers, R. S.: Bullous pemphigoid responding to sulfapyridine and the sulfones, Arch. Dermatol. 113:610, 1977.
9. Katz, S., et al.: Herpes gestationis: An update, Obstet. Gynecol. 49:733, 1977.
10. Ackerman, A. B., et al.: Herpes gestationis, Arch. Dermatol. 112: 1543, 1976.
11. Keaty, C., Jones, P. E., and Lamb, J. H.: Progesterone therapy in dermatoses of pregnancy (herpes gestationis), Arch. Dermatol. 63:675, 1951.
12. Costello, M. J., and Buncke, C. M.: Dermatitis herpetiformis (Duhring) successfully treated with promacetin, Arch. Dermatol. 72:348, 1955.
13. Fosnaugh, R. P., Bryan, K. G., and Orders, R. L.: Pyridoxin in the treatment of herpes gestationis, Arch. Dermatol. 84:90, 1961.
14. Lever, W. F.: *Histopathology of the Skin* (5th ed.; Philadelphia: J. B. Lippincott Co., 1975), p. 141.
15. Kirsch, N., et al.: Dapsone-induced motor polyneuropathy, Arch. Dermatol. 112:1158, 1976.

SUGGESTED READING

Kimmig, J., and Jänner, M.: *Pocket Color Atlas of Dermatology* (Chicago: Year Book Medical Publishers, Inc., 1975).

Fitzpatrick, T. B., et al.: *Dermatology in General Medicine* (New York: McGraw-Hill Book Co., 1971).

Cutis

Archives of Dermatology

7 / Diseases of the Mouth

The mucous membrane of the mouth has no sebaceous or sweat glands, is thin and has many mucous glands. Saliva coats it at all times. Normal bacterial flora in the mouth do not produce disease, except perhaps in Vincent's infection.

Oral hygiene in general means care of the teeth and gums; this field rightfully belongs to the dentist. The ripe red strawberry tongue of scarlet fever, the smooth shiny tongue of the Plummer-Vinson syndrome and the pale flabby tongue of late pernicious anemia all should be easily recognizable by the trained dermatologist, as should gumma, chancre, myxedema, the dry furred tongue of uremia, and the swollen life-threatening angioneurotic edema of the tongue. Gum changes such as the hypertrophic gingivitis of pregnancy and Dilantin dosage; the blue line from bismuth, mercury or lead; pigmentation from "amalgam tattoo" or Addison's disease; the ulcerative erosion of pemphigus and leukemia; and the bleeding of pyorrhea or scurvy may have importance in the management of a dermatologic entity. The oral mucosal changes of lichen planus and lupus erythematosus may be diagnostic. Relief of any symptoms involves treatment of the main disease, hence recognition is important.

Dry Mouth

Often the patient complains, and yet while an incipient Sjögren's syndrome may be suspected, dry mouth can never be diagnosed. Symptomatic relief taxes the physician's therapeutic ingenuity. Glycerin and honey lozenges (Pine Bros.), chewing gum, lemon juice or flavored liquid petrolatum held in the mouth periodically may help. Potassium iodide saturated solution in water taken three times a day starting with small doses, for example 3 minims, and increased if there are no contraindications to its use, or pilocarpine hydrochloride, 5 mg taken three times a day, may stimulate salivary gland secretion before meals. Antihypertension medication may be a factor here. Roger and Gallet lip pomade controls dry lips.

Burning Mouth

Mild warm mouthwashes, e.g., liquor aromaticus alkalinis NF diluted 50-50 with water, or diluted Lavoris, are occasionally helpful. On occasion, Compazine, 5 mg taken orally three times a day, also relieves the distressing sensation. Avoidance of certain rather strong denture cleansers which may contain sodium perborate is essential, and denture sensitivity should be checked out. Malocclusion or ill-fitting dentures occasionally lead to "tongue thrusting" and a sore tongue.

Antihistamines such as diphenhydramine (Benadryl) elixir and chlorpheniramine (Chlor-Trimeton liquid) may be used as a mouthwash before meals if discomfort is great enough. Syrup of Phenergan is excellent for this purpose. In rare instances, Xylocaine 0.5% in solution or ointment form can be used. In severe cases viscous Xylocaine 1% can be beneficial.

Sensations of foulness in the mouth can be dealt with by using either Lavoris or Cepacol (cetylpyridinium chloride) mouthwashes diluted with water or peroxide.

Diabetes, sinusitis, uremia, blood diseases or other systemic illnesses may have to be considered.

Angular Stomatitis (Perleche)

Removal of the cause ideally clears this condition. Quite often there is a simple explanation such as lollipops or toothpaste sensitivity, with drooling because of adenoids or "long-in-the-tooth"—that is, bony recession of the gum producing overlap in the bite and fissures at the mouth corners, which can be corrected by a dentist adjusting the bite. Otherwise anemia or B-complex deficiency (which I have never really been sure as causing this) have to be considered. Quite often *Monilia* is a secondary invader, and Mycolog or 1% hydrocortisone in Mycostatin cream or Vioform hydrocortisone lotion 1%, or 3%

ammoniated mercury ointment, or in extreme cases 10% balsam of Peru in petrolatum at night, or Silicote cream at night if the patient is a drooler, can be most helpful. Occasionally painting the cracks, if they are deep, with 10% silver nitrate solution is also helpful.

Aphthous Stomatitis

Recurrent ulcerations that are red and painful but heal without scars are probably caused by *Streptococcus sanguis*. There is often a familial tendency, and precipitating factors include fatigue, psychic stress, allergy and menses, so that constitutional factors are important. Treatment with antibiotic suspensions four times a day, held in the mouth before swallowing, comfort and speed healing. Kenalog in Orabase gives instant comfort, as do intracutaneous injections of steroid suspension. Oral decadron suspension daubed on with a cotton swab or gauze sometimes does as well as or better than Kenalog in Orabase, and Topsyn gel can be used with similar success. A dye-free diet may be valuable as well. Flagyl taken orally has a nebulous effect and currently is not popular.

Superficial cautery of the surface with 10% silver nitrate or 25% trichloracetic acid coagulates the sensitive raw area. A short, limited, rapidly tapered course of steroids taken orally may clear the condition in emergencies. Antibiotic anesthetic lozenges, (e.g., Hydrozets), or Lactinex tablets, four tablets taken four times daily in milk, gamma globulin injected intramuscularly, repeated cowpox vaccinations and antihistamine mouthwashes all have their advocates, indicating that physicians do not know much about this condition yet. If you can find the "trigger" and eliminate it, that often is successful.

Herpes Simplex

This viral disease, when occurring for the first time (primary complex), can be severe with lymphadenitis, fever and constitutional symptoms. There may even be meningo-encephalitis or visceral disseminated herpes simplex (acute herpetic gingivostomatitis) ushered in with prodromal malaise, then gingivitis and scattered vesicles which rupture to leave ulcerations and last about 24 hours and heal. Treatment here is symptomatic with mouthwashes, rest, aspirins, fluids, highly nutritious egg-nog-type drinks, and relief of oral discomfort with either viscous Xylocaine or Kenalog in Orabase and ice cream. Gamma globulin treatment helps.

Secondary Herpes Simplex

This occurs usually on the skin or at the junction of the skin and mucous membrane of the lips, and is usually triggered by sun, fever, wind, trauma, psychic stress and other causes. Treatment with Herplex (Allergan) iododeoxyuridine applied during the earliest sensory warning time sometimes helps; usually there is a burning sensation before the blisters appear, and then the treatment should be applied every 5 minutes for the first hour and every hour for the first 2 or 3 days; this may abort the herpes. If there is no satisfactory outcome, then Cortef, 2.5% every hour, or intracutaneous Kenalog, 5 mg/cc for the first 24 hours, will help. Cowpox vaccinations weekly for the patient have definite value and suppress frequent attacks. Red dye (neutral red 0.1%) or proflavine dye treatment is controversial, but occasionally very effective. The dye is rubbed into the ruptured vesicles and a Wood's lamp is shined for 2 minutes at a 6-in. distance. This can be repeated at home using fluorescent bulbs at 6 in. for 15 minutes. It must be borne in mind that dye and light therapy is not approved by the FDA. Freezing with ether-soaked swabs for 5 minutes every 6 hours is reported to be helpful. Two percent buffered glutaraldehyde solution is occasionally helpful.

Herpes Zoster

Oral lesions can occur if the second (maxillary) or third (mandibular) division of the trigeminal nerve is involved. Ruptured vesicles on the tongue, gums or palate make chewing uncomfortable. Intramuscular administration of Kenalog, 60–80 mg immediately, repeated in 5 days, heals quickly and prevents scarring in the inflamed ganglion, preventing postherpetic neuralgia. There are many other varieties of treatment.

Herpangina

Acute oropharyngitis caused by the coxsackie virus group A involves the posterior pharynx. Treatment is as for herpes simplex. Its short duration often makes treatment unnecessary.

Hairy Black Tongue

Hairy black tongue tastes terrible, feels raspy and looks scary, but is essentially harmless, often related to antibiotic or vitamin B ingestion. (See p. 210, PCAD.) Scrubbing with a toothbrush (with or without meat tenderizer) or painting with a 5% solution of podophyllin in 95% alcohol weekly usually clears it.

Leukoplakia

The mucosal equivalent of senile keratosis on the skin, this thickened white patch can usually be removed by electrodesiccation and curettage, or painting with silver nitrate or 100% trichloracetic acid when *dry*. Examining the patient every 6 months to ensure a lasting cure is essential, since all leukoplakia clinically is premalignant. Mouth biting, smoking, rough teeth and ill-fitting dentures have to be corrected. Vitamin A, taken orally, 150,000 units daily for 3 months on, 2 weeks off, or vitamin A-soluble tabs, e.g., Disp-A-Tabs (Person & Covey), sucked daily seem to help. The risk of malignant change is probably slight. Liquid nitrogen cryotherapy is effective.

Moniliasis (Thrush)

Candida albicans can be easily cultured and often is easily recognized clinically, especially in babies. (See p. 78, PCAD.) Treatment of choice is the oral suspension of Mycostatin, 60 cc, four squirts a day, sluiced around in the mouth and swallowed. It is commonly seen in people taking methotrexate, birth control pills and antibiotics, and in diabetics or those debilitated. Sodium caprylate (naprylate), taken three times a day and kept up for 2 or 3 weeks with vitamin B complex taken orally or subcutaneously by injection, seems to have definite value, too. Severe systemic cases have been treated with systemic lotrimin recently.[1, 2]

Vincent's Stomatitis

Periodontoclasia and gum disease in general favor development of this disease, so dental prophylaxis is good for those who can afford it. Treatment with penicillin peroxide mouthwashes, proper instruction in brushing and gum massage and the use of Stimudents to clean between the teeth and keep the gums tight is important.

Fordyce's Disease

Aberrant sebaceous glands in the mouth require no treatment. Persons with scrotal tongue or geographic tongue need reassurance. Glossitis rhomboidea mediana should be clinically recognizable, but it is unimportant. Torus palatinus requires no treatment and may be a handy thing to hang a denture on someday. Dental sinus (from an old tooth) under the chin, or a retained root, a periapical abscess pointing in the infraorbital region, must not be forgotten. Fissured granuloma (epulis fisseratum), a granulomatous pad where the denture rests on the labioalveolar sulcus, can be removed by electrosurgery; remove the denture until it heals. Mucous cyst of the lip can be excised using an eye-clamp (chalazion clamp) under local anesthesia. Mixed tumor of the palate, while not as common here as in the parotid and submaxillary glands, must be referred to a good surgeon. Hypertrophic lingual papillae can be very annoying, catching on a tooth while talking. They can be easily destroyed with 100% trichloracetic acid on a toothpick applied while the tongue is dry. Moeller's glossitis is a painful tongue with absent filliform papillae in irregular red patches on the tip and lateral surfaces. Injection of Kenalog benefits. The condition is chronic. A stone in Stensen's duct producing a painful parotid swelling should be referred to an oral surgeon or an ear-nose-and-throat man. Behcet's syndrome, with ulceration of the genitals, mouth and uveitis, so-called aphthosis, is usually seen in young women in their

30s. It is difficult to treat, and perhaps gamma globulin, repeated small transfusions and copious antibiotic local treatment may assist recovery. Lidex ointment locally is useful.

In electrogalvanic lesions, currents can pass between dissimilar metals in differing types of fillings in the teeth, especially if the saliva is copious. Andrews describes an ammeter useful for testing an ulceration defying diagnosis.[3]

Cheilitis

Cheilitis is usually an allergic reaction to lipstick (also coffee, oranges, lemons, nail polish, toothpaste, mouthwash, lip biting, sun and wind) or lipstick and sunlight. Treatment is to remove the suspected causes and use no lipstick. Use 2.5% Cortef ointment every 3 hours and later add the unscented Almay lipstick. In the sun, A-Fil sunstick, or for women the Arex sunstick that looks like a lipstick, is very helful.

Cheilitis glandularis exudes mucus, which forms a glossy film on the lips and in the familial form is precancerous. Treatment is with the enzyme ointments, e.g., Varidase, Elase, Chymar and Biozyme ointments; remove the cause if possible or excise.

Desquamative Gingivitis

Occasionally a dermatologist will run across this rare entity, which is difficult to classify and treat. Some patients will later develop lichen planus, and some will develop a benign mucous membrane pemphigoid. Short courses of oral steroid treatment seem to be the best way to handle this distressing condition.

REFERENCES

1. Meade, R. H., III: Treatment of chronic mucocutaneous candidiasis, Ann. Intern. Med. 86:314, 1977.
2. Ipp, M. M., Boxall, L., Gelfand, E. W.: Clotrimazole, Am. J. Dis. Child. 131:305, 1977.
3. Andrews, G.: Personal communication.

8 / Hair

Embryologically the hair follicle appears to form from a downward growing bud of epithelium in about the third month of gestation, depicting its epidermal origin. Lanugo and vellus hair is present at birth, and in due course falls out; normal hair, especially on the scalp and eyebrows, commences to grow thereafter within several months. Most hair follicles appear to reach maturity when a person reaches the age of 10. Thereafter, hair follicles continue to grow (anagen), then have a period of normal growth (late anagen), shrink up (catagen), cast out the small "club hair" and have a rest (telogen phase) for 7 to 10 months, then "reawake" and start another growth. In humans, this cycle may take several years, and about 80% of all hair follicles are active at any given time.

There is no molting season, and a normal adult loses about 60–70 hairs a day from scattered sites. Montagna has shown that hair growth perceptibly slows in the presence of moderate starvation in mice.[1] Undoubtedly, comparable stresses in humans can affect the hair growth pattern. Since the "fight or flight" alarm reaction in an animal causes some muscles to contract, making the hair rise, the ears go flat and the mouth corners pull back, with the eyes opening wide, it is not hard to envisage a taut muscle in a round-headed human who has had a hard day at the office, blanching out the top of his scalp. Plucking hair out will not make hair grow faster or slower; and neither will shaving, although hair may appear coarser from the blunt-cut ends.

Androgens, whether testicular, adrenal or ovarian, stimulate hair growth on the ears, nose, moustache, beard, axillary and pubic areas. Body hair seems to be androgen-dependent, too, though hair on extremities seems to be more a matter of heredity. Scalp hair, as well as eyelash and eyebrow hair, seems to be independent of a healthy pituitary, but dependent on either testosterone or estrogen. Male-pattern baldness can be produced in hereditarily predisposed eunuchs by testosterone injections.

Alopecia in the Female

Alopecia is a worrisome problem, which with neglect by the dermatologic therapist, may end up in the hands of the quack. Since the Ogilvie sisters with their "angora hair" that never stopped growing, feminine humanity has been getting less hairy. There is a definite increase in female alopecia, and probably the multiplicity of faddy diets and assorted stressing hair manipulations is partly to blame. Civilization with its attendant indoor living, artificial environment, lack of exercise, as well as the everyday tensions of noise, speed and crowding, add to the lessening of hair growth. (See pp. 132 and 133, PCAD.)

ALOPECIA FROM DRUGS.—This is fairly well documented as resulting from (1) heparin and other anticoagulants such as Coumadin, (2) nitrogen mustard, (3) folic acid antagonists, (4) colchicine taken intravenously, (5) thallium and vitamin A, and (6) birth control pills, e.g., Enovid, usually after several years. This alopecia is usually reversible. There may be some hair loss with appetite-suppressant drugs, but this is merely a suspicion.

ALOPECIA FROM FEVER.—Temperatures higher than 103 F for a long time, such as in typhoid fever, lead to defluvium.

ALOPECIA FROM SYPHILIS.—This is a moth-eaten patchy hair loss in late secondaries.

POSTPARTUM ALOPECIA.—Presumably the hair loss that occurs in women in the third or fourth month after childbirth is due to the adjustment for the gestation period when no hair enters the telogen phase, hence there is an apparent compensating increase in the number of hairs entering the resting phase, with a comparative increase in hairfall, usually self-correcting within 6–9 months.Attention to the possibility of anemia and hyperthyroidism may be needed in addition and should be checked out.

NEWBORN ALOPECIA.—Fine hairs get rubbed off by the constant friction of the baby against the mattress. In any event, all the birth hair is replaced within 6 months.

ALOPECIA FROM ANEMIA.—A low level of serum iron has in the past been linked with thinning hair in women. Certainly a woman with a hemoglobin value of 50% can grow hair with alacrity when this is corrected. Ferrous sulfate, three grains taken three times a day, or Trinsicon is the treatment of choice.

ALOPECIA FROM CRASH DIETS.—Whether from hormone adjustments inherent in the state of starvation induced in those who lose 25 lb in a month, or from other reasons, certainly crash diets can be a very real cause of hair loss in young models and middle-aged women. Reassurance, proper diet with vitamin B complex supplement, massage, and iron if necessary generally correct this within 3 months.

ALOPECIA SYMPTOMATIC OF HORMONAL CHANGE.—Examples of causes are diabetes (rare), hyperthyroidism (common) or hypothyroidism (common), which can be detected by the usual tests and corrected.

TRAUMATIC ALOPECIA.—This is often the easiest to diagnose, but the hardest to correct, since the patient will not give up the traumatic manipulation of the hair too readily. Nylon brushes, pony tails tautly pulled, braids tightly woven, overuse of the hair dryer, and rollers with brushes worn overnight too tightly, especially if the girl is tall, may do their damage unnoticed for many months until suddenly bald scalp shines out and the call for help is heard. Real *trichotillomania* seems to be less common in girls than in boys, and often a tender giveaway is to gently ask the patient to show you how he does it. Most of them will oblige.

ALOPECIA FROM STRAIGHTENING OR OVERWAVING.—In the black patient, the practice of straightening kinky hair with an alkaline grease, such as Madame Walker or Dixie Peach, and a hot pressing iron will often lead to the hair becoming brittle through overcooking. Breakage will leave short stubble, especially over the back of the scalp. Strict avoidance of this practice for many months will produce normal hair. A type of frontal parietal alopecia is seen in small girls, where the hair is pulled taut in small braids.

The "crew-cut" in overwaved (cold wave) hair is often the result of applying a cold wave too soon after a platinum bleach. This leads to brittleness and breakage, and although purely temporary, is often the source of plaintiffs' suits.

PRESSURE ALOPECIA.—Known to brain surgeons for many years, pressure alopecia has lately been seen in women undergoing operations in the lithotomy position, especially if surgery lasts longer than 6 hours. The pressure on the unpadded scalp is sufficient to cut off the blood supply long enough to cause complete defluvium in the pressed-upon area in 10–20 days. The hair grows back in 9 to 10 months. The patients often suspect that they have been dropped while unconscious, for the day after the operation the affected scalp is swollen and sore as if bruised. Reassurance and explanation are all that are needed, though sympathy and emotional support may not be enough to prevent the customary lawsuit. A tight band on a wig worn for longer than 6 hours, especially in the frontal region, may also lead to a small strip of pressure alopecia.

ALOPECIA AREATA.—This is moderately easy to diagnose with generally a good prognosis except in marginal ophiasis (poor). It can be treated by a variety of methods. Intracutaneous injection of dilute suspensions of Kenalog is the method of choice. This can be done with ethyl chloride (fluoroethyl) spray prior to the quick insertion of 1 cc/sq in. (50-50 dilution with water). Repeat it monthly for 3 months, and if this does not grow hair, then switch to phenol painting or other stimulant treatment, e.g., cold quartz lamp. If emotional strain is a factor, various mild sedatives are occasionally effective. Often the personality of the patient is the one factor that cannot be altered. Many patients give a family history. Some families get ulcers, some get alopecia areata, some get ulcerative colitis.

Alopecia areata probably belongs among the manifestations of neurosis, and psychiatry occasionally can give rapid and instructive cures. Occasional cases progress to alopecia totalis or universalis.

Current interest in autoimmune diseases has fostered many investigations here. Successful treatment of a patient who had had alopecia universalis for 10 years, using DNCB, 0.001% daily within 3 weeks (after sensitization), was reported.[2]

TICK-BITE ALOPECIA.—This affects persons in the western states and resembles the moth-eaten secondary syphilis alopecia, or alopecia areata. No treatment is needed beyond getting rid of the tick.

ALOPECIA MUCINOSA.—Microscopically mucinous edema of the hair follicles occurs, and clinically small inflammatory plaques occur on the scalp or face with hair loss. These may be idiopathic or symptomatic of lymphoma. Superficial x-ray therapy benefits some patients. Spontaneous involution may occur in other cases.

CONGENITAL ALOPECIA.—Congenital alopecia has to be recognized if only to assure the sufferer that treatment is of no avail. Symptoms are ectodermal defect, monilethrix or beaded hair, that snap off and pili annulati (ringed hair with dark and light bands because of air in the hair). Trichorrhexis nodosa may occur because of excessive manipulation, e.g., brushing and bending the hair.

FAMILIAL MALE-PATTERN ALOPECIA.—Diffuse hair loss is a very common and insidious thinning of the vertex and frontal scalp in young or middle-aged women who have both male and female relatives demonstrating partial baldness. There is often seborrhea.

SCARRING SCALP DISEASES.—Discoid lupus erythematosus, pseudopelade and folliculitis decalvans (sycosis of the scalp) all produce scarring. The latter sometimes respond to Betadine shampoo, systemic antibiotics over a long period of time, and locally applied antibiotic creams at night as well. Perifolliculitis capitis abscedens et suffodiens is a tunneling pyoderma-like hidradenitis, and it responds to similar treatment. Lupus erythematosus and pseudopelade respond disappointingly to Kenalog spray and antimalarials, although these do occasionally seem to arrest the progression. Acne necrotica miliaris responds to treatment as for folliculitis decalvans. Coup de sabre (scleroderma), x-ray or thermal burns and scars as a result of a postfuruncular state, or kerion after tinea, may be permanent. Warty birthmarks can be excised in a linear fashion, producing cosmetic improvement.

SEBORRHEA CAPITIS.—This is probably the single most common cause of hair loss in women, and often is extremely stubborn and hard to control. The case of the woman with the perpetually oily scalp and thinning frontal hair will continue to plague the conscientious physician for many years. Although androgens undoubtedly play a part in its cause, little can be done. Antiseborrheic measures, including proper diet (e.g., low cholesterol), exercise regimes, cleanliness, sea and sun and vitamin B complex taken orally, plus the local use of steroid lotions (Texacort or 1% hydrocortisone in propylene glycol), a 5-minute massage at night with kneading of the scalp over the skull and avoidance of stress are all helpful measures. Lichen planopilaris is a rare variety of lichen planus affecting the scalp. It is also recalcitrant.

Hirsutism in the Female

At puberty and the menopause, as well as during pregnancy, there may be temporary spurts in hair growth, which often are self-correcting. There are certain families who are hirsute, and all their endocrine studies are normal. There are other cases of hirsutism, however, associated with acne, menstrual disorder, obesity and even, on occasion, hypertension, where an endocrine explanation has to be considered. Cushing's syndrome, adrenal virilism, polycystic ovary (Stein-Leventhal syndrome), ovarian tumors and basophilic adenoma of the pituitary are some of the entities producing hirsutism. Elevation of the urinary 17-ketosteroid level indicates that an endocrine test is needed.

Treatment

Shaving with an electric razor is often suitable for elderly women with bristles. Depilatories, applied for a definite time and then washed off, destroy the hair chemically, though they can be irritating to the skin. *Plucking* is the usual method, although poor eyesight and inaccurate plucking may lead to inflamed papules and scarring. *Electrolysis* is tedious with the galvanic current, and the diathermy can leave pits. However, a skilled operator can achieve satisfactory results if the work is repeated carefully. *Wax depilatories* strip the hair off by pulling it out. *Bleaching* with peroxide and ammonia, equal parts, produces transparent bleached hair that sometimes is acceptable cosmetically. (See Formulary, no. 41.)

Alopecia in the Male

In addition to the causes already listed, male-pattern baldness seems to be dependent on an adequate androgen level and a hereditary predisposition. Eunuchs do not show baldness even though it is familial, unless given androgen therapy. The effect of sebum in depressing hair growth has been experimentally shown and appears clinically evident; there is a good probability that sebum production is related to androgen level, too.

Treatment

Treatment of male-pattern baldness involves local measures to reduce the seborrheic component, as well as systemic general measures to build up the health of the patient, who may be fat, flabby and sedentary. These measures include outdoor exercise, vitamins, an adequately nutritious diet, and above all else, a balanced outlook toward work and recreation. Actors traditionally massage their scalps with their heads hanging over the edge of the bed in a dependent position, facilitating the circulation. This is awkward, but 5 minutes of kneading massage, with the elbows resting on a table so the shoulder muscles can come into play and the fingers moving the scalp around on the skull in such a way as to stimulate muscle relaxation and increase blood flow to the vertex of the scalp, can be beneficial if done regularly. The best time is toward the end of the day when fatigue and taut scalp muscles combine to blanch out the vertex of the scalp. The margins of the scalp should be manipulated. There are no holes in the head and the blood vessels approach the scalp from behind and in front of the ears and above the eyebrows, so the marginal area should be massaged. Producing a relaxed scalp after an aggressive day *may* help the patient to retain his hair a little longer.

Management of seborrhea capitis includes using selenium sulfide suspension, lathering in well for 3 minutes after a preparatory shampoo, then rinsing well and shampooing again with a bland shampoo; this to be done three times a week at first, tapering the frequency gradually. In cases of difficult or intractable seborrhea capitis, sulfur oil (see Formulary, nos. 28, 29, 30), P & S Liquid or one of the other antiseborrheic shampoos such as Ionil, Meted, Alvinine, Sebulex, or Capitrol, leaving them in the scalp for longer periods, may suffice. Many pleasant hair dressings such as Sebucare (Westwood), Scadan (Dome) and steroid lotions such as Aeroseb HC (Allergan Labs.) or the Texacort scalp lotion (Texas Pharmacal), which are essentially hydrocortisone with a little hexachlorophene in propylene glycol, are very helpful.

Stimulating tonics such as Almay's Resorcitate, which is an alcoholic lotion with salicylic acid and resorcin monoacetate, is very satisfactory treatment for brunettes, while mercury bichloride, salicylic acid and tincture of capsicum in alcohol will not stain blonde or gray hair. Sebucare has an advantage when used with gray hair in imparting a pleasant sheen to the hair.

REFERENCES

1. Montagna, W.: *The Structure and Function of the Hair* (New York: Academic Press, 1956), p. 182.
2. Dunaway, D.: Alopecia areata: Case report, Arch. Dermatol. 112: 256, 1976.

SUGGESTED READING

Rook, A., Wilkinson, D. S., and Ebling, E. J. G.: *Textbook of Dermatology* (Oxford: Blackwell Scientific Publications, 1968).

9 / Fungus Diseases

Fungal diseases can be divided into superficial, deep and systemic.

Superficial

TINEA VERSICOLOR.—Tinea versicolor is caused by the *Malassezia furfur.* It seems to be increasingly common, especially in people who habitually lie on sandy beaches in the Caribbean. It usually affects the upper trunk and produces a variegated hyper- or depigmentation. (See p. 77, PCAD.) Selenium sulfide shampoo, using Abbott Selsun two or three times a week and leaving it on overnight, is very helpful; and if the areas are localized, Whitfield's ointment, 3% sulfur-sal and Whitfield's "ointment" in an alcoholic solution are effective preparations. Twenty percent or a saturated solution of sodium hyposulfite (or sodium thiosulfate) is the classical remedy, but has an unpleasant odor. When people perspire in hot communities, it is unpleasant for their friends.

Another preparation is Akrinol cream (Schering), which is actually a very greasy acrosorcin type of ointment, but is very effective. This can be rubbed on twice a day also. Tinver lotion (Barnes-Hind) is a pleasant lotion suitable for daytime use. The amino-acridine preparation, Akrinol, is to be rubbed on at night. Patients should be advised to either bathe with Fostex cream once a day or use a good strong soap, e.g., Stiefel's Salicylic Acid & Sulfur Soap, once a day at least and to wear T-shirts so they will not reinfect themselves from their clothing. The T-shirts can be discarded daily and boiled for 10 minutes. (See Formulary, no. 25.)

The problem of cure is largely due to the fact that the small fungus can get down into the hair follicles, and when a clinical cure appears to have been achieved, the infection may still be present in the depths of the hair follicles. Then, when the patient perspires excessively, the organism comes back up onto the surface again and reinfects, and the clinical infection is obvious. The patient should be instructed therefore to continue to treat himself for at least a month *after* all signs of clinical infection have disappeared.

TINEA NEGRA.—This disease, caused by the *Cladosporium wernecki* or *mansonii* (these are synonyms for *Hormodendron),* occurs in Brazil, Cuba, Panama, Puerto Rico and India. In the Western Hemisphere, it involves only the palms. There are brown or black asymptomatic annular lesions, which usually respond to keratolytics, e.g., 3% sulfur-sal.

PIEDRA.—Trichosporosis causes nodes on the hair which are white, brown or black. There are essentially two varieties—white and black. It occurs in patients in the tropics, with occasional cases in the temperate zones, mostly on the scalp. It does not fluoresce under Wood's light. Usually the treatment is shaving, or formalin or mercury preparations.

TRICHOMYCOSIS AXILLARIS.—Small yellow-red or black axillary spots form; and treatment is with an alcoholic solution of formaldehyde 2%, or a sulfur 5% ointment. It fluoresces under Wood's light, and clothing is usually stained by the colored sweat. Oral antibiotics and antibiotic vanishing creams are a somewhat more elegant way to clear these patients.

ERYTHRASMA.—Erythrasma is caused by a gram-positive *Corynebacterium minutissimum,* occurring in humid climates. (See p. 78, PCAD.) It fluoresces with a coral red color and responds to systemic antibiotics, especially erythromycin, tetracycline and Chloromycetin; and occasionally in widespread cases, this is the only way you can cure them. Penicillin and griseofulvin do not help, and generally keratolytic ointments are sufficient to clear them.

Dermatophytes

Ringworm fungi consist of *Microsporum, Epidermophyton* and *Trichophyton.* Human serum inhibits the growth; this is diminished in blood dyscrasia and possibly also in schizophrenia. There is evidence to suggest that the infections are self-limiting, and in individuals who lack this "serum factor," the mycelia proliferate in the dermis in the living tissue and not just in the keratogenous zone, which is a nonliving keratinized structure. Individuals may get granulomas;[1] e.g., women who shave their legs may get a hair follicle granuloma.

TINEA CAPITIS.—Tinea capitis is caused by any dermatophyte except *Epidermophyton floccosum* and *Trichophyton consentricum.* Microsporums usually fluoresce with a bright green color, chiefly *M. canis,* and *M. audouini.* (See p. 77, PCAD.) These usually clear at puberty, except for a small percentage of favus and endothrix *Trichophyton* infections, e.g., the tonsurans and violaceum infections. Chronicity is associated with a lack of inflammatory response, and while kerion is curative in many cases, it is extremely unpleasant.

T. tonsurans, T. violaceum and *M. gypseum,* contracted from soil and animals, do *not* fluoresce and *can* affect adults. Most other microsporums affect children, but not adults. Occasionally in the tropics, *T. rubrum* can produce tinea capitis, and then it is endothrix. Cultures should always be made to identify the fungus. Rapid diagnosis can be made by placing epilated hair on a glass slide, applying a few drops of 10% KOH, placing a coverslip on top, heating over an alcohol lamp and examining with a low-power microscope directly.

Griseofulvin is curative for most of these microsporums and tinea capitis. For persons weighing less than 30 lb, the dose is 0.5 gm per day; 50 lb and over, 0.75 gm per day; and 100 lb and over, 1.0 gm a day at least.

Many people with cases of tinea tonsurans have to be kept on this treatment for 3 or 4 months.

TINEA BARBAE.—This is often mistaken for a bacterial folliculitis at first. *M. canis* has a positive reaction to Wood's light, but other fungi do not and have to be identified by cultures of epilated hair. Generally *T. mentagrophytes* produces dry inflammatory nodules, while *T. rubrum* and others produce more chronic infections similar to sycosis barbae. (See p. 73, PCAD.) Treatment with griseofulvin for several months clears almost all cases.

TINEA CORPORIS.—Annular or polycyclic marginated scaly erythemas, occasionally plaques suggesting psoriasis, and less often granulomatous nodules are found. Verrucous lesions are rare.

TINEA CRURIS.—This disorder is generally monilial if the scrotum is involved, otherwise the classic jock itch with the distinct margin can be caused by *E. floccosum*, *T. rubrum* or *T. mentagrophytes*. (See p. 75, PCAD.)

TINEA OF THE HANDS AND FEET.—Tinea is vesicular if caused by *T. mentagrophytes* and dry, branny and scaly if caused by *T. rubrum*. Occasionally monilia will produce a margin halfway up the palm.

TINEA UNGUIUM.—Onychomycosis is a disease causing detached and heaped-up nails. The diagnosis is more accurate with KOH examination of the scrapings. Again, griseofulvin is the treatment of choice (4–6 months for healing fingernails and 14–16 months for toenails). (See Formulary, no. 25E).

Local Treatment

Local treatment of dermatophytes makes up probably about 10% of a physician's practice. Griseofulvin has certainly helped in the management of these cases, particularly the *T. rubrum* cases, but it is still amazing how many people do not seem to get complete clearing with oral griseofulvin. Micronizing the powdered tablet or capsule and administering this along with a fatty meal greatly assist in absorption. The side effects of occasional headache and occasional depression and nausea can generally be dealt with, but local treatment is still the crux of the management of most dermatophytes, particularly athlete's foot. Undecyclenic acid, 20% powder or cream, is effective. Propionic acid and tolnaftate or Tinactin (Schering), either cream or solution, are effective if rubbed on a dry area twice a day at least and rubbed in thoroughly. Halotex and Micatin cream and Lotrimin cream are effective remedies.

Whitfield's ointment, which is 6% salicylic acid and 12% benzoic acid in a suitable base, usually lanolin or vaseline, though we can cut the strength and use it in USP hydrophilic ointment, is very effective in treating the blistering type of dermatophytosis. Three percent sulfur, 3% salicylic acid in a suitable base, and occasionally anywhere from 2% to 5% ammoniated mercury in a suitable base are also suitable although more confined to the more chronic types of dermatophytosis. In acute blistering types of *T. mentagrophytes* athlete's foot, soaks and Burow's solution or potassium permanganate, or some astringent type of wet dressing that shrivels the blisters and helps to pass the disorder from the acute stage to the more amenable-to-therapy second stage, is necessary. Very often steroids will assist this; the preparation with which I have had success consists of the following:

Salicylic acid	3%
Pyrogallic acid	3%
Benzoic acid	3%
Thymol iodide	2%
In collodion to make	100%

This should be mixed well ahead of time and kept for a month or so; when thoroughly dissolved in the collodion, it can be painted on the areas of involvement at weekly intervals. I have had superior results with this, although it is rather strong and dangerous and should be given only to very capable patients. Painting it on in the office at intervals of 1–2 weeks can be an extremely effective method of holding the *T. mentagrophytes* type of acute blistery athlete's foot under control. It is also useful in the splits in the fourth toe webs. (See Formulary, no. 25.)

Treatments for nail infections consist of Onychophytex (Unimed Labs.) 2% thiobendazole in DMSO, and Verdefam liquid (Texas Pharmacal), which is also useful on glabrous skin. Sometimes 3% chrysarobin in chloroform, 3–5% thymol in chloroform and salicylic acid in tincture of merthiolate can be very useful in the management of onychomycosis. One percent 5-FU in propylene glycol (Fluoroplex—Herbert) is helpful. Generally speaking, in the dry branny type of dermatophytosis, 3% sulfur-sal is as effective as any treatment, and in the more acute blistering type of *T. mentagrophtes* one-foot type, undecylenic acid powder in the morning and half-strength Whitfield's ointment at night are effective treatment.

For the treatment of *tinea cruris,* similar preparations can be used. Do not use Desenex preparations in the groin; it is extremely uncomfortable. Castellani's paint is one of the remedies that I rely on. If this is painted on the tinea cruris every day for 3 weeks, cure is almost invariable. Caldesene powder (Maltbie) is a calcium undecylenate preparation, does not sting the scrotum, and is a suitable remedy, also having mild antimonilial effects. Vioform hydrocortisone lotion or cream is also an effective remedy when rubbed on two or three times a day for tinea cruris. (See Formulary, nos. 17, 18, 25.)

If the strong suspicion is that you are dealing with a monilial intertrigo or tinea cruris, gentian violet, although messy, is effective. If the condition is very inflammatory, Burow's soaks followed by 1% hydrocortisone in mycostatin cream four times a day, or Lotrimin cream (which also seems to be effective in treating all varieties of tinea) twice a day is often very effective.[2]

In *tinea capitis*, generally a mild antibiotic ointment, in an effort to lessen the likelihood of kerion formation, is satisfactory as a rule. Also 2% ammoniated mercury ointment may be used, since it is mildly fungicidal. I caution patients to have the hair on the infected regions shaved so that they do not leave small pieces of infected hair all over the house; and the head should be shampooed two or three times a week in order to also remove infected spores. A stocking cap made from an old nylon stocking should be worn in the house so that the head does not leave contaminated hair on the furniture. This cap can be freshly applied each day and boiled at the end of the week.

For *tinea of the beard,* vioform in its various forms, plus Quinolor compound, is often effective. Sometimes plucking the hair is necessary. Oral griseofulvin is most effective.

Dermatophyte ids on the hand are very often effectively controlled by treating the source on the feet and by 1% hydrocortisone lotion rubbed in on the fingers frequently. Sometimes systemic steroids are extremely effective in reducing the intensity of the id reaction. Five percent thymol in chloroform is an excellent remedy for tinea of the nails, but repeated debridement with the electric drill is a helpful method of controlling it, too.

The best culture media for all purposes is mycosil agar (Scott Labs.) which is Sabouraud's agar with additional cyclohexamide and chloramphenicol to suppress unwanted contaminating bacteria and molds. This can be obtained in small bottles or agar slants, whichever appeals to the dermatologist. It is easier to get a scalpel into the agar slant than into the small bottles, although a small curette can be used to implant the fungus scrapings. They can be incubated at room temperature in the office and identified by a mycologist at any hospital or bacteriology laboratory or identified by the practicing physician. Other sources of culture media can be obtained through the nearest antibiotic manufacturer.

Yeast Infections

CANDIDIASIS.—Moniliasis is saprophytic yeast with pathogenic mycelial forms. Susceptibility to it is increased by taking steroids, antibiotics, hormones such as birth control pills, radiation, cold and mucin. Thirty-nine percent of normal vaginas have it as a saprophyte. Diabetes and pregnancy increase its pathogenicity.

Serum contains an anti-*Candida* factor which is reduced in lymphoma and leukemia. Mycostatin and amphotericin B can be used prophylactically in antibiotics, e.g., mysteclin F and tetrastatin, to lessen the incidence of flares following destruction of normal bacteria in the intestine.

CANDIDA OF SKIN.—Candidiasis can be the result of an endotoxin produced, say, from an intertrigo, which when injected intravenously into mice, gives hair loss. There are candidal granulomas, which are the result of mycelial invasions of the dermis, and intense local treatment with gentian violet or Mycostatin creams and ammoniated mercury may be necessary.

ORAL CANDIDIASIS IN THE NEWBORN.—This occurs because of contamination through the maternal birth canal. Prophylaxis consists of 100,000 units of Mycostatin given in 1 cc water on the second day. It usually produces white friable grayish plaques on the month, occasionally perleche, and occasionally in the hypopharynx and diaper area. If it is bad enough, Mycostatin, 100,000 units per cc given at the rate of 4 cc four times a day for 7–14 days, usually is sufficient. Occasionally amphotericin B, 80 mg/cc, is necessary three times a day for 3–28 days.

CANDIDIASIS OF THE ESOPHAGUS, INTESTINE AND PERIANAL REGION.—For a severe esophageal infection, intravenous injection of amphotericin B is necessary for candidal enteritis; 50 mg amphotericin B four times a day, or 250,000 units of Mycostatin four times a day is necessary for about 9 or 10 days. Mucocutaneous candidiasis was cleared using clotrimazole (Lotrimin) in a 3-year-old girl.[3]

PERIANAL PRURITUS WITH CANDIDA.—This condition can be relieved by mixing 1% hydrocortisone in Mycostatin cream, or you can mix triamcinolone with Mycostatin cream and give oral Mycostatin, Vitamin B Complex and yogurt.

CANDIDAL VAGINITIS.—Candidal vaginitis can be treated with Mycostatin suppositories or Gyne-Lotrimin vaginal tablets, amphotericin B, or Trichomycin locally. Another preparation to which I am partial is "A.V.C. Improved" (National Drug), which is an allantoin sulfonamide preparation that seems to be quite effective not only in treating *Candida* of the vagina, but also occasionally for complicating bacterial or *Trichomonas* infections. Flare-ups are apt to occur before and after menstrual periods and, of course, women should be warned about taking care of them at such times. (See Formulary, no. 25.)

ACRODERMATITIS ENTEROPATHICA.—These patients are prone to *Candida* infections; probably the organism is not causative, but is saprophytic in such a degree that the absorption of the endotoxin causes some of the hair loss seen in this condition. The treatment consists of oral Mycostatin, as well as oral suspension for the mouth and Diodoquin. The usual dose of Diodoquin is 2.4–2.6 gm daily (650 mg tablets—

Searle) for the average 15-kg child. Once the condition clears up, this dose may be discontinued or reduced, but it would probably have to be reinstituted after an interval.

The introduction of zinc therapy has revolutionized the treatment of this entity. The exact dosage is difficult to assess, though several authors recommend 200 mg zinc sulfate taken three times a day. Zinc gluconate does not upset the gastrointestinal tract quite as easily; as little as 50 mg taken twice a day can be effective. Remember that zinc nullifies tetracycline.[4-6]

DEEP CANDIDAL GRANULOMA.—This is treated best by intravenous injections of amphotericin B.

SUPERFICIAL CANDIDA INFECTIONS.—These can be treated with 20% aqueous sodium caprylate compounded by a good pharmacist, Chlordantoin, Mycolog or Mycostatin creams, gentian violet, Castellani's paint and, best of all, Lotrimin cream are useful.

CANDIDA INFECTIONS OF THE NAIL.—Monilial paronychia, commonly seen in barmaids, barmen, housewives, pastry cooks and bakers, fishmongers, cooks and chefs, can be extremely chronic. Sometimes it is also seen in waitresses who have to wipe off tables with wet cloths and masons whose hands are wet with cement.

The treatment of choice is 20% sodium caprylate solution, since it is capable of penetrating the paronychial fold. Other remedies are 10% resorcin and 70% alcohol, 3% chrysarobin in chloroform and gentian violet, some of which can be applied with a toothpick poked under the nail fold. Additional treatments are 1% iodine in chloroform, 5% thymol iodide in chloroform, salicylic acid in merthiolate and Lotrimin lotion. Sometimes when there is a great deal of inflammation and improvement has been very difficult to attain, superficial x-ray therapy, using doses of 75 rad, shielding closely to the fingernail paronychial area once a week for 4–6 weeks, is extremely effective. This is not to be used as a routine treatment but reserved for really difficult, problem patients—e.g., a diabetic bartender with 6 children. Patients should be instructed to keep their hands out of water as much as possible and not to get flour poked in around the fingernail area. If they are going to wear rubber gloves, persons should not put their hands in extremely hot water so their fingers will sweat inside the gloves, and not wear gloves for more than 10–15 minutes. Patients should be encouraged to do their work in spurts and be fast and less thorough than usual. Many of them dawdle at their job and get their hands thoroughly soaked; this should be discouraged.

Disseminated Candidiasis

This occurs usually in patients suffering from a serious primary disease or in those who have undergone surgery and antibiotic treatment. The diagnosis should be prompt, and treatment as a general rule is with intravenous injection of amphotericin B, approximately 1 mg/kg daily for about a month. In some cases, perhaps there is a vitamin B-complex deficiency along with this.

Major Systemic Mycoses

CRYPTOCOCCUS (TORULA HISTOLYTICA OR CRYPTOCOCCUS NEOFORMANS).—This is contracted mostly from pigeon-contaminated soil inhalation. The skin lesion is a small circular papule or nodule exuding thick pus. Biopsy is diagnostic.

NORTH AMERICAN BLASTOMYCOSIS (BLASTOMYCES DERMATITIDIS).—A granulomatous skin condition is secondary to systemic infection, usually in farmers.

SOUTH AMERICAN BLASTOMYCOSIS (BLASTOMYCES BRASILIENSIS OR PARACOCCIDIOIDES BRASILIENSIS).—This results in ulcerating granuloma of mucosa. Diagnosis is by direct examination of scrapings under the microscope. Sulfadiazine treatment suppresses it.

COCCIDIOIDOMYCOSIS (COCCIDIOIDES IMMITIS), VALLEY FEVER.—Inhalation of soil dust in the San Joaquin Valley in California produces valley fever in 40% of the people, a short-lived pulmonary infection with recovery. Some develop erythema nodosum, which spontaneously disappears.

HISTOPLASMOSIS (HISTOPLASMA CAPSULATUM).—Pulmonary granulomas result from contact with bird excreta and often bats.

SPOROTRICHOSIS (SPOROTHRIX SCHENCKII).—This disease is found mostly in agricultural workers. A skin inoculation usually leads to a chancre with a chain of lymphatic nodules. The diagnosis is made by seeing the cigar-shaped bodies on direct examination of scrapings, skin tests and serology. Treatment is by potassium iodide saturated solution, up to 40 drops taken three times a day for 6–8 weeks.

All of the above can be treated with amphotericin B injected intravenously in varying doses up to about 2.0 gm total daily dose. Texts on the deep mycoses should be consulted before attempting treatment.

ACTINOMYCOSIS (ACTINOMYCES ISRAELI).—Symptoms are lumpy jaw with sulfur granules from draining sinuses. Treatment is with penicillin in large doses. In general, any antibiotic used against gram-negative organisms is effective in treating actinomycosis. Sensitivity tests should be done. (See p. 79, PCAD.)

NOCARDIOSIS, MYCETOMA, CHROMOMYCOSIS, MUCOMYCOSIS, ASPERGILLOSIS, GEOTRICHOSIS AND RHINOSPORIDIOSIS.—All these affect the skin and require specialized care. They are perhaps better dealt with in specialized texts.[7-11]

INFECTIONS OF THE EYE AND EAR.—These are occasionally secondary to steroid eyedrops. Treatment with Mycostatin, Trichomycin or amphotericin B is recommended. Eyedrops are effective.

EXTERNAL OTITIS.—When not simply seborrheic, the outer ear canal may harbor secondarily opportunistic organisms, mainly saprophytic rather than causative. Often diseases caused by *Pseudomonas* will require skilled treatment, however, and then it helps to lower the pH of the ear canal with Burow's soaks and 2% hydrocortisone in Aerosporin otic

(Burroughs & Wellcome), which contains 1% glacial acetic acid. It effectively lowers the canal's pH. Colimycin eardrops also are very effective. I avoid Cortisporin because neomycin sensitizes the ear canal.

Chemotherapy of Fungus Diseases

MYCOSTATIN.—Mycostatin is also called Nystatin (named after the New York state laboratory in which it was developed). It is derived from an actinomycete found on a dairy farm in Virginia. It is a polyene, which is a group or class of antifungal antibiotics discovered in recent years with multiple chromophore groups, e.g., fungichromin, candicidin, trichomycin, homycin and amphotericin B.

Mycostatin has no effect on bacteria and is not toxic to viruses. It has a long shelf life in the dry powdered form, loses 25% of its activity in 6 months and lasts about 4½ years in the refrigerator. If it is mixed, it lasts only about 2 weeks, even in the refrigerator, and it is not absorbed in the gastrointestinal tract at all. It is active against *Trichomonas vaginalis, Leishmania donovani* and *Candida* and also suppresses contaminants in tissue-culture studies. It acts by damaging the cell membrane to produce cessation of intracellular glycolysis. Resistance to it develops slowly, if at all. Mycostatin can be given intravenously, but it produces severe toxic symptoms when taken intramuscularly, with pain and muscle destruction, so it is too toxic for systemic use. It is apparently not sensitizing, so it can be used topically in the eye, skin, ear and other areas.

AMPHOTERICIN B.—This drug was obtained from soil in the region of the Orinoco River in Venezuela. It is stable for long periods of time when stored away from air and light. When dissolved in isopropyl alcohol, it loses its effect rapidly, depending on the pH. It is effective against *Leishmania braziliensis* and *L. donovani,* as well as *Blastomyces dermatitidis, Coccidioides immitis, Histoplasma capsulatum, Cryptococcus neoformans* and *Candida albicans.* It enters the leukocytes. Orally it has no really toxic symptoms, although there is mild gastrointestinal irritation.

Dogs are intolerant to intravenous doses of amphotericin B. They get melena and gastrointestinal hemorrhages. Humans taking doses of 1 mg/kg/day in an intravenous drip occasionally have fever, chills, headache, nausea, vomiting, anorexia or phlebitis. However, impaired kidney function is the most common side effect. The vehicle for intravenous drip is 5% glucose in water, 1,000 cc in 6–8 hours. Usually on the first day the patient is given 10 mg; the second day, 25 mg; the third day and each day thereafter, 50 mg.

Sodium chloride and procaine should not be used intravenously because they precipitate the amphotericin. Ten mg heparin in the vial will usually inhibit phlebitis. Antihistamines given orally lessen the chills and fever, and Compazine lessens the nausea.

GRISEOFULVIN.—This is the metabolic product of a mold (penicillin griseofulvin—Dierdkx). In 1958 it cured an experimental infection in a guinea pig caused by *Microsporum canis*. Blank treated *Trichophyton rubrum* the next year, and this led to a cure.[12] Griseofulvin acts mostly in a fungistatic manner, but under conditions of active growth it can be fungicidal (inhibits nucleic acid synthesis). It works on dermatophytes *(Trichophyton, Microsporum* and *Epidermophyton floccosum),* but not on erythrasma or tinea versicolor.

Fungi can develop a degree of adaptation to griseofulvin, perhaps by a change in permeability to the drug, they can develop metabolic antagonism, or they can develop a method of detoxifying it. Nobody is really sure. Some *T. rubrum can* develop resistance!

The drug reaches the horny layer by a process of diffusion and is incorporated into the keratinized tissue, probably in the interstices of the keratin lattice. It is detected in the base of the stratum corneum in 48 hours, but it does not pass the placental barrier.

Usually a headache, gastrointestinal upset, occasional rashes, thirst, incoordination, insomnia, feeling of irritability, occasional light sensitivity and potentiation of alcohol are the most noteworthy side effects.

Impressionable or "artistic-creative" personalities may suffer side effects more intensely than more average patients, but generally the drug is more effectively therapeutic in such patients as well. One well-known painter cured his toenail within 6 weeks of treatment, although he had to go to bed while taking the drug! It took a year to grow out clear naturally.

POLYENE ANTIBIOTICS (FROM STREPTOMYCES).—Trichomycin is topically effective for *Candida* or *Trichomonas* infections. Pimaricin is good only for suppressing yeasts; candicidin is effective for treating *Candida* infections.

REFERENCES

1. Majocchi, D.: Sopra una nuova tricofizia (granuloma tricofitico): Studi clinici e micrologici, Bull. Acad. Med. Roma 9:220, 1883.
2. Spiekermann, P. H., and Young, M.: Clinical evaluation of clotrimazole, Arch. Dermatol. 112:350, 1976.
3. Ipp, M. M., Boxall, L., and Gelfand, E. W.: Clotrimazole, Am. J. Child. 131:305, 1977.
4. Neldner, K. H., and Hambidge, K. M.: Zinc therapy of acrodermatitis enteropathica, N. Engl. J. Med. 292:879, 1975.
5. Hirsh, F. S., Michel, R., and Strain, W. H.: Gluconate zinc in acrodermatitis enteropathica, Arch. Dermatol. 112:475, 1976.
6. Campo, A. G., McDonald, C. J.: Treatment of acrodermatitis enteropathica with zinc sulfate, Arch. Dermatol. 112:687, 1976.
7. Rebow, G., and Caplan, D.: *Dermatophytes: Their Recognition and Identification* (Coral Gables, Fla.: University of Miami Press, 1970).
8. Conant, N. F., et al.: *Manual of Clinical Mycology* (Philadelphia: W. B. Saunders Co., 1954).
9. Ash, J. E., and Spitz, S.: *Pathology of Tropical Diseases* (Philadelphia: W. B. Saunders Co., 1945).
10. Duldorf, G.: Symposium, New York Academy of Medicine (Springfield, Ill.: Charles C Thomas, Publisher, 1962).
11. Hazen, E. L., Gordon, M. A., and Reed, F. S.: *Laboratory Identification of Pathogenic Fungi, Simplified* (3d ed.; Springfield, Ill.: Charles C Thomas, Publisher, 1970).
12. Blank, H., and Roth, F. J. J.: The treatment of dormatomycoses with griseofulvin, Nature (London) 182:476, 1959.

10 / Venereal Diseases

Syphilis

While the Oslo study by Bruusgaard indicated that 60–70% of untreated patients went through life with little or no inconvience,[1] still 30–40% suffered serious inconvenience, so that the diagnosis and treatment are very worthwhile.

There are essentially three stages in syphilis: the primary (chancre), the secondary (florid rash and dissemination) and the late (gumma, aneurysm, tabes, paresis). There is a latent stage of anywhere from 2 to 40 years after the second state, during which flare-ups of the latent infection can lead to actual clinically infectious relapses. Insufficient or irregular treatment favors relapses. Figure 10–1 shows the natural history of untreated syphilis.

Primary

This stage is characterized by chancre or indurated ulcer, which may be insignificant, on the penis, vulva, lip or anus following 18–21 days after exposure. (See pp. 189–191, PCAD.) It may be delayed by intercurrent antibiotic treatment of another infection. The diagnosis is by darkfield examination of the chancre fluid for treponomas under the microscope.

Secondary

The second stage is characterized by a florid symmetric coppery erythematous macular exanthem that almost always involves the palms, soles and mucous membranes and is accompanied by general lymphadenopathy 3–6 weeks after the appearance of the chancre. (See pp. 192–196, PCAD.)

Relapsing secondaries occur during the latent period in untreated or insufficiently treated patients and are characterized by indolent polymorphic grouped skin or mucosal lesions that are often annular or corymbose (satellites around a central

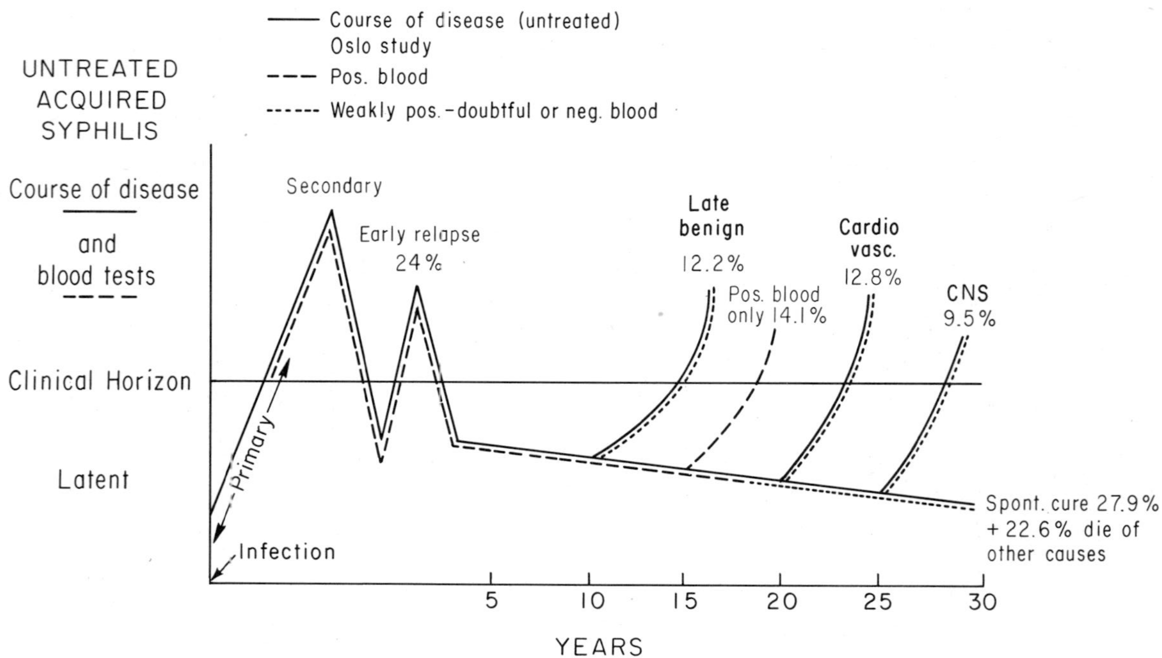

Fig 10–1.—The natural history of untreated syphilis and the incidence of clinical disease in the 1934 Oslo study. Thirty-five percent of the subjects showed spontaneous seroreversal and no manifestations of syphilis. (From Morgan, H. J., South. Med. J. 27:18, 1933. Used by permission.)

large lesion), very occasionally pustular (the pox) or rupial (oyster shell-like) and often near a mucous membrane orifice such as the mouth or nostril. Their appearance is preceded by a rise in the serologic titer.

Latent syphilis is characterized by an absence of symptoms. Meanwhile the serology is positive, and invasion of the cardiovascular or central nervous system may silently occur. Early latent syphilis is less than 2 years' duration, whereas duration of longer than this is considered late latent syphilis. Almost all central nervous system (CNS) invasion occurs before this second year (most within 6 months) so that lumbar punctures should be performed as soon as the diagnosis is made. A baseline chest x-ray to use for future comparison of the width of the aorta is useful since cardiovascular or CNS syphilis can proceed in the presence of a negative Venereal Disease Research Lab Test (VDRL) in 20% of patients.

Late

Late syphilis is characterized by an asymptomatic period in most patients, although 25% will develop symptoms of gumma, aortitis, tabes or paresis if untreated early. In the skin, nodular serpiginous copper-colored firm, scaly or smooth lesions may appear and progress slowly over the years. Gummata may occur singly or as disseminated kidney-shaped patches with punched-out ulcerations. Interstitial glossitis or mucosal gummatous ulceration can also occur. (See pp. 196–199, PCAD.)

Passive transfer of antibodies will give an infant positive serology for several months even if healthy. Diminishing titers indicate the biologic false positive reaction, whereas a rising titer is very suggestive of luetic infection. Snuffles, frontal bossing, tender bones, periostitis or epiphysitis on x-ray, an enlarged spleen, or occasionally skin lesions may suggest syphilis in the young infant, who *can* be seronegative for up to 6 months.

Diagnosis of Syphilis

Biologic false positive reactions will occur in persons with infectious mononucleosis, lymphogranuloma venereum (LGV), leprosy, recent vaccination and rheumatoid arthritis, as well as in terminal cancer patients. In cases of questionable VDRL, it is well to remember that "positive in high dilutions" suggests true positivity, and the *Treponema pallidum* immobilization test (TPI), which is slow, may have negative results in 15–20% of definite secondary syphilis cases. The fluorescent treponemal antibody absorption test (FTA-ABS) gives positive results in almost every case of syphilis whether successfully treated or not and whether seronegative or not, and even earlier than the VDRL 50% of the time, *but* it is a sensitive test and can give false positive reactions in persons with lupus erythematosus and in terminal cancer patients. Many cardiovascular and CNS syphilis patients will be seronegative and give positive FTA-ABS test results.

Treatment

Penicillin has revolutionized the treatment of all forms of syphilis. In the days of arsenic treatment, fear of the Jarisch-Herxheimer reaction (presumably an intensification of symptoms because of the release of the antigenic protein when the spirochete was destroyed), causing swelling of the coronary ostia in cardiovascular syphilis and thereby leading to coronary occlusion, usually led to the "softening" or "mild preparation" of the patient with bismuth for a few weeks before starting arsenic treatment. While many therapists feel this is unnecessary with penicillin, caution is in order when treating cases of optic atrophy or severe CNS lues or suspected aortitic patients. In one patient where inadvertent ECGs were done three times in one day shortly after penicillin was introduced, there was classic T-wave inversion of the coronary occlusion type, although symptoms were mild.

Successful therapy requires a high enough level of penicillin over a long enough period of time to eradicate the spirochete. Whether *every* spirochete is killed is an academic question, and it is most likely that such does not occur. Probably enough spirochetes are killed so that the body's natural defenses can handle the remnants thereafter. Benzathine penicillin G gives adequate levels over long periods.

Table 10–1 gives an adequate program of treatment for average cases. In cases of optic atrophy, interstitial keratitis and more severe forms of symptomatic neurosyphilis, however,

TABLE 10-1.—TREATMENT SCHEDULE FROM THE CENTER FOR DISEASE CONTROL

TYPE OF SYPHILIS	PENICILLIN TREATMENT	ALTERNATE TREATMENT
Early syphilis Primary Secondary Early latent Pregnancy	Benzathine penicillin G, 2.4 million units IM weekly × 2, total 4–8 million units, or penicillin and aluminum monostearate	Tetracycline, 0.5 gm 4 times a day for 20 days, total 40 gm Erythromycin, 0.5 gm 4 times a day for 20 days, total 40 gm
Late syphilis Latent Benign	Benzathine penicillin G, 2.4 million units IM weekly × 3, total 7.2 million units	Tetracycline, 0.5 gm 4 times a day for 30 days, total 60 gm Erythromycin, 0.5 gm 4 times a day for 30 days, total 60 gm
Neurosyphilis and cardiovascular syphilis	Aqueous procaine penicillin G, 2.4 million units every 2 days × 6, total 14.4 million units Benzathine penicillin G, 2.4 million units IM weekly × 5, total 12 million units	Tetracycline, 0.5 gm orally 4 times a day for 30 days, total 60 gm Erythromycin, 0.5 gm orally 4 times a day for 30 days, total 60 gm
Congenital syphilis Less than 77 lb	Aqueous procaine penicillin G, 50,000 units/kg body weight IM daily for 14 days If neurosyphilis has been excluded by CSF exam, Benzathine penicillin G, 75,000 units/kg body weight divided into two injections at 1-week intervals	Tetracycline, not recommended for children under 12 because of adverse effects on teeth Erythromycin, 20 mg/kg body weight divided into four doses for 2 weeks
More than 77 lb	Same as late latent treatment	Tetracycline, same as late latent treatment Erythromycin, same as late latent treatment

the Presbyterian Hospital schedule, which is closer to 25 million units over 10–14 weeks in 20–28 injections, is preferable.

All patients who refuse cerebrospinal fluid (CSF) lumbar puncture (LP) should be treated as having asymptomatic neurosyphilis (at least 12 million units over 6–8 weeks). Usually after this course, the CSF cell count will return to normal (less than 6) in 6 months and the serum protein level will normalize in one year. Follow-up requires a serologic test for syphilis (STS) every 6 months for 2 years and then yearly thereafter, plus a chest x-ray.

Cephaloridin (Loridine–Lilly), 0.5 gm given intramuscularly daily for 10 days, appears to be effective.[2]

In questionable penicillin allergy, scratch or conjunctival tests using 5 units per cc of aqueous penicillin can be read in 20 minutes, and if negative, an 0.02-cc intracutaneous injection of the 10,000 units of aqueous solution can be used. If results are negative, the patient may be treated. If pseudopods, wheals or flares occur, then the patient is allergic, and one of the other drugs must be used.

"Pre-Pen" (Kremers-Urban) benzylpenicilloyl-polylysine, is new on the market as a method of testing for penicillin allergy.[3]

Oxygen should be on hand in every office where penicillin is used. An airway and an oxygen mask plus a tourniquet of the arm, if injected, help in anaphylaxis. Subcutaneous or intravenous epinephrine, as well as intravenous Benadryl or aminophylline and later steroid suffice in most moderately severe reactions. It is a very frightening experience, so be prepared!

Other Venereal Diseases

Chancroid (soft chancre)

The incubation period of *Hemophilus Ducreyi*, which stains with methylene blue, is 2 to 7 days. Chancroids appear as tender and usually multiple punched-out genital ulcers with unilateral lymph gland enlargement (which suppurates if untreated). (See p. 202, PCAD.) The diagnosis is by staining the direct smear to find the "school-of-fish" arrangement of the organism, which is gram negative. The intracutaneous skin test with ducrey vaccine has positive results *after* the second week.

The following treatment is usually curative: sulfa (Gantanol–2 gm daily for 14 days, Madribon–2 gm daily for 14 days, sulfadiazine–4 gm daily for 7–14 days, and Gantrisin—4 gm daily for 14–21 days) or streptomycin (1 gm daily for 7–10 days). Erythromycin, Aureomycin, tetracycline, Terramycin or Chloromycetin (2 gm daily for 14 days) is also curative. Occasional cases need treatment of up to 4 weeks, with local soaks and antibiotic locally assisting.

Granuloma Inguinale

The incubation period is 1–12 weeks and is caused by the *Donovania* granulomatis. "Closed safety pin" inside the cytoplasm of cells stains with the Wright stain. Scrapings (not smears) show the organism. The disease consists of progressive granulomatous ulceration with fleshy edges, almost invariably in blacks. The lesion is not very uncomfortable, and there is usually no regional lymph node involvement.

Treatment should be with tetracycline, Chloromycetin or streptomycin (all 2 gm daily for 21 days—or 1 gm four times a day for 7 days).

Lymphogranuloma Venereum

This disease, with incubation 5–20 days, is characterized by a "bubo" leading to a sinus that usually drains a long time, finally producing convoluted scarring. (See p. 203, PCAD.).

In the male, there is unilateral inguinal adenopathy following an insignificant lesion on the genitals. A good treatment is sulfadiazine, 4 gm daily for 21 days. In the female, adenopathy is more apt to occur in the pararectal nodes, producing rectal stricture. The best treatment is tetracycline, 2 gm daily for 3 weeks.

Treatment is as for granuloma inguinale, although tetracycline, sulfa and chloromycetin can be used (in decreasing order of choice).

The LGV complement fixation test is highly specific and shows positive results early in the infection. The Frei test (antigen is hard to get; try Hollister-Stier) intracutaneously, 1/10 cc, is read in 72 hours. Infiltration of more than 7 mm is a positive reaction.

Herpes Progenitalis

Symptoms are grouped vesicles on opposed surfaces, which often ulcerate early and heal rapidly. They recur, and if you can elucidate the trigger and eliminate it (e.g., wine, cheese, chocolate), this is the best management. (See the sections on viral diseases and herpes simplex, and p. 82, PCAD.).

Acidophilus milk or Lactinex tablets (Hynson, Westcott & Dunning) may, by altering the local environment, have some effect. Lupidon-G (Herbal Chemie) is a vaccine used in Germany requiring weekly injections for a year. Application of solvents, such as 70% alcohol, acetone and ether, may destroy the lipoprotein envelope around the infectious viral particles. Condoms should be worn during intercourse. Smallpox vaccination here does not seem as effective as in oral or facial herpes. Neosporin powder or Vioform hydrocortisone lotion usually heals the attack, and occasionally Castellani's paint is helpful.

Balanitis Erosiva

A long foreskin leads to moisture, which with retained smegma produces irritation and a bright red glans. Occasionally the foreskin becomes edematous, leading to phimosis. Yeasts or Vincent's spirillum, along with other bacteria, thrive in this milieu, and mild cleansing and soothing wet dressings with 0.25% silver nitrate, or Burow's or boric acid solution, help. Antibiotic dusting powder or hydrocortisone Mycostatin lotion, with or without Vioform, and occasionally aqueous gentian violet are of assistance here. I generally suggest Phisoderm for normal skin as a washing agent. Balneol (Westwood) is useful also as a gentle cleanser. Ointments are often aggravating here unless cleaned off occasionally. One-half strength Carbofuchsin is occasionally curative.

Recent reports from Helsinki have mentioned a type of treatment that is successful where there is a lot of moisture, e.g., a long foreskin, using beads of a dextran polymer called Debrisan (Pharmacea) which is dusted on like salt twice a day. It cleans things up in short order.[4] One case of balanitis xerotica obliterans was successfully treated with 2.5% testosterone propionate in an ointment.[5]

For venereal warts, see the section on warts.

REFERENCES

1. Bruusgaard, E.: Über das schicksad der nicht spezifisch behondelten luetiker, Arch. f. Dermat. v. Syph. 157:309, 1929.

2. Glicksman, J. M., Short, P. K., and Knox, J. M.: Parenteral cephaloridine treatment of patients with early syphilis, Arch. Intern. Med. 121:342–44, 1968.
3. Parker, C. W.: Drug allergy, N. Engl. J. Med. 292:957, 1975.
4. Lassus, A., Karvonen, J., and Juvakoski, J.: Dextran polymer particles (debrisan) in the treatment of penile ulcers, Acta Derm. Venereol. 57:361, 1977.
5. Pasieczny, T. A. H.: The treatment of balantis xerotica obliterans with testosterone, Acta Derm. Venereol. 57:275, 1977.

SUGGESTED READINGS

Domonkos, A. N.: *Andrews' Diseases of the Skin* (6th ed.; Philadelphia: W. B. Saunders Co, 1971).

Acta Dermato-Venereologica

11 / Antibiotics

The empiric discovery of the effect of quinine on protozoan malaria in Peru, which was brought to Europe in the 17th century, might be said to be the beginnings of modern chemotherapy. Ehrlich's discovery of an effective organic arsenical in 1906 and the development of Prontosil in 1935, which led to the discovery of other sulfonamides, paved the way for Fleming's discovery of penicillin in 1929, which gave Chain and Florey the opportunity to usher in the antibiotic era in 1940 with therapeutic penicillin.[1]

Antibiotics interfere with bacterial metabolism, and the precise point of interference differs. Some (penicillin, streptomycin, erythromycin and novobiocin) are bactericidal, while others (chloramphenicol, sulfonamides and tetracyclines) are bacteriostatic. *Pseudomonas* and *Proteus* organisms are resistant to most agents, and an increase in gram-negative infections seems to be occurring in the skin.

Specifically resistant strains of bacteria probably occur spontaneously as a result of mutation. If the inhibiting effect of the sensitive strain majority is removed by continued antibiotic treatment, then we *select* a drug-resistant strain. In the case of streptomycin, this is fast, whereas with penicillin it occurs slowly. Table 11–1 lists the susceptibilities of most of the organisms affecting the skin.

Substitution infection, e.g., as with penicillin, may clear the organisms initially responsible for the infection, but the lesion may become reinfected from the environmental organisms, which very often in hospitals may be resistant and lurking in abundance. The displacement colonization of nursery personnel's nostrils with harmless *S. aureus* (502A strain) can effectively *prevent* spread of a resistant strain in nursery epidemics, and the work of Shinefield[2] and Light[3] proves this. (See the section on staphylococcal infections.)

TABLE 11-1.—BACTERIAL SENSITIVITIES

	PENICILLIN	TETRACYCLINE	KANAMYCIN	COLISTIN	ERYTHROMYCIN	VANCOMYCIN	CHLOROAMPHENICOL	RISTOCETIN	STREPTOMYCIN	SPIROMYCIN	TRIACETYLOLEANDOMYCIN	LINCOMYCIN	CLINDOMYCIN	OXACILLIN	CLOXACILLIN	KEFLEX
STAPHYLOCOCCUS	⊕	+	+	−	⊕	+	+	+	−	+	+	+	⊕	+	+	⊕
RESISTANCE TO STAPHYLOCOCCUS			+		+		+						+	⊕	⊕	+
STREPTOCOCCUS	⊕	+	+	−	+	+	−	+	−	+	+	+	+	+	+	+
ACTINOMYCIN	+	−	−	−	+	−	−	−	−	−	−	−	+	−	−	−
PNEUMOCOCCUS	+	+	−	−	+	+	−	+	−	+	+	+	+	+	+	+
T. PALLIDUM	+	+	+	−	+	+	−	+	−	−	−	−	−	+	+	−
MYCOBACTERIA	−	−	−	−	−	−	−	+	−	−	−	−	−	−	−	−
TUBERCULOSIS			VIOMYCIN						+	CYCLOSERINE-CAPREOMYCIN						
GC	+	+	−	−	+	−	−	−	−	−	−	−	−	+	+	−
MENINGOCOCCUS	+	+	−	−	+	+	−	−	+	+	−	−	−	−	−	−
PSEUDOMONAS	−	−	+	⊕	−	−	−	−	−	−	−	−	−	−	−	−
PROTEUS VULGARIS			+					NOVOBIOCIN								
PROTEUS MIRABILIS			+					NOVOBIOCIN								
PSITTACOSIS–LGV	+	+	−	−	+	+	+	−	−	−	−	−	−	−	−	−
RICKETTSIAE	−	+	−	−	−	−	+	−	−	−	−	−	−	−	−	−
AEROBACTER AEROGENES (PYOCYANEUS)	−	−	+	+	−	−	−	−	−	−	−	−	−	−	−	−
ENDAMOEBA HIST.	−	−	−	−	−	−	−	−	−	−	−	−	−	−	−	−
HELLERIA	−	−	+	−	−	−	−	−	−	−	−	−	−	−	−	−
SERRATIA	−	−	+	−	−	−	−	−	−	−	−	−	−	−	−	−
KLEBSIELLA	+	−	?	⊕	−	−	+	−	−	−	−	−	−	−	−	−
TYPHOID	−	−	−	−	−	−	+	−	−	−	−	−	−	−	−	−
E. COLI	−	−	+	+	+	−	+	−	−	+	−	−	−	−	−	+

⊕ = Very susceptible
\+ = Susceptible
− = Not susceptible

Superinfection, e.g., destruction of normal gut and respiratory tract flora by broad-spectrum antibiotics, allows resistant strains to "take over," and occasionally a serious enterocolitis occurs *(Proteus, Pseudomonas, S. aureus, Monilia).*

When a drug has been used in a community for some time, the relative proportion of organisms resistant to it should increase. This *has* occurred, though to nothing like the extent feared.

To control drug resistance, avoid half-hearted treatment. If treatment is to be prolonged, consider combined therapy, such as streptomycin *and* isoniazid for tuberculosis. If there is an underlying surgical problem, correct it with speed. Prevent substitution by controlling cross-infection. Avoid using broad-spectrum antibiotic agents for trivial infections, and if sensitivity tests indicate an organism of low susceptibility to any of the available antibiotics (e.g., *Pseudomonas*), use a combination (e.g., polymyxin and tetracycline) for synergistic effect. In general, antagonisms between antibiotics do *not* occur in vivo.

Bacterial and cryptococcal opportunism is an increasingly complicating factor in the management of bacterial infections. Increasing incidence of serious infection is being reported from the *Klebsiella* Enterobacteriaceae group—*Herellea, Serratia, Aeromonas* and others. Specific identification may be lifesaving.[4]

The Penicillins

The penicillins are all derived from 6-aminopenicillanic acid. Procaine penicillin G by injection is the method of choice in treating those infections caused by sensitive strains of *S. aureus, Streptococcus*, pneumococcus, gonococcus or meningococcus, diphtheria, actinomycosis, *T. pallidum*, and the psittacosis-LGV group. Oral penicillin has much less effect than injected penicillin. Table 11–2 lists the antibiotic penicillins.

Penicillin Reactions

These reactions can occasionally be extremely severe. In any questionable state of allergy to penicillin, its use should be avoided. There is reason to believe that oxacillin and meth-

TABLE 11-2.—ANTIBIOTIC PENICILLINS

1. Penicillin G
   a. Parenteral penicillin.—Comes as crystalline potassium, crystalline sodium, procaine aqueous, procaine aqueous fortified, procaine in oil with 2% aluminum monostearate (PAM); useful in treating syphilis
   b. Oral penicillin.—Comes as procaine penicillin G potassium tablets, e.g., Pentids K pen G
2. Penicillin V.—Is stable when taken orally; potassium salt is better absorbed, e.g., Pen-Vee K (Wyeth), V cillin K (Lilly); Compocillin-VK (Abbott), 125 or 250 mg tablets
3. Benzathine penicillin.—Used in long-acting penicillin by injection, e.g., Bicillin (long-acting)
4. Semisynthetic penicillins. Those orally effective against penicillinase-producing strains are:
   a. Sodium oxacillin (Prostaphlin-Bristol, Resistopen—Squibb)
   b. Sodium nafcillin (Unipen—Wyeth)
   c. Sodium cloxacillin (Tegopen—Bristol)
   d. Sodium dicloxacillin (Dynapen—Bristol, Veracillin—Ayerst)
   e. Sodium methicillin (Staphcillin—Bristol, or Dimocillin—Squibb); used intramuscularly only

   Those inactivated by penicillinase include:
   f. Phenothicillin (Synicillin, Maxipen, Seropen)
   g. Ampicillin (Polycillin, Penbritten, Omnipen); very effective against gram-negative bacilli, e.g., *Proteus mirabilis* and *E. coli, Salmonella, Shigella* (*not* against *Klebsiella, Aerobacter* or *Pseudomonas*)
5. *Penicillin O* (Cirocillin—Upjohn).—Less apt to produce allergic reaction

icillin do *not* produce the same kind of sensitivity reactions in patients hypersensitive to penicillin G, although in 25% of people there *is* cross-sensitivity. Allergic people are the poorest risks.

Allergic reactions to penicillin are usually urticarial, although purpura, pericarditis, toxic psychoses and hematemesis due to an urticaria-like reaction of the gastric mucosa can occur. More common is a delayed serum sickness reaction. If anaphylaxis occurs, it is fatal in enough of the victims that an airway and oxygen tank should be in every physician's office, just in case.

When penicillin is given in large amounts (especially in cases of renal damage), cortical irritation can occur, including convulsions. Methicillin has significant nephrotoxicity.

Penicillin passes into the cerebrospinal fluid (CSF) poorly, although when 5 million units of crystalline penicillin is given intravenously, it leads to therapeutic concentrations in the CSF within 5 minutes.

Penicillin O is reportedly much less sensitizing than penicillin G, although it has to be given frequently.

Penicillinase (Schenlabs), 800,000 units in 2 cc water given deeply intramuscularly, is an effective way to destroy allergy-causing penicillin depots, although antihistamines and sometimes steroids are usually required in addition. Penicillinase itself can produce severe allergic reactions, and this should be borne in mine.

Broad-Spectrum Antibiotics

TETRACYCLINES.—These antibiotics, which penetrate the CSF poorly and are derived from fungi of the *Streptomyces* genus, include Tetrex (Bristol), Achromycin (Lederle), Tetracyn (Pfizer), Mysteclin (Squibb) and Panmycin (Upjohn). They also include chlortetracycline (Aureomycin—Lederle), oxytetracycline (Terramycin—Pfizer), dimethyl-chlortetracycline (Declomycin—Lederle), methacycline (Rondomycin—Wallace), Minocin (Lederle) and Vibramycin (Pfizer). They are all highly active against gram-positive and gram-negative organisms (except *Proteus* and *Pseudomonas*) and active against *T. pallidum* and rickettsiae. They are the most active of the antibiotics against psittacosis and the LGV group of viruses. However, many strains of *Staphylococcus* and *E. coli* are resistant. Declomycin is phototoxic, but allergy is uncommon. Gastrointestinal disturbances occasionally result from the destruction of the ordinary gut bacteria and replacement with *Monilia,* but Mycostatin, Bacid, yogurt, *Lactobacillus* or B-complex vitamins can assist this. The tetracyclines stain the osseus structures and the teeth of the unborn when given to pregnant women (during the last trimester chiefly) or newborn infants, and if denatured by heat or age, can lead to detached nails or a syndrome causing excessive urination and drinking of water, which is extremely infrequent (Fanconi's syndrome—tubular reabsorption failure). Declomycin kills some strains of *Proteus* and *Pseudomonas*. Other side effects are moniliasis, diarrhea, urticaria and erythema multiforme.

The tetracyclines are bactericidal when taken in large doses.

NOVOBIOCIN (ALBAMYCIN—UPJOHN).—This is effective against gram-positive bacteria, occasionally *Proteus*, and has a relatively high toxicity.

ERYTHROMYCIN.—Erythromycin has a range of activity similar to that of penicillin. It is relatively free of side effects except for occasional nausea, which often can be avoided or removed by switching to the erythromycin base, which does not have the enteric coating.

SPIROMYCIN, OLEANDOMYCIN, CARBOMYCIN, RISTOCETIN, CHLORAMPHENICOL, LINCOMYCIN, VANCOMYCIN AND STREPTOMYCIN.—These are seldom used in dermatology.

CLINDAMYCIN (CLEOCIN—UPJOHN).—Despite a bad reputation for producing serious diarrhea, clindamycin is extremely useful in twice-daily doses (on an empty stomach, with nothing to eat for an hour before or after) for patients with severe acne, including conglobate acne. It hits some gram-negative and anaerobic organisms, mainly gram-positive cocci.

KANAMYCIN (KANTREX—BRISTOL).—This is used especially against staphylococcal infections that are resistant to other antibiotics. It is related to neomycin and cross-reacts. It is given intramuscularly, 500 mg every 6 hours, to an adult, and resistance develops rapidly. It produces nephrotoxicity and eighth nerve damage. It is *not* absorbed from the gut, but can be used for preoperative gut sterilization. In a healthy adult, less than 1.5 gm per day in divided doses should *not* produce ototoxicity. The maximum *total* dose, however, should not exceed 20 gm, although this figure is debatable. It should not exceed 15 mg/kg body weight per day. It is effective against most strains of *Proteus vulgaris, P. mirabilis, pseudomonas aeruginosa, aerobacter aerogenes, Endamoeba histolytica,* all coliform organisms and many staphylococci. It is used principally in resistant staphylococcal infections. Sensitivity tests should guide you, however.

COLISTIN (COLYMYCIN OR POLYMIXIN E—WARNER CHILCOTT).—This antibiotic is injectable only, very rapidly bactericidal, and the specific antibiotic for infections with *Pseudomonas* (but not *Proteus*). It is very effective in treating pathogenic *coli* infections, but is essentially used against gram-negative bacilli. Resistance appears very slowly, and colistin cross-reacts with only Polymyxin. Gut absorption is minimal. The dose is 150 mg given intramuscularly once or twice a day. Side effects include parasthesias around the mouth, vertigo and ataxia, which are exacerbated with renal impairment. It is nephrotoxic, and excellent in treating external otitis locally.

CEPHALOTHIN (KEFLIN—LILLY).—This substance is bactericidal and resistance develops slowly. It shows no cross resistance with any other antibiotic and is active against resistant *Staphylococcus, P. mirabilis, E. coli, Klebsiella, Aerobacter, Streptococcus hemolyticus* and *T. pallidum (Pseudomonas* are *resistant*). Dose is 2–4 gm given intramuscularly for 24 hours (and it hurts). Side effects include pain on injection, so you must move the sites and give deeply intramuscularly. Maculopapular rashes have occurred. Sensitivity tests should guide its use. Cross sensitivity with penicillin is not uncommon.

KEFLEX (LILLY) (CEPHALEXIN).—Sensitization to Keflex is about the same as to Keflin, though Keflex is acid stable and effective orally without regard to meals. There are a few strains of *Staphylococcus* that are resistant, though. There is partial cross allergenicity with penicillin, so caution is in order. Side effects include diarrhea, genital moniliasis, hives and occasional anaphylaxis. Treatment is from 1 to 4 gm daily in divided doses, usually 250 mg three times a day after meals. Keflex is supplied as pulvules of 250 and 500 mg, and tablets of 250 mg. Oral suspensions can be 125 mg or 250 mg per teaspoon.

Local Antibiotics

POLYMYXIN.—Actually this is a group of polypeptide antibiotics produced by *Bacillus polymyxa* and called A, B, C, D and E. A, C and D are nephrotoxic, and B and E can be given parenterally with caution. However, its major use is in ointments or eardrops where it is extremely effective against *Pseudomonas,* pyocyaneus and other gram-negative organisms. It possesses considerable surface activity and is rapidly bactericidal. It is of little value against *Proteus* organisms. (See Formulary, nos. 23, 24.)

BACITRACIN.—This is usually 500 units per gram. It is from *B. subtilis* and is nephrotoxic, but not absorbed from the gut. It is inactivated by ions of heavy metal, so it should not be mixed with mercury or zinc ointments. Peroxide also inactivates it. It is a little unstable in aqueous solutions, but stable in ointments. It is effective against gram-positive organisms having the same range as penicillin and is *not* very sensitizing in the skin. Resistance emerges slowly. It inhibits *Endamoeba histolytica, T. pallidum,* and Vincent's fusospirochetes.

NEOMYCIN.—This is usually 5 mg/gm. It has the same range as streptomycin more or less, mostly against gram-negative bacilli (also gram-positive), but it is useful in ointments and occasionally in bowel preparation; otherwise it is too toxic for systemic use. It shows some cross resistance with streptomycin and kanamycin. It is effective against *Pseudomonas* in high concentrations and is occasionally sensitizing, especially in the ear, the eye and occasionally the skin. I have seen it sensitize in the groin and around the rectum with marked regularity, especially in powdered form. It seems to potentiate monilial infections in these areas. It is stable in solutions, lotions and ointments.

TYROTHRICIN.—This is usually 0.5 mg/gm. It is from *B. bovis* and is a mixture of two polypeptide antibiotics, gramicidin and tyrocidin. It is highly active against gram-positive organisms. It has hemolytic properties, hence is only suitable for surface application, and it *has* been considered to be sensitizing, although I think neomycin is more so.

GENTAMYCIN (GARAMYCIN—SCHERING).—This is a sulfate, related to neomycin and kanamycin and has wide effectiveness on the skin against *Pseudomonas, Aerobacter, Proteus, E. coli, Staphylococcus* and some mycobacterial tuberculosis strains. Resistance appears slowly. Systemic toxicity includes eighth nerve damage and kidney damage, and it is used mostly in neonates—less in the general population. Hence it is suitable for skin use. Apparently local use has no side effects. Ophthalmic solution is 0.3%, and the cream for the skin is 0.1%.

FRAMYCETIN (SULFATE).—This is effective against gram-positive cocci and gram-negative bacilli. Resistance appears slowly. It has systemic toxicity, so is useful on the surface in solution and ointments in 2–3% concentrations.

CHLOROMYCETIN CREAM (CHLORAMPHENICOL—PARKE-DAVIS).—This cream is effective against a wide range of gram-negative and gram-positive organisms. It is pleasant to use, and if sensitivity develops, the systemic use of this drug is only a remote possibility, so no harm is done.

ERYTHROMYCIN OINTMENT (ILOTYCIN—DISTA).—The ointment is effective against gram-positive organisms as well as some gram-negative organisms. It is chiefly used for erythrasma (0.01%).

QUATERNARY AMMONIUM COMPOUNDS.—These surface agents, e.g., Zephiran (Zephiran is *not* effective against *Pseudomonas*), benzalkonium chloride, tincture of iodine or tincture of merthiolate, dilute potassium permanganate, dilute silver nitrate and sulfonamide ointments (ophthalmic), are also effective local agents. Furacin ointment, which is a nitrofurazone preparation that is popular among surgeons in the treatment of varicose ulcers, has probably been responsible for more exacerbated varicose ulcers and widespread eczematization than any other agent. The use of hexachlorophene in soaps and occasionally Phisoderm, such as Gamophen soap and Phisohex, may have a place in the cleansing of the skin, although experimental work in the early days seemed to indicate that if this was not continued consistently without the use of any other cleansing agent for more than 7 days, the bacterial suppressant effect was completely zero. Therefore I think that the occasional use of these soaps is of no use at all. If you are going to use them, you have to use them consistently and all the time. Hibiclens (Stuart) is an effective antibacterial skin cleanser.

BETADINE.—Betadine is colored, though nonstaining and nonstinging, povidone-iodine. It is a water-soluble antiseptic cleanser, and can be used as an antiseptic soap. It should be left in contact with the skin for about 3 minutes. It comes in a shampoo as well (Purdue—Frederick).

Sulfonamides

Sulfonamides are bacteriostatic, but inhibited by pus. Side effects include rash, nausea, fever, blood dyscrasia, Stevens-Johnson syndrome and renal irritation.

GANTRISIN (SULFISOXAZOLE).—Two tablets of 0.5 gm given four times daily is the dose usually preferred. It has good absorption, activity and renal solubility. Other sulfonamides include Gantanol (sulfamethoxazole), Madribon (sulfadimethoxine), sulfadiazine, sulfaguanidine and Sulfasuxidine; the latter two are used in treating intestinal infection. Sulfacetamide is useful in treating skin and mucous membrane infections. Sulfacet R (Dermik), a lotion used for acne, and Unguentum Salumyd Opthalmic (Schering) and Metamyd Opthalmic are useful for blepharitis. Sulfathiazole is useful in 5% ointment, especially in treating acne necrotica miliaris. It is much less sensitizing than the other sulfonamides.

SULFAPYRIDINE.—This is very useful in treating acrodermatitis continua and dermatitis herpetiformis, also perhaps in pyoderma gangrenosum. It is probably immunosuppressive in addition to its normal sulfa activity. Response is rapid.

Sulfones

The response to sulfones is slow.

PROMIN (PARA-DIAMINODIPHENYLSULFONE).—Promin is used intravenously in the treatment of leprosy in doses of from 2 gm to 5 gm, usually daily for 6 consecutive days, omitting treatment on the 7th day. It also is provided topically as a 5% jelly.

PROMIZOLE.—This is usually administered orally, 1–2 gm, three times a day for leprosy.

DIASONE (ABBOTT).—Diasone is sodium sulfoxone USP. The tablets come in 0.165 gm. The usual dose is one tablet taken three or four times a day, although it can be given up to a full dose of 3 gm daily. Toxicity is low. Anemia may occur, but disappears during therapy as a rule. Occasionally it has to be discontinued because of gastrointestinal symptoms. It seems better tolerated in dermatitis herpetiformis than sulfapyridine.

DAPSONE (DIAMINODIPHENYLSULFONE, DDS, AVLOSULFON—AYERST).—Dapsone comes in 100-mg tablets. The dose varies anywhere from one-half tablet a week to four tablets a day. Cyanosis, nausea, headache, tachycardia, and occasionally psychoses and depression occur as toxic manifestations of the use of this drug. Generally speaking, the people look and feel blue, but very often they can tolerate the slight cyanosis of the lips because the anemia that occasionally results is about the only long-term toxic side effect, and this can generally be corrected by the oral administration of iron for several months. It is a wise precaution to have white cell counts done, although hemoglobin seems to be the main target of this drug. It is a very good suppressive in treating dermatitis herpetiformis.

PROMACETIN (ACETOSULFONE—PARKE-DAVIS).—Promacetin is manufactured in 0.5-gm tablets. Initially, to get dermatitis herpetiformis under control, 3–4 gm daily are required, but the maintenance dose is usually between 2 and 3 gm in divided doses. Promacetin is much less toxic than some of the other sulfones, although drug rashes of the morbilliform or erythema multiforme type have been reported by Costello and Buncke.[5] Iron deficiency anemia develops after continued use; and it is advisable to administer iron preparations concurrently, constantly or occasionally and have the blood checked periodically.

Management of Staphylococcal Cases

When dealing with penicillin G-resistant organisms, generally you should start with Erythrocin, next cephalothin, then Prostaphlin (sodium oxacillin), after that kanamycin and vancomycin, and chloramphenicol last.

Coagulase-positive *and* coagulase-negative organisms *can* cause disease. An antibiotic cream should be applied to the groin, axilla and nostrils morning and night after a Phisohex scrub to reduce the carrier state, which is often found in a member of the family as a hidden source of infection. Control of the environment by washing doorknobs, telephone receivers, and light switches plus hand washing is important. The question of bacterial antitoxins, bacterial antigenic complexes and toxoids is still up in the air, although they do offer some help. Long-continued sulfonamide treatment, particularly with Gantrisin, seems to be a method of control when all else seems to fail.

Certain bacteria can increase their penicillinase production many times after a short exposure to penicillin. They may later revert to a sensitive type.

There is some evidence to indicate that drug resistance can be transferable from one organism to another, although this is clinically not too important.

In conclusion, we may say that in clinical practice resistance is due to the selection of resistant mutants. Fast resistance develops in the cases of streptomycin and novobiocin. Slow resistance develops in the cases of polymyxin, bacitracin and neomycin. Intermediate resistance may develop with tetracycline and chloramphenicol. The longer the time of administration, the greater the resistance.[6]

Staphylococcal Infections

Staphylococcal infections form localized abscesses in which rapid necrosis occurs. Additional destruction of tissue follows the thrombosis of neighboring capillaries.

The organisms are versatile chemical factories, as shown by their ability to defy many new antibiotics. They can persist in the crevices of the body and multiply when opportunity presents. Immunity, if it does occur, is transient and poor in quality.

Indiscriminate use of antibiotics has often removed all susceptible (possibly protective) staphylococci from the anterior nares (where they are carried), and the void (especially in a hospital) is being filled with hardy strains resistant to many antibiotics. These have caused epidemics in hospitals, and a new disease (postantibiotic staphylococcal enteritis) is being seen.

Staphylococcus aureus of phage type 80 or 81 is being isolated in increasing frequency in hospitals all over the world and is responsible for practically all of the outbreaks of staphylococcal sepsis in newborn nurseries and hospital personnel. The strains are resistant to almost all commonly used antibiotics. (See Formulary, no. 24.)

In general, pigment-producing power is a sign of pathogenicity, e.g., *aureus* over *albus* (although occasionally it takes time for it to produce pigment), as is the ability to coagulate plasma—"coagulase positive." The production of hemolysins also indicates pathogenicity. Virulence can be tested in small laboratory animals by the antigen-antibody flocculation tests. Sensitivity tests can be carried out by either tube dilution or disk sensitivity tests (less accurate) to pick the best antibiotic. Most general population strains are penicillin sensitive. It is most unusual for a *staphylococcus* organism to change its antibiotic sensitivity during treatment. When this appears to happen, usually the original strain has been replaced by another with different antibiotic sensitivities. "Resistance to everything" does not mean a more *virulent* strain, just a *selected* strain, usually from a hospital, where most antibiotics have been used.

Individual strains emerge with characteristics different from those of the preceding generation and siblings, and these changes are passed on to their descendants. The changes occur spontaneously, e.g., a few bacterial individuals will be resistant to tetracycline and their descendants will also be resistant. In addition, certain factors favor mutation; hence, they are "mutagenic," e.g., peroxide, ferrachloride, phenol, antibiotics, x-ray and ultraviolet light. Lederberg and Lederberg[7] showed that resistant bacteria exist in a population before contact with the antibacterial agent involved, so that in clinical practice after a period of treatment, although the first phase of the infection has been controlled, a relapse occurs in which the antibiotic that was sufficient at the start is no longer effective. In epidemiology, after an infection is considered to be cured, we may encounter resistance to the same treatment when the infection is transmitted to another person, even though the strain is known to be the same. Adaptation can also occur in that bacteria can adapt to new conditions, modify their characteristics and transmit these new characteristics to future generations even after removal of the inducing agent, for example, subinhibiting doses of antibiotics. There is some evidence to indicate that there is such a thing as transferable drug resistance from one bacteria to another, e.g., from resistant *E. coli* to a sensitive *Shigella.*

At birth, staphylococci are not found in the nose or skin, but within 2 weeks almost every child has them. Any infection occurring is likely to be in the eye. After a month, the carrier rate falls, and at 6 months it falls to 23%, only to rise thereafter to 70% in adults. Only about 30% of the population carry potentially virulent staphylococci in the nares; and a higher percent, of course, occurs in hospital personnel or in long-term hospital patients.

Control of Staphylococcal Infections in Hospitals

It is unlikely that a dermatologist would be called upon for expert knowledge in the event of an epidemic of staphylococcal infections, but some information on this score can be helpful in the management of family infections. The peak period of staphylococcal infections in hospital patients appears to be about 10 days after admission, and most patients are home by then. Carriers can usually be identified by a simple nasal swab and culture using the phage type to select the "dangerous" carriers.

Handwashing is most important with hexachlorophene soaps; and in the United Kingdom an antiseptic hand cream called "Hibitane" (I.C.I. and Stuart Labs.) is used; this has helped to cut down resident flares. It is also available as a liquid soap (Hibiclens).

Staphylococcal Diseases of the Skin

In infants, we see sweat gland infections in the immature glands of the scalp (periporitis staphylogenes). They respond to 6 weeks of systemic antibiotic treatment.

NEONATAL MASTITIS.—This disease develops in about the 8th or 10th day of life and can destroy breast tissue; hence, it is important to women. This should be treated as an emergency with systemic antibiotics.

IMPETIGO NEONATORUM.—This varies from small pustules to bullae and responds to local antibiotic therapy and cleansing (oil-free) as a rule. In cases where there is a more severe spreading pyoderma, Ritter's disease may be suspected; systemic penicillin treatment, local antibiotic cream and antiseptic baths will usually be needed. Remember that there are no papillae in the epidermis of a newborn, and subepidermal infection can spread rapidly to almost exfoliative proportions. Impetigo neonatorum must be differentiated from Leiner's disease (seborrheic buttocks) and congenital syphilis, which involves the palms and soles.

IMPETIGO.—Causes of this are approximately 80% staphylococcal, 6% streptococcal and 14% mixed (mostly phage type 71). As a rule, you do not catch impetigo from the same staphylococcus that causes boils. The sores are usually honey-yellow "stuck-on" crusts, and they usually start around the nose. (See pp. 62–64, PCAD.) It can follow herpes simplex or an upper respiratory infection and is very contagious in newborns and young adults. The occasional case of nephritis is enough to lead one to treat this urgently. The usual treatment is systemic penicillin with local antibiotic cream and occasional peroxide, daubing on boric acid or Burow's soaks to remove crusts. Occasionally a choice of antibiotic cream will have to be influenced by the type of infection that seems to be occurring in the community. For instance, in some areas, polysporin, bacitracin and neomycin creams are not as effective as Chloromycetin.

BOCKHART'S IMPETIGO.—This is a superficial follicular pustular infection, which very often complicates pediculosis or scabies and can generally be treated by simple washing with Phisohex or Betadine and the application of antibiotic creams.

ACNE NECROTICA MILIARIS.—This acne is a discrete isolated itchy crusted scalp folliculitis in which systemic antibiotics are usually helpful. Unguentum Quinolor helps either alone or in combination with Vioform cream. Mercury bichloride 0.1% in 70% alcohol helps also. Microcrystalline sulfathiazole ointment 5% is effective, and a Phisohex or Betadine daily shampoo is perhaps the most effective of all remedies. Constant local treatment is the secret of success here, plus building up the patient's general condition.

INFECTIOUS ECZEMATOID DERMATITIS.—So-called pustular eczema or superficial *Staphylococcus* dermatitis (jungle rot) usually has an explosive onset of a papulopustular asymmetric widespread, occasionally oozy and often extremely itchy dermatitis in circumscribed patches, usually on the exposed area and often preceded by severe digging and scratching. Allergy, overtreatment, debility, autosensitization and psychosomatic factors are all involved. Antibiotic-steroid combination treatment plus soaks and 1% hydrocortisone in bactracin ointment usually cures the patient.

TUNNELING INFECTIONS.—Hidradenitis suppurativa results from deep infections in the apocrine glands, which are found in the axilla, groin, perianally and around the nipples. The abscesses that form resemble perifolliculitis capitis abscedens et suffodiens and acne conglobata in the indolent nature of their sinus formation. They often have to be deroofed surgically and sinus tracts laid open. Phisohex washes and neomycin lotions, perhaps neosporin lotions or spray (Burroughs Wellcome), internal antibiotics and occasionally staphylococcal toxoid and estrogens are the treatment at our disposal, although surgery has given the best results and very often excision of the central portion of the axilla is a cosmetic procedure of great value to the patient. In the scalp and face, diluted Kenalog injected intralesionally helps immensely. Long-continued antibiotic therapy is needed. In rare cases, suppression of apocrine activity by x-ray therapy is helpful, but only in desperate situations and by those experienced and skilled in its use.

FOLLICULITIS KELOIDALIS.—This disease is usually seen on the nape of the neck in people who wear tight collars, e.g., chefs, motorcyclists and policemen, or people who sweat a great deal on the back of their heads. This is one of the therapeutic challenges of the age. The condition can be treated by liquid nitrogen freezing, with antibiotics internally and either intracutaneous Kenalog injections or the Dermajector needle. In rare or desperate situations, skilled x-ray therapy after electrosurgery has value.

SYCOSIS BARBAE.—Sycosis barbae usually involves the upper lip at the start. There is a sort of continuous marginal spread of the infection to involve adjacent hair follicles. Plucking out a hair from the region usually shows it to have quite a lot of white sheath surrounding the follicle bulb. It is more common in Europe than it is in this country, and it is tediously and rebelliously chronic. A remedy of some merit is equal parts of Unguentum Quinolor and Vioform cream with systemic antibiotics plus local epilation technique. There is very often a seborrheic background, and the patients seem to have diminished resisting powers, so any systemic improvement that can be given to them, such as vitamins and iron, and search for general health hazards such as focal infections in the teeth or tonsils, are a very marked help in improving their ability to overcome this infection.

FOLLICULITIS.—This is commonly seen in hairy individuals with oily or dirty occupations. It can also be seen secondary to suntan oils used on sunburned skin on hot days. Anything oily on the skin, from moisturizers to hair dressings, may provoke this. Usually simple local treatment with cleansing measures, wet dressings or baths and antibiotic creams will clear the eruption quickly.

Folliculitis of the beard with boggy induration sometimes turns out to be due to *Trichophyton mentagrophytes* and cultures should always be made for fungus. Bacterial cultures and sensitivity tests, of course, should be done, too.

PILI INCARNATI.—This is a condition in which the beard hairs turn in and grow into or under the epidermis. It is known as "ingrown hairs" and is often quite stubborn in black skin. It can be dealt with by increased care in preparation for shaving. The only thing that softens hair is water; the beard should be washed first with soap and water to remove the collection of skin oil that coats the hair, and water should be allowed to remain in contact with the beard hair for at least 3 minutes before shaving. I have found the use of the Buff-Puff while washing before shaving to be of great assistance in prevention of pili incarnati.

FURUNCLES AND CARBUNCLES.—These are probably the most common staphylococcal entity. Generally speaking, incision and drainage, ordinary simple treatment with antibiotics internally, local hygiene, cleansing with Phisohex, changing clothes routinely, avoidance of friction and irritation by secretions of dressings and adhesive tape, avoidance of occupations involving exposure to grime and oils, and insuring that the patient is not a diabetic and that his diet is not too rich in such foods as chocolate and sugar often suffice to control the outbreak. When there seems to be a carrier in the family, it very often turns out to be an asymptomatic spouse. In these instances, a search for the focal point of the infection should be made, perhaps by phage typing. Members of the family should be instructed to anoint their nares, inguinal and rectal areas, as well as axillary areas, with antibiotic creams after washing with Phisohex or Betadine twice a day. Clothing should be sterilized by washing with strong detergents after frequent changes, and effort should be made to avoid contaminating door knobs, telephone receivers and other articles commonly handled.

Staphylococcus toxoid has its advocates in the management of long-continued susceptibility to furuncles. I prefer a bacterial antigenic complex (Hoffman Labs.). It seems to me that some resistance can be developed by its use. There are no recent papers on its use that are very convincing, however. Autogenous vaccines using the killed cells suspended 1 billion per cc have many adherents, and gamma globulin when given alone is not much help but perhaps has synergistic effect when given along with antibiotics. The proper choice of antibiotic and the long-continued use of this is probably the best approach along with the local control of the carrier state.

Twenty percent of the cases of staphylococcal septicemia seem to occur in patients who are already taking cortisone, so the use of steroids in patients in *Staphylococcus*-susceptible surroundings should be viewed with caution.

PYODERMA GANGRENOSUM.—This entity is not a bacterial infection but is probably viral or a vasculitis. Recent reports of successful therapy of this stubborn disease with Lamprene (British) or clofazimine, 100 mg taken three times a day, with rapid healing in 3-14 days, sound very encouraging.[8] Side effects sound minor (red urine and dry skin).

STAPHYLOCOCCAL BEDSORES.—In the development of bedsores, the length of pressure is more important than the degree of pressure. Vasomotor factors appear to be the main ones. If the skin is soaked in moist body discharges, it is more likely to get infected and lead to bedsores; *Pseudomonas, Proteus* and *Staphylococcus* are the major organisms. Sponge-rubber doughnuts, the skin being kept dry, the mattress or the sheet overlying it being kept taut so that wrinkles do not press into the areas of skin, and occasionally the use of a bland ointment to lubricate very dry skin are helpful. Avoidance of soap and the use of magnesium carbonate as a powder, since it does not cake, are often helpful. Skilled nursing care, frequent movement of patients and padding in the proper places are the best method of care. Occasionally immune globulin or gamma globulin is helpful along with efforts to build up the patient's general health with iron and vitamin B, plus an enforced high-protein diet. Tincture of benzoin is good in treating early cases.

Occasionally debridement with enzyme ointments (Varidase or Elase) for a few days is helpful, then there should be a switch to Chloromycetin cream or Garamycin cream applied twice a day with dry, sterile dressings and twice-daily compressing with Burow's solution for 10–15 minutes (in addition to the pressure-avoidance techniques). The "egg crate" sponge-rubber cushion or the special cushions made for wheelchair paraplegics can prevent and assist as well. The "sheep skin" stretched taut under the buttocks is also helpful in providing small pockets of air to buoy up the skin from excessively continued pressure, and the oscillating mattress, for those who can afford it, is another aid. An air cushion for the wheelchair that is extremely useful for paraplegics is called the ROHO balloon cushion (ROHO Research and Development Co.). Its value resides chiefly in that one can tie any number of small protuberances in any location, to give a hollow in which the decubitus sits. This has been very effective.

The benzoylperoxide paste method of Doctor Pace of London, Ontario, can be amazingly effective if applied well.[9] A 20% paste should be applied directly to the ulcerated area and covered with a gauze pad the exact size of the ulcer around which Lassar's paste is applied to protect the skin; on top of that an occlusive dressing is applied and fixed in place. This is changed every 12 hours, and healthy tissue appears very soon. It is said the 10% benoxyl lotion works as well, though purists may use benzoylperoxide (Syosset Labs.), 20% ointment or paste.

OTITIS EXTERNA.—Most of these are caused by *P. aeruginosa* (26%), *S. albus* (22%), *S. aureus* (15%), *E. coli* (8%) and *Proteus* (6%). Swimming and tropic heat appear to be the predisposing factors, with trauma often the precipitating cause, and very often poking at the ear with an instrument such as a bobby pin. Treatment is generally to clean out the wax and debris and dry it. Packing with sterile gauze wick soaked in aluminum acetate or Burow's solution is good treatment. A home remedy is vinegar dropped in the ear six to eight times daily; later an alcoholic solution of gentian violet is very helpful, but best of all is polymyxin solution. My preference is for 2% hydrocortisone in Aerosporin otic solution (Burroughs Wellcome), since it contains no neomycin and is essentially a mixture of polymyxins. (See Formulary, no. 23g.) This can be applied by the patient, who comes into the office and has the ear syringed out once in a while using 1:10,000 aqueous metaphen solution. After this, if the ear is not dry, 2% hydrocortisone in Terramycin powder is insufflated with a powder insufflator. This appears to control most external otitis cases that have been stubbornly resistant to many other treatments. In many cases, I feel sure neomycin sensitivity has played a part. Colymycin S otic has neomycin and hydrocortisone and is often very effective.

BLEPHARITIS.—Staphylococci are the usual cause, and the patient may suffer from recurrent sepsis in other areas, often with an underlying seborrhea or seborrhea capitis. Three percent ammoniated mercury ointment, or 10% sodium sulfacetamide ophthalmic ointment with a check on the phage type to see if it is the same as in the nose, and then treating the reservoir, are effective treatment. Zinc sulfate eyedrops, 0.25–0.125%, though old-fashioned, help.

Modern Treatment

Treatment depends on adequate knowledge of family sepsis and the source of infection, perhaps acquired from a hospital stay or from the general community; we expect resistance if from the former. If the infection is recurrent, look for the carrier area (80% in the nose, 20% in axilla groin and the spouse's nose). In severely ill people, after the cultures, treatment with penicillin, erythromycin or oxacillin should be instituted immediately. Aseptic procedures will prevent spread to other individuals and to other areas in the same patient. Dressings should be occlusive and contaminated clothing changed. Intravenous injections of glucose should be avoided, as should periods of fasting. In staphylococcal enteritis, watch for potassium depletion.

Local applications, such as iodine USP, which is very useful in surgical preparation, and Zephiran, which is a cationic surface active agent 1:750, are not effective against *Pseudomonas*, and soap is antagonistic to it. Tincture of merthiolate is very effective, as are other mercurials. Acriflavine is an occasional antiseptic of value. Ammoniated mercury ointment USP 5% is occasionally useful in the treatment of toe-web cracks, and 2% ammoniated mercury ophthalmic ointment is helpful in managing ophthalmic infections. One-quarter percent acetic acid is bactericidal in wet soaks. Enzyme ointments such as streptokinase, and streptodornase (Varidase) help to lyse fibrinogen and purulent exudates, although they are allergenic, as is trypsin enzymatic ointment. A local antibiotic such as Bacitracin USP, which usually comes 500 units per gram is an excellent topical and ophthalmic ointment. Tyrothricin, which comes in 0.5 mg/cc, is a moderately effective topical and intranasal antibiotic for local use. Neomycin (5 mg/gm) is another excellent topical ophthalmic or spray local antibiotic. Neomycin is occasionally sensitizing, and Bacitracin is probably the least sensitizing of the group. Surgical treatment by incision and drainage after localization are matters of judgment and are frequently the only answer. (See Formulary, nos. 23, 24.)

Other Bacterial Infections

STREPTOCOCCAL INFECTIONS.—These include *erysipelas*, which usually produces fever and bright red swollen cheeks near the nostrils, which are usually the source. (See p. 64, PCAD.) Erysipelas responds to penicillin, wet dressings and antibiotic cream in the nares. *Chronic recurrent erysipelas* (and chronic recurrent cellulitis) can be more of a therapeutic challenge, with chronic lymphedema and repeated debilitating attacks of high fever. This responds, sometimes dramatically, to *Streptococcus* toxin injections (Hollister-Stier) in desensitizing doses plus antibiotic treatment long continued. *Ecthyma* can be difficult to treat when insects, e.g., sand flies, are continually attacking the patient, but in general antibiotics given locally and systemically with cleansing measures plus peroxide will pull the patient through. The *granuloma pyogenicum* tumor (once thought to arise from infected wounds) requires removal. (See p. 175, PCAD.) *Streptococcal intertrigo* and *paronychia, perleche* and *streptococcal acrodermatitis* are other more common varieties of streptococcal infection. The latter, producing a blister pyoderma, responds best to systemic penicillin treatment.

RECALCITRANT PUSTULAR ERUPTIONS

Dermatitis repens (*acrodermatitis of Hallopeau*).—This usually starts around the tip of a finger or toe, at the side or under the nail. Many cases appear to be due to *P. aeruginosa*, though others appear to be a special variety of host response to the particular bacteria involved. Local treatment with 1% Vioform hydrocortisone cream and oral sulfonamides, especially Gantrisin, seem to clear most cases.

Pustular bacterid of Andrews-Barber.—This is a stubborn recurrent condition often strangely related to dental foci and clearing with removal. It can on occasion defy careful study. Local treatment involves steroid creams and on occasion grenz ray; antibiotic or sulfa may be taken internally in addition to foci removal.

ERYTHRASMA.—Peculiar bacteria produce a marginated scaly erythema in the flexures. (See p. 78, PCAD.) Therapy is usually successful with bacitracin creams locally and Erythrocin orally. (Diagnosis is by pink fluorescence with the Wood Lamp.)

DERMATITIS VEGETANS.—Moist, exuberant verrucous vegetations in the folds of the body, especially the axillae and groin, occur in neglectful and debilitated patients. Therapy with neomycin solution soaks 0.1%, or potassium permanganate soaks 1:8,000, plus either oral or intramuscular administration of antibiotics, occasionally curettement under local anesthesia and gamma globulin intramuscularly will usually clear this. Rarely, x-ray therapy in the hands of experts is effective.

DESERT SORE AND TROPICAL ULCER.—These are seen where the climate is hot and keeping clean is a problem. These chronic nonhealing ulcers occasionally grow from diphtheroids, though most are staphylococcal and streptococcal. The usual local and systemic antibiotics clear all except the diphtheria cases, which occasionally require diphtheria antitoxin injected around the ulcer (4,000 units or so).

ERYSIPELOID OF ROSENBACH.—This is seen in fish handlers, and produces a purplish erythema on the hands. (See p. 65, PCAD.) It requires penicillin for at least 10 days.

BERULLI ULCER.—This tropical condition, which relentlessly chews away at the surrounding flesh, produces an ever-widening ulceration. It is caused by a *Mycobacterium* organism and requires special culture techniques. Usually, it does not respond to antibiotic treatment but requires surgical debridement.

SYNERGISTIC GANGRENE (MELENEY).—Microaerophyllic nonhemolytic *Streptococcus* plus *Staphylococcus* organisms combine to produce this remorselessly progressive undermining ulceration, which usually starts in the edge of surgical wounds. Zinc peroxide paste used to be the treatment of choice, but bacitracin and systemic antibiotic treatment seems to have made this dreaded complication less common.

SWIMMING POOL GRANULOMA.—This is caused by *Mycobacterium balnei* and seems to occur mostly in persons who clean out fish tanks. Favorable responses to oral minocycline treatment have increased the optimism with which these cases are treated now. Debridement with electrodesiccation and curettage, cryotherapy with liquid nitrogen, intralesional steroid injection or surgical excision may be used with success. Often an abrasion on the elbows sustained at the edge of a swimming pool leads to the formation of group of nodules that may ulcerate. They do not respond to para-aminosalicylic acid, isoniazid (INH) or streptomycin. Bactrim tablets (Roche) are effective also.

RARE INFECTIONS.—Infections with Hellerea (sensitive to erythrocin usually), *Pasteurella* (sensitive to penicillin usually) and *Listeria* (sulfonamides), *Salmonella* (Chloromycetin) and other organisms occur and often produce bizarre, boggy, granulomatous abscesses. In any unusual appearing skin lesion, a culture from the depth of a biopsy, not only for deep fungi but for bacteria as well, is occasionally surprisingly rewarding. Sensitivity tests usually determine the choice of antibiotic.

REFERENCES

1. Chain, E. B., Florey, H. W., et al.: Penicillin as chemotherapeutic agent, Lancet 2:226, 1940.
2. Shinefield, H. R., et al.: The Ohio epidemic, Am. J. Dis. Child. 105:655, 1963.

3. Light, I. J., et al.: Use of bacterial interference to control a staphylococcal nursery outbreak, Amer. J. Dis. Child. 113:291, 1967.
4. Cryptococcal opportunism (Editorial), N. Engl. J. Med. 279:102, 1968.
5. Costello, M. J., and Buncke, C. M.: Dermatitis herpetiformis (Duhring) successfully treated with promacetin, Arch. Dermatol. Syphilol. 72:348, 1955.
6. Lorian, V.: *Antibiotics and Chemotherapeutic Agents in Clinical and Laboratory Practice* (Springfield, Ill.: Charles C Thomas, Publishers, 1966).
7. Lederberg, J., and Lederberg, E. M.: Replica plating and indirect selection of bacterial mutants, J. Bact. 63:399, 1952.
8. Michaëlsson, G., et al.: Clofazimine: A new agent for the treatment of pyoderma gangrenosum, Arch. Dermatol. 112(3):344, 1976.
9. Pace, W. E.: Treatment of cutaneous ulcers with benzoyl peroxide, Can. Med. Assoc. J. 115(11):1101, 1976.

12 / Acne

Acne, the curse of the teenager, can also occur in adults and in the newborn (probably because of the stimulation in utero) and occasionally starts at age 8 or 9. (See pp. 129–132, PCAD.) The development of the sebaceous glands and the general toughening of the childish skin at this time reflects nature's attempts to provide protection from the elements that primitive man encountered. At ages 12–14, boys and girls were expected to make their own way and catch their own food. There is no acne among the tribes along the Amazon. I believe this is a disease of civilization, and it responds very well to summer outdoor living. In general, estrogens decrease sebaceous gland activity and androgens increase it. While the adrenals can convert progesterone into androgen, progesterone has little to do with the pathogenicity of acne. In women, androgens are produced by the ovaries (markedly so in polycystic ovaries), the placenta and adrenals, and in men by the testes and adrenals. Norethynodrel (Enovid) has an inherent estrogenicity and no discernible androgenicity. Norethisterone, on the other hand, does *not* have inherent estrogenicity and has been reported to aggravate cases of acne.[1] It takes 10 mg per day or more of norethindrone to stimulate sebaceous gland activity, while norethandrolone and methandrostenolone both increase sebaceous activity.[2] Birth control pills, high in estrogen then, would be the choice for acne control, especially for treating the steatoma-like sebaceous overactivity variety.

Oral contraceptive preparations are listed in Table 12–1 in order of increasing estrogen content (ethinyl estradiol and mestranol are about equal in milligram potency; there is no satisfactory basis for comparing the milligram potencies of the various progestogens).

TABLE 12-1.—ESTROGEN AND PROGESTOGEN CONTENTS IN ORAL CONTRACEPTIVES

ORAL CONTRA-CEPTIVE	ESTROGEN		PROGESTOGEN	
Loestrin (Parke-Davis) 1/20	Ethinyl estradiol	20 μg	Norethindrone acetate	1 mg
Norlestrin (Parke-Davis) 1/50	Ethinyl estradiol	50 μg	Norethindrone acetate	1 mg
Demulen* (Searle)	Ethinyl estradiol	50 μg	Ethynodiol diacetate	1 mg
Norinyl (Syntex) 1/50	Mestranol	0.05 mg	Norethindrone	1 mg
Ortho-Novum (Ortho)	Mestranol	0.05 mg	Norethindrone	1 mg
Enovid 5* (Searle)	Mestranol	0.075 mg	Norethynodrel	5 mg
Enovid E* (Searle)	Mestranol	0.1 mg	Norethynodrel	2.5 mg
Ovulen (Searle)	Mestranol	0.1 mg	Ethynodiol diacetate	1 mg

*These usually help cure acne; sometimes the others may not. Ortho-Novum is often better tolerated.

It is occasionally noticed that some of the more androgenic preparations, such as Norlestrin and Ortho-Novum, may aggravate acne and even produce mild hirsutism. A certain amount of trial and error for each individual is therefore necessary to pick out the best contraceptive. Patients on the pill should have a yearly Pap test.

Oily seborrhea and acne often go hand in hand, and there is often a family tendency. The varieties of acne are: comedone acne, papular acne, acne excoriee des jeunes filles, acne pustulosa, atrophic acne, indurated acne, cystic acne, acne cachecticorum, acne conglobata (tunnelling), acne keloid, tropical acne, acne neonatorum and chloracne (occupational).

Treatment

Diet

Although many dermatologists allow patients to eat anything, we usually advise patients to avoid chocolate and cola of all kinds and to drink milk very sparingly. Bromides and iodides should be avoided (some chocolate may be made by a process using bromides).

General Measures

Antiseborrheic measures help, especially shampoos and occasionally Mycolog or other steroid-antibiotic cream combinations for treating facial seborrhea. Also, routine, regular and frequent cleansing of the skin with soap and hot water using the fingers three times a day and attention to general health are especially needed in the patient with cachectic acne.

Local Measures

Sulfur in its various forms is the traditional remedy, whether used in a soap (such as the Stiefel soaps) or in the standard, double, triple or even quadruple-strength lotio alba for application at night. Mills and Kligman showed sulfur (*except* lotio alba and Vleminckx solution) to be comedogenic.[3] Sulfur and resorcin combinations in various percentages are available as makeup-tinted lotions and creams, such as Clearasil, Acnomel, Fostril and Resulin, and can be extemporized in a shake lotion. Sulfur makeup, such as Liquimat, can be used if resorcin is an irritant. Quite often a chapping itching dryness of the neck or face results from too long continued or too widespread use of sulfur preparations, and the irritation may be at some distance from the site of application. If the patient applies it well before bedtime, at least 1/2 hour, then the spreading to the distant sites may be minimized (such as when the patient turns his head on the pillow). A well-made lotio alba is of great benefit in treating acne, and when fresh, is superior to many of the so-called ethical proprietaries. (See Formulary, nos. 27, 28.)

Some pharmacies put out a two-bottle lotio alba kit; the lotion is always fresh since the patient mixes it himself directly before applying it. If the pharmacist uses first-class ingredients, the preparation compounded locally can be extremely effective however. The patient should be told to refill the prescription after about 6 weeks, since the effectiveness is lost after that time. Periodically the lotio alba can be made stronger. (See Formulary, nos. 1 and 9.) The gentle desquamating effect of the polysulfides and the shriveling effect on the comedones are of value.

Benzoyl peroxide has a somewhat more dramatic effect and is available in a lotion called "Benoxyl" (Stiefel) (10% sulfur in Benoxyl lotion does a good job, too) or Persadox (Texas Pharmacal). Other benzoyl peroxide gels are very effective.

These preparations are a real advance in local treatment of acne. Tolerated better than retinoic acid, they have antiseptic as well as desquamative powers. They come usually as 5% or 10% benzoyl peroxide preparations. (See Formulary, no. 27.)

Sulfacetamide plus sulfur and resorcin in Sulfacet lotion (Dermik) is also helpful. Skin-colored lotions are popular with girls; some boys object to them, and for them the vanishing lotions are superior. The preparations that are commercially available are too numerous to mention, but these are the leading ones.

Occasionally a very fair-skinned patient will be unable to tolerate many of the drying medications, unless a "moisturizer" is applied to alleviate the dryness. This can be a problem, especially since much perioral dermatitis can be directly traced to overuse of moisturizing creams.[4] At such times, simple makeup may be used during the day; some fairly safe ones are Clinique "pore minimizer," Revlon "Natural Wonder," Estee Lauder "Fresh Air," and Max Factor "Super Unshine." Such patients may benefit from the topical antibiotic preparations listed below. If too drying, there can be a slight increase in the amount of propylene glycol.

	Ilosone powder (acid stable from the capsules)	500 mg
	Propylene glycol q.s. ad	25 cc
or	Ilosone powder	500 mg
	(Westwood) Desquam-X 10	
	Cordran cream aa q.s. ad	25 gm
or	Erythromycin base filmtabs (Abbott)	3 tabs
	Sodium lauryl sulfate	0.2%
	Sebanil (Texas Pharmacal) q.s. ad	30.0

or Erythromycin filmtabs (Abbott) 3 tabs
E Solve lotion (Syosset Labs.) ad 30.0

Shake label.

Cleocin phos (from caps) 0.3
70% alcohol with 10% propylene glycol to make 30.0
This may be filtered or not.

or Cleocin HCl (ampule for IV use) 0.3
90% Alcohol
Distilled water aa q.s. ad 30.0

All these are to be shaken before use and applied by rubbing in gently with the fingertip.

Vleminckx solution or magma alba, a pastier thicker collection of polysulfides like a gel, is often of use directly on the skin in treating nodular or cystic acne, although a hot compress of it is more effective. Vleminckx solution also comes in plastic packets and can be dissolved in a pint of water (Vlem-Dome – Dome Co.) or can be ordered as a prescription. (See Formulary, no. 27.) This will tarnish silver, and jewelry should be removed. Also, of course, it has a smell of rotten eggs and should be done with the window open and the door closed, but it works in cystic acne.

Other local measures, such as special soaps, e.g., Gamophen, Dial, Phisohex, Acne-Aid Detergent (Stiefel) and Neko (1 or 2%, Parke-Davis), are occasionally helpful. Lava is another moderately strong soap. Beauty grains, oatmeal granules, and in the case of the Acne-Dome cleansers (Dome), soybean preparations, are all useful in treating comedone acne. Brasivol (Stiefel), an abrasive cleanser, in fine, medium and rough textures, as well as Pernox (Westwood), with tiny polyethylene spheres in a sulfur soap, are useful when patients can tolerate a little rougher measure. A so-called dry wash sulfur soap called Proseca (Westwood) is useful for girls with tiny comedones on the nose. It is rubbed in dry, left on 15 minutes and then washed off with water. Fostex Cake and Fostex Cream are sulfur and salicylic acid soaps. Aveeno bar is an oatmeal type of soap. There are many such. An antibacterial cleanser found extremely effective in Britain is available in the United States as Hibiclens (Stuart Labs.).

Retin-A cream or lotion 0.05% (Johnson & Johnson) has been relentlessly advocated by Kligman for the treatment of acne.[5] It has special value in treating comedone acne if the patient can be taught to use it carefully. Avoidance of sun, other strong cleansers and overtreatment is essential. The manufacturer's instructions should be read thoroughly and the patients selected. Initial use of the 0.025% gel three nights a week for 3 hours only may avoid reactions.

Surgical Measures

Removal of comedones is almost a necessity, and it should be done with care, especially in the middle of the cheek (Fig 12–1). Following removal, ultraviolet light treatment will help to lessen the amount of posttraumatic swelling. Intralesional steroid injected carefully *into* cysts (to avoid atrophy that occasionally results from tissue injection) will hasten resolution. The 5 mg/cc intralesional Kenalog, if diluted 10 mg/cc 50–50 (or weaker) with Xylocaine or saline, lessens the risk of atrophy, which fortunately is almost always temporary on the face. Scarring however, from a cyst neglected too long and which is not temporary, should not be confused in the mind of the patient with steroid atrophy. The patient should be advised not to wait too long when a large cyst appears. Sometimes several injections are required at intervals for flattening. At other times, incision and curettement using a fine-eye curette, followed by insertion of pure liquid phenol on a cotton-tipped toothpick, plus pressure, will flatten a stubborn cyst. Doctor Pipkin of San Antonio[6] injects liquid phenol, keeping alcohol wipes handy to catch the excess. Alcohol, if quickly applied, will prevent the overflowing phenol from "burning" the surrounding skin. The Dermaject also helps. Other stubborn cysts require liquid nitrogen or dry ice application.

Carbon Dioxide Slush Treatment

Using powdered dry ice in a gauze bag made by unfolding three 4 × 4-in. gauze pads dipped in acetone and sulfur just

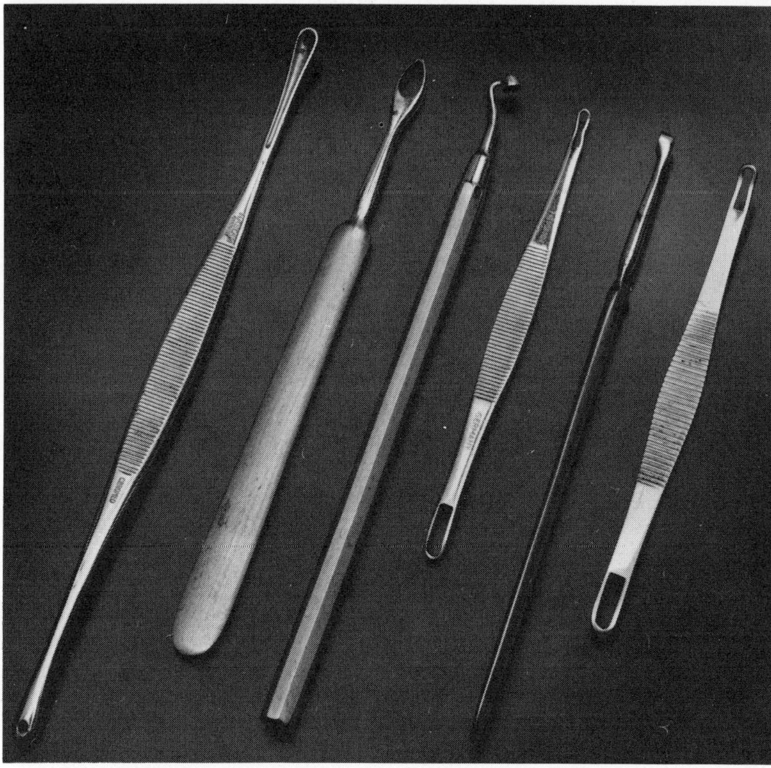

Fig 12–1. —Varieties of comedone extractors.

before it is applied to the skin, with a sliding motion to produce a faint temporary frostbite of the affected region, is extremely effective in treating the scarring nodular acne conglobata, especially in very fair skins. Some of its effect may be rearranging collagen bundles in the connective tissue, apart from the freezing and peeling superficial effect, which gives a much smoother look to the hitherto hills and valleys, pits and ridges of severe acne. It can be done on a Wednesday, and patients start to look terrible on Friday, but are fine by Monday again. We do it every 2 weeks for six times, although it can be done more often. We find after six treatments that the rate of improvement perceptibly slows. Many dermatologists feel this treatment is not helpful, possibly because they are innately too cautious in its use. I still use it, though I must confess less than formerly now that we have liquid nitrogen. The value of cryotherapy in the treatment of scars (and dermatofibroma) indicates there is therapeutic merit in the modality.

Ultraviolet

Many patients benefit from periodic ultraviolet lamp treatments. A cheap lamp at home is of help if the patient understands the inverse square law, so that the distance is constant—say, 18 in. in the case of a Westinghouse or G.E. reflecting surface ultraviolet bulb, and then vary the time. Patients should do it sitting in a chair wearing goggles; and only three times a week. Explain that they can't tan, because most of them try to get a tan. The Hanovia mercury vapor lamp is the best. A cold quartz lamp for peeling scars or cysts is of some help in managing tough acne problems, and usually we hand-hold it over the cheek at about 2 in. away for 1¼ to 1½ minutes.

Scalp Care

Selsun and Dara shampoos seem to be the best, although other preparations, such as Ionil or Sebulex shampoo or the insertion of various remedies overnight and then washed out in the morning, are satisfactory. Attention to the scalp is essential, however. (See Formulary, no. 28.)

Systemic Treatment

Tetracycline, which operates by reducing the amount of lipase in the sebaceous secretion or by altering the skin flora, some of which might be instrumental in producing irritant triglycerides, wax esters and free fatty acids in the pore, can be extremely effective. Often after initial success, control wears off gradually. This can be especially true if sporadic dosing is involved. It is good practice to start off with three or four doses daily and gradually reduce to twice or once a day, depending on the progress. It takes 4–6 weeks to assess the effectiveness, and if little improvement occurs, the patient may be switched to Declomycin (prone to make a patient susceptible to severe sunburn), Terramycin, Rondomycin, Vibramycin, Erythrocin or sulfa, such as Gantrisin.

Cleocin can be dramatically effective when used in treating the severe nodulocystic acne that nothing else helps. The incidence of pseudomembranous colitis (somewhere between 1:10,000 and 1:100,000 or more) may be slightly higher in persons who use this antibiotic than in others, but it has been unfairly maligned by scare publicity after an epidemic of bacterial diarrhea in an old men's home in California some years ago. Current information indicates that a *Clostridium* organism resistant to Cleocin causes the diarrhea; vancomycin may prevent this strain from surviving. If severe diarrhea occurs, it is a hospital problem and can be successfully treated. Patients and their families must be warned. The medication seems to cause less trouble if taken on an empty stomach, that is, nothing should be eaten for an hour before or after taking medication. One dose twice a day is adequate for many patients with severe acne, who later can be maintained on one dose daily. I fortunately have not had any problems in the years I have used it.[7]

Minocin or Vectrin (minocycline) is often extremely effective in a dosage of 50 mg given two or three times daily. Dizziness is hardly ever a side effect from this dosage.

Keflex can be a good treatment for severe acne and should not be forgotten. The same is true of ampicillin, which often will do wonders for patients who have had a change in their skin flora after long continued antibiotic treatment. Occasionally megadoses of tetracycline will be useful. In stubborn cases culture of the pus and sensitivity tests, or autogenous vaccines, are helpful. Vaccines seem to be in disrepute among some physicians, although they can be of the greatest help at times.

Vitamin A in doses of 100,000 units daily in the winter helps some patients with acne, especially comedone and cystic acne. We skip it in the summer. We give a short break of about 2 weeks' rest every 3 months in the administration of vitamin A. Not every dermatologist agrees that this is helpful, but I believe it is useful in treating comedone acne. Pseudotumor cerebri (headache and double vision) has to be watched for in overenthusiastic pill-takers.

When difficulty is encountered in the taking of antibiotics, the patient can often be induced to continue with additional advice. Where the enteric coating on E mycin, for example, causes indigestion, switching to the Erythromycin Filmtab (base by Abbott) will usually remove this problem. Where tetracycline capsules cause trouble, the tablets are better tolerated. Patients taking tetracycline should be warned of the effect of milk in preventing absorption, and they should be warned *not* to take the tetracycline at bedtime, since the horizontal position seems to favor the development of a mild esophagitis (heartburn). Where monilial vaginitis is a problem, yogurt, acidophilus milk (Lactinex tablets or Bacid), vitamin B given orally, Gyne-lotrimin vaginal inserts nightly for a week or more plus oral Mycostatin with the antibiotic dose can achieve toleration.

In severe necrotic, conglobate or cystic acne, oral steroids given in short courses may get difficult problem patients "over the hump," although we use it less and less. Avlosulfone (dapsone) treatment, 50 mg every other day by mouth, occasionally suppresses cystic acne. For acutely inflamed acne, occasionally the application of a steroid lotion with immediately following wet compresses of, e.g., dilute boric acid solution can be extremely helpful.

Treatment with premenstrual estrogen in girls who have regular cycles, e.g., Premarin, 2.5 mg daily for 10 days premenstrually, as recommended by Torre, is useful. Contraceptive pills, using estrogen-dominant ones where possible, and being fully aware of the drawbacks (such as weight gain, nausea, chloasma) and the dangers (such as thrombophlebitis, pulmonary embolism and "strokes") and avoiding them in those with family history of clotting abnormalities, are useful too, but the risk is sometimes too great.

Hypoglycemic agents and thiazide diuretics given premenstrually have had their devotees. The antibiotics or the contraceptive pills (which usually do not start working until after 3 months) are the best.

Treatment of Scars

Dermabrasion and sandpapering help cure the icepick scars, although less of this is being done today. Carbon dioxide slush treatment is almost always helpful. Cross-hatching scarification occasionally is helpful, and chemical peeling with either 25% trichloracetic acid or phenol is effective in skilled hands. Plastic surgeons do small sections at a time, covering with adhesive. Phenol (buffered or not) "marbleizes" the underlying connective tissue, which smooths wrinkles as well as pits. Punch and suture, or drill and Gelfoam for small deep pits occasionally are helpful.

Betanaphthol paste is advocated by Sam Peck and is a helpful way of doing chemical peeling.[8] The following paste is recommended by him:

Betanaphthol	10
Sulfur precipitate	20
Soft soap ad q.s. to	100
Petrolatum ad q.s. to	100

Apply for one-half hour weekly. On the first occasion, do it for 10 minutes to get the reaction. This is an intense peeler. (See also Formulary, no. 32.)

Acne Rosacea

Rosacea is a term used to describe a chronic condition characterized by diffuse inflammation of the central portion of the face with seborrhea, telangiectasia and acneform eruptions. It appears to be the result of repeated flushing, which in most instances is related to frequent intake of hot spicy foods, e.g., hot coffee, tea, soup, or alcohol. Anything too hot, too cold, too sweet, too sour or too spicy aggravates the condition, although on occasion an infected tooth or tonsil, or gross indigestion seems to be the underlying mechanism. Blepharitis and conjunctivitis can occur, as can spongy gums and a tendency to sinusitis. Occasionally *Demodex* may be the cause.

Management

Treatment involves correction of the diet, with removal of hot spicy foods, location of any dental infection and its correction, and usually tetracycline, 250 mg daily for 6–8 weeks. Relapse is common, although it may be minimized by the subsequent administration of dilute hydrochloric acid, such as

Acidulin capsules (Lilly), ½ hour before lunch and supper for many months. Usually some modification in the patient's way of life is necessary to develop a lasting cure; and this may require some discussion of the patient's habits. Menopausal females often respond to estrogen treatment. Spontaneous cure after partial gastrectomy has been seen.

For local treatment, Lacksen's salve applied at night is helpful:

Salicylic acid	0.9
Sulfur ppt.	0.9
Quinolor compound ointment (Squibb)	1.5
Aquaphor q.s. to	30.0

One-half percent hydrocortisone in Sulfacet R lotion (Dermik), Kenalog-S lotion and Mycolog cream are all helpful. Occasionally a 25–40% sulfur paste at night is helpful treatment. Vioform (a little less irritating than Quinolor) can be effective with or without hydrocortisone 1%. Other resorcin-sulfur combinations can be useful, as can ultraviolet and x-ray therapy in skilled hands. A winter vacation in the sun can be very helpful.

If rhinophyma occurs, cutting-current reshaping after maxillary nerve block and infiltration across the bridge of the nose and under the nostrils can be performed by the heroic. Dermabrasion is very bloody, and electrocutting is very smelly. The results are worth it, however.

For the patient with blepharitis, Unguentum Salumyd, which is 10% sodium sulfacetamide ophthalmic ointment, or the same with steroid (Metimyd Ophthalmic suspension) is very helpful. Correction of seborrhea capitis also is essential.

Perioral Dermatitis

This has also been known as photosensitive seborrhea and follicular seborrhea and has been shown by the British to result from incidental (and apparently habit forming) use of fluorinated steroid creams. I believe that fluoridated toothpaste and numerous other factors may aggravate this; patients will relapse less often if they can be less messy with their toothpastes and, best of all, avoid the stronger fluoridated ones. Tetracycline administered orally in small doses for a few weeks, plus the use of *mild* soap-and-water cleansing, hydrocortisone lotion, or on occasion Mycolog cream (despite the Kenalog in it) seem to be helpful. The "constitutional" aids, e.g., vitamin B, sea and sun and outdoor exercise, also assist in clearing this.[9]

REFERENCES

1. Jackson, M. C. N.: Oral contraception in practice, J. Reprod. Fertil. 6:153, 1963.
2. Strauss, J. S., and Pochi, P. E.: *Clinical Endocrinology* (2d ed.; New York: Grune & Stratton, Inc., 1968).
3. Mills, O. H., and Kligman, A. M.: Is sulphur helpful or harmful in acne vulgaris, Br. J. Dermatol. 86:620, 1972.
4. Abele, D. C.: Moisturizers and perioral dermatitis, Arch. Dermatol. 113:110, 1977.
5. Plewig, G., and Kligman, A. M.: Vitamin A acid in acneiform dermatoses, Acta Derm. Venereol. (Suppl.) 74:119, 1975.
6. Pipkin, J. L.: Meeting of American Academy of Dermatology, Dallas, Texas, December, 1977.
7. Basler, R. S. W.: Potential hazards of Clindamycin in acne therapy, Arch. Dermatol. 112:383, 1976.
8. Domonkos, A. N.: *Andrews' Diseases of the Skin* (6th ed.; Philadelphia: W. B. Saunders Co., 1971).
9. Mellette, J. R., Aeling, J. L., and Nuss, D. D.: Fluoride toothpaste, a cause of perioral dermatitis, Arch. Dermatol. 112:730, 1976.

13 / Leprosy

There are essentially two types of leprosy. The serious *lepromatous* type, with loads of bacteria in the skin and negative results on the lepromin test, has little nerve involvement. The leonine facies and involvement of the skin, lymph nodes, spleen, bone marrow and nerves characterize this anergic type. Skin nodules, plaques and infiltration are found in the *open* cases.[1] (See p. 72, PCAD.) An excellent discussion of leprosy may be found in the textbook by Moschella, Pillsbury and Hurley.[2]

The less serious *tuberculoid* type, with scant bacilli in the skin and positive results on the lepromin test, has more nerve involvement than skin involvement. Macules of anesthesia, thickened nerves and a hyperergic good prognosis are found in the *closed* cases.

There are *indeterminate* and *dimorphous* groups showing unstable features; classifying them may be difficult since they often swing one way and then later the opposite. When the lepromin test and the bacteriologic findings agree with the histopathology, then the case can be classified.

Treatment

Dapsone or DDS (diaminodiphenylsulfone) is the medication of choice in treating all forms of leprosy. The Cochrane schedule is as follows:

1st 2 weeks – 25 mg twice a week (50 mg per week)
2nd 2 weeks – 50 mg twice a week (100 mg per week)
3rd 2 weeks – 75 mg twice a week (150 mg per week)
4th 2 weeks – 100 mg twice a week (200 mg per week)

The importance of minimal initial doses and gradual increase cannot be overemphasized. The Committee on Therapeutics of the International Congress of Leprosy recommended the above dosage schedule in 1963. Higher doses or more rapid increases lead to lepra reactions or toxicity with disastrous results. Clinical cure may require 3–6 years. The medication is bacteriostatic. Routine complete blood cell counts and urine tests and if possible iron, vitamin B_{12} and a high-protein diet should be encouraged.

Other Sulfone Drugs

Diasone (sodium sulfoxone), 0.165 gm, is equivalent to DDS, on a ½ tablet (DDS) for tablet (Diasone) basis.

Promin (sodium glucosulfone) should be given intravenously 5 gm per week in divided doses (1 gm per day given five times weekly) or three times a week, then rest a week.

Madribon (sulfadimethoxine) is effective in treating tuberculoid leprosy.

Sulphetrone—three or more 0.5-gm tablets should be given daily. The dosage is difficult to determine because it is poorly absorbed.

Ciba SU-1906 (diphenyl thiourea) may help in treating the "sulfone-resistant" cases. The maximum starting dose is 2 gm daily, and there is a 2-year limit.

Treatment of Lepra Reaction

Reactions of the erythema nodosum type may be extremely difficult to treat and may tax the resources of the physician.

For a *mild reaction,* reduce the specific medication dose to half and give antihistamines or antimalarials. If the reaction persists, stop the sulfone treatment temporarily.

For a *moderate to severe* reaction, stop the antileprous medication immediately and treat with sedatives, antimalarials or antihistamines. (Empirically, penicillin, streptomycin and blood tranfusions help some cases.)

For a *severe reaction,* treat with steroids. However, the rebound phenomenon on discontinuance is a *real* hazard, and steroids should be used only to permit continuance of the badly needed specific medication. Cochrane says other medication, such as Ciba SU 1906 or Madribon, may be given for a few months before trying to reinstitute sulfone therapy.[3]

The proper balance between the amount of antileprous

medication required *and* the amount that the patient in reaction will *tolerate* is the most difficult aspect of management.

In dapsone-resistant patients, particularly those with the lepromatous types of leprosy, the dose of dapsone can be increased to 600 mg per week. However, the use of combined ethionamide (Trecator—SC Ives) and rifampin (Rinactane—Ciba) is currently under study, and B 663 (Geigy) Lamprene is useful in treating cases of reactive leprosy, being less likely to lead to lepra reactions, and is often considered the next step in the treatment of sulfone-resistant lepromatous cases.

REFERENCES

1. Canizares, O.: Diagnosis and treatment of leprosy in the U.S., Med. Clin. North Am. 49:801, 1965.
2. Moschella, S. L., Pillsbury, D. M., and Hurley, H. J.: *Dermatology* (Philadelphia: W. B. Saunders Co., 1975), p. 808 ff.
3. Cochrane, R. G., and Davey, T. F.: *Leprosy in Theory and Practice* (2d ed.; Bristol, England: John Wright & Sons, 1964).

14 / Seborrheic Dermatitis and Psoriasis

Seborrheic Dermatitis

A first cousin to psoriasis, this condition causes greasy salmon-pink scales on the sternum and in the nasolabial folds, with the scalp, hairline and ear folds occasionally involved. Inguinals, inframammary and axillary folds, the navel, pubic area and eyebrows are often involved. The patient experiences itching, especially on the scalp, where it can cause hair loss. The condition can be intractable in diabetics and in patients with Parkinson's disease. It is usually a spring, fall or wintertime disease, being benefited by sunlight and outdoor living. There may be a familial predisposition, and it seems to occur most commonly (at least in my experience) in fair-skinned blue-eyed people who love cheese, milk, cream and butter and who are sedentary and do not eat much meat. Osler used to say that the gall-bladder wards were filled with fair, fat females who were forty and flatulent. The same people seem to get seborrhea. (See p. 35, PCAD.)

Treatment

It is essential to project some understanding of the mechanics of the disease's development to the patient, who in all probability will have to battle the condition all his life and therefore should have weapons to use. Avoidance of a too sedentary life, avoidance of long-continued "stewing strain," avoidance of eggs, cheese, cream and butter, and wintertime daily doses of vitamin B complex all are extremely helpful in loading the constitutional factors in the patient's favor.

Local treatment consists chiefly of scalp care and, in *severe cases*, 7.5% sulfur mixed with salicylic acid 1%, castor oil 10% and olive oil to 100%. This mixture should be left on overnight, shampooing in the morning, and doing this about every four days. Shampooing with Selsun (selenium sulfide suspension) and Dara shampoo three times a week, gradually tapering, plus Sebucare or Resorcitate scalp lotion (salicylic acid and resorcin monoacetate in alcohol—Almay) in brunettes, will often correct the scalp condition, as will tincture of cantharides scalp lotion in blondes. (See Formulary, no. 28.) Occasionally a stubborn seborrhea capitis appears that defies all skill. Steroid lotions with 1% hydrocortisone in propylene glycol, Synalar solution 0.01%, or Kenalog lotion will help. Diasporal cream (Doak), which is sulfur and salicylic acid in a carbowax base, is washable and quite effective when rubbed in one, two or even three nights before shampooing. (See Formulary, nos. 28, 29.)

Several antiseborrheic shampoos are on the market, e.g., Ionil (which incorporates Zephiran), Meted (which is Texas Pharmacal's sulfur with a wetting agent), Sebulex (Westwood), Selsun (Abbott), and Capitrol (Westwood—which may yellow gray hair), all of which have to be lathered in well and left in contact with the scalp for varying periods of time. Usually this has to be done two or three times a week and left in much longer than the manufacturers recommend before rinsing out. If no headway is being made, one must suspect psoriasis.

For treating involvement of the glabrous skin, ointments or creams of antibiotic-steroid combination work best, e.g., hydrocortisone in polysporin ointment, Chloromycetin in Aristocort cream or Mycolog cream (bear in mind its sensitizing properties).

Other remedies for tender facial skin include Sulfolac cream (Kelgy), Sulfur-Sal ointment (3% of each) or Sulforcin lotion (Texas Pharmacal), and on occasion 3% sulfur in Aristocort cream.

Sometimes 5% sulfur in zinc paste can be very useful, and on occasion 2% ammoniated mercury in a variety of creams can help, as well as Vioform hydrocortisone lotion 1%, or Vioform cream 3%. (See Formulary, no. 28.)

Systemic treatment, e.g., ultraviolet lamp treatment administered three times a week to the face and scalp, or to the whole body if needed, can be efficacious. Crude liver used to be given deeply intramuscularly by injections.

Occasionally in treating rough tender skin, a sulfur soap is helpful, as is vitamin A taken internally. At other times 1% hydrocortisone lotion and Neutragenia soap may be needed. Many who claim they can't use soap will tolerate Oilatum (Stiefel).

For treating marginal blepharitis, sulfacetamide ophthalmic ointment (Schering—Unguentum Salumyd) and metimyd ophthalmic preparations (Schering), which contain neomycin, are very effective.

Psoriasis

The varieties of psoriasis are: *acute guttate,* which usually follows an acute upper respiratory infection, commonly a strep throat; *inveterate,* involving patches on the elbows, knees, scalp and over the sacrum; *flexural,* involving the creases, with fissures and adjacent red raw moist regions; *Pustular,* of the generalized Zumbuch type; *pustular,* of the palms and soles (Andrews-Barber type); and *psoriatic erythroderma.* (See pp. 23–26, PCAD.)

The Common Kind of Discoid Plaques on Elbows and Knees

Response to tars is the best treatment measure here, and a representative number are listed below. The tars must be rubbed in, preferably after a warm bath, whether they are crude coal tar in a paste or ointment, liquor carbonis detergens in a cream, or Tar-Doak in a lotion.

Salicylic acid	0.6	Crude coal tar	0.3 (to 0.9)
Phenol	0.6	(or Zetar)	
Liquor carbonis detergens	6.0	Lassar's paste (plain)	
USP Hydrophl-ic Ointment q.s. ad	60.0	q.s. ad	30.0

or Tar-Doak Lotion (Doak)

Other mercurial preparations, e.g., 5–30% ammoniated mercury in the scalp with 3% salicylic acid in an ointment base (avoid creams) or Riasol or Siroil, which are mercurials, also help.

Tar paints, such as crude coal tar 2% in any good aromatic solvent (which is difficult to make), Zetar 100%, Stokes' modification of Sabouraud's ointment (see Formulary, no. 29), the Doak Company's Tar Distillate, or Wright's Liquor Carbonis Detergens, can be painted on. They can also be rubbed into the scalp vigorously, say, on a Friday night and then shampooed out either Sunday night or Monday morning. Estergel (Westwood) and Psorigel (Owen), recently introduced tar gels, have value especially in the scalp since they wash out easily. They can be mixed with either Topsyn gel or Lidex ointment, 50-50, to enhance their effect.

Ultraviolet lamp treatment, whether using a box or a Hanovia lamp, is effective, too. Often the modified Goeckerman treatment of painting on the tar or rubbing on Balnetar prior to stepping into the sunlamp box is helpful.

Intracutaneous injections of 50-50 Kenalog in distilled water are especially useful for treating nails and for inveterate small plaques, although atrophy may be a problem.

Steroid creams, such as Synalar, Kenalog, Cordran, Aristocort, Lidex, Halog, and Diprosone, and occluding with Saran wrap (a method that leaves much to be desired), has been popular on occasion. (See Formulary, no. 22.)

Steroid-impregnated tapes, such as Cordran tape, follow the same principle and can be left on for 12–24 hours.

The best remedy of all is probably a vacation at the seashore where there is lots of sunlight.

Methotrexate, which is a folic acid antagonist that depresses the bone marrow, is a remedy that can be used at times. (See also Formulary, nos. 10–12, 15–17, 22.) Methotrexate is used by 52% of dermatologists in the treatment of psoriasis, 66% of whom prefer the iii tabs. every 12 hours for three doses per week, as opposed to i twice a day for 5 days each week (using 2.5-mg tablets).[1] Platelets and white blood cell counts must be watched carefully. A diabetic family history is a contraindication. Either pregnancy or impaired liver or kidney function is an absolute contraindication. Apthae, gastrointestinal bleeding, perianal erosions and heart failure as well as frightening depression of the level of bone marrow (which usually rebounds) are the common side effects. Liver biopsy is not done as much as the lawyers would like, but physicians should be wary of alcoholics. The serum glutamic oxaloacetic transaminase monitoring is adequate protection for ordinary patients. Two courses given one week apart will usually clear a patient for 4–8 weeks, occasionally longer. Sedation, sensible diet and avoidance of overwork and strain are helpful factors, too. Mycophenolic acid, an inhibitor of purine synthesis, has therapeutic effectiveness, though powerful side effects.[2] I must confess I almost never use methotrexate now that long-wave ultraviolet is more readily available for treating severe psoriasis.

Radiation and grenz rays are again helpful, though caution must prevail.

Acute Guttate Psoriasis

This occurs almost invariably after an upper respiratory infection or tonsilitis. Tonsilectomy prevents recurrent attacks in many patients. The following are helpful: vitamin A in large doses, ultraviolet light, 2% ammoniated mercury cream, Riasol (which consists essentially of mercury soap 0.5%, phenol 0.5% and cresol 0.75% in a lotion base), Siroil (which consists of mercury oleate 0.4% and cresol about 1% in a lotion base) and Alphosyl (which is 2% allantoin and 5% coal tar extract in a lotion base). Another is Tar-Doak lotion. The baths, such as Balnetar, Almay and Zetar, are helpful.

Most people believe that guttate psoriasis goes away by itself, although it sometimes needs a little push.

Flexural Psoriasis

Triamcinolone cream seems to be the leading method of control here, and for deep fissures 10% silver nitrate painted on with a swab is helpful. A tense life-style is one of the aggravating factors.

Pustular Psoriasis of the Extremities

Gantrisin or tetracycline taken internally, antibiotic-steroid local ointments, e.g., 1% hydrocortisone in bacitracin ointment, radiation with grenz in small doses, and a search for a focus of infection on the basis of the theory that it is related to Andrews bacterid, are often helpful. Vioform, mercury, tar and antibiotic-steroid combinations are the drugs used locally. Antimetabolites are effective but have to be used with caution.

Zumbuch Pustular Psoriasis

Antibiotics and antimetabolites are about all a physician can offer these patients. The patients have an extremely poor prognosis. Long-wave ultraviolet light treatment has favorable effects.

Erythroderma

Antimetabolites are probably the best measure here, but sometimes when steroids are used, the condition can be cleared, although very often in order to bring about the clearing, the patient has to take so much steroid that there is a risk of steroid diabetes or some other side effect that is extremely undesirable.

Living in the Florida Keys, where there is an offshore breeze, or in the desert in Arizona or some such measure will often clear these patients with erythroderma, although it is an uphill struggle all the way.

The sunlight at the Dead Sea, being below sea level, produces tanning *without* burning because of the filtering effect of the atmosphere. Psoralen used with ultraviolet A (PUVA), with Oxsoralen given orally 2 hours before, offers promise as a treatment. It must be continued, however. PUVA, as described by Parrish and Fitzpatrick, has proved valuable in treating stubborn, severe psoriasis, but the expense is limiting. Recent reports of success using black light, after 50 mg methoxsalen is given 2 hours before, are encouraging. Seven tubes, each 91.6 cm long, were used twice a week with slow improvement in 14 weeks or so.[3-5] Topical colchicine in concentrations of 0.5–1.0% was used by Kligman et al.[6, 7]

REFERENCES

1. Bergstresser, P. R., Schreiber, S. H., and Weinstein, G. D.: Systemic chemotherapy for psoriasis, Arch. Dermatol. 112:977, 1976.
2. Marinari, R., et al.: Mycophenolic acid in the treatment of psoriasis, Arch. Dermatol. 113:930, 1977.
3. Parrish, J. A., Fitzpatrick, J. B., et al.: Photochemotherapy of psori-

asis with oral methoxsalen and long wave ultraviolet light, N. Engl. J. Med. 291:1207, 1974.
4. Esther, J. R.: Letter: Photochemotherapy using ordinary black light, Arch. Dermatol. 112:564, 1976.
5. Mizuno, N., et al.: Methoxsalen and irradiation: Treatment for postulosic palmaris et plantaris, Arch. Dermatol. 112:883, 1976.
6. Kligman, A. M., et al.: Topical colchicine therapy for recalcitrant psoriasis, Arch. Dermatol. 111:33, 1975.
7. Gaylarde, P. M., and Sarkany, I.: Letter: Colchicine therapy for psoriasis, Arch. Dermatol. 112:556, 1976.

15 / Mycosis Fungoides: Light-Sensitive Diseases

Mycosis Fungoides

Early-stage mycosis fungoides is the erythema, eczema or parapsoriasis "en plaque disseminee," which in a later stage becomes infiltrated and lichenified and still later becomes tumorous and even ulcerated. A reticulum cell is the basic source of this lymphoma, which terminates as a variety of lymphosarcoma as a rule. (See pp. 163–164, PCAD.)

Treatment

Radiation treatment with ultraviolet light is occasionally enough, when given early on, to provide several years of control. Sea and sun are the therapy, and the patient should enjoy them in the summer.

Electron beam therapy, as practiced by John Fromer and his group at the Lahey Clinic, does not depress the level of bone marrow and provides great relief in many cases, although it must be repeated.[1] Grenz ray and x-ray therapy in small doses to localized areas is very effective; grenz rays are preferable in view of the eventual dangers of continued x-ray treatment. Weekly treatments for four or six weeks usually suffice.

Cytotoxic agents such as *cytoxin* (cyclophosphatine), 200 mg given intravenously, slow drip, daily and subsequently 50 mg given daily orally with dose control of hematologic and bone marrow status by frequent laboratory examinations, are needed. Depression of the level of bone marrow, nausea, diarrhea and alopecia are side effects.

Methotrexate, either in once-a-week doses of 25–50 mg or 2.5-mg doses given twice a day for five days, then resting for two days and resuming for five more days, has occasional success. Depression of the level of bone marrow, nausea, vomiting, diarrhea, ulceration of the mucous membranes and alopecia are signs to stop treatment at once. Blood studies must be done. Platelet counts are usually depressed first. Methotrexate may aggravate diabetes.

Chlorambucil (Leukeran), 2–6 gm per day in courses of 4–6 weeks, *triethylene melamine* (TEM), 5 mg weekly for 4 weeks, and *nitrogen mustard* can be used. Steroids assist in handling complications of treatment in mycosis fungoides, but otherwise should be held in reserve. Triacetyl azauridine treatment shows promise.[2]

Topical nitrogen mustard therapy or *mustargen HCL* (Merck, Sharp & Dohme) is another treatment.[3] A solution of 10 mg nechlorethamine hydrochloride in 50 cc saline, that is to say, one vial dissolved in 50 cc water, equals 29 mg/100 cc of solution. This should be used fresh, applying it to the cleansed skin with gauze sponges held in forceps. The application is made to the entire body even though the lesions do not involve the entire body, and the person painting should wear rubber gloves since sensitization to nitrogen mustard can occur. The skin should be kept moist for 15 minutes, then dried with a towel. Three hours later the patient takes a soap-and-water bath; the application is done daily for 6–8 days and then weekly. The family can do this.

Best results occur in treating the early erythematous or eczematous stages, and the itching is relieved. The patients did not ever seem to become unable to tolerate the painting in my small series. In the tumor stages, local nitrogen mustard treatment, in combination with either x-ray or chemotherapy internally, seems to be the method of choice. There appears to be little systemic toxicity. Help from oncologists is usually needed.

Discoid Lupus Erythematosus

Discoid lupus erythematosus consists of a persistent localized erythema, usually on the face, but can occur on the extremities and scalp, often with adherent scales, patulous follicles with keratin plugs, and usually followed by atrophy. The cause is unknown, but the condition is aggravated or induced by sun. Butterfly lesions are typical. Spontaneous cure occurs, often *without* scars. However, in the scalp the patches usually leave scars that destroy the hair and look like pseudopelade. The erythrocyte sedimentation rate is usually elevated, and there may be leukopenia. (See pp. 142–143, PCAD.)

Treatment

LOCAL TREATMENT.—Steroid aerosol spray (Kenalog preferred) given three times a day and then gradually less often; Synalar HP (high potency) or Valisone 0.1% under occlusion or even without occlusion; and the Cordran tape are all partially and often wholly effective in clearing the lesion. Intracutaneous Kenalog injection, carbon dioxide snow application, painting with pure phenol and mild lotio alba application also help. Avoiding sun with blocking makeups, e.g., Solar Cream or A-Fil Cream, is essential.

INTERNAL TREATMENT.—The antimalarials, introduced after World War II, have markedly suppressive effects. Atabrine, 100-mg tablets, stain the skin yellow. Aralen (Chloroquine), 250-mg tablets, Plaquenil, 200-mg tablets, and Camoquin, 200-mg tablets, are varieties. The most effective treatment is a combination of Chloroquine 65 mg, Atabrine 25 mg, and Plaquenil 50 mg, called Triquin (now removed because it was a "fixed combination"). A good pharmacist can make it in a capsule size. Dosage varies from six to one daily, usually three times a day initially, dropping to as low a maintenance dose as can be found later. The major side effect of irreversible retinopathy somewhat discourages its free use, although there is probably a dose relationship; if small doses are used for a short time, no great risk is seen. Opacities in the cornea appear to be reversible when the antimalarials are stopped, and other side effects such as nausea, diarrhea, drug rash (often like lichen planus), lightening of the hair and aplastic anemia have to be taken into account.

Other methods of treatment include gold sodium thiosulfate given intravenously starting at 5 mg and increasing to 50 mg weekly for 6–10 weeks.

Polymorphic Light Eruption

Polymorphic light eruption, a condition that can be confused with discoid or systemic lupus erythematosus, although it is usually itchy (photoallergy always itches; phototoxic reactions may or may not itch), comes on in early spring or summer, affects light-exposed areas, and is usually papular or plaque-like. It starts 18–24 hours after exposure and goes away in 2–4 days if the patient is kept out of the sun. If the patient continues to expose himself to bright sun (e.g., parking lot attendants), the eruption will start appearing in the covered areas. It has to be differentiated from lupus erythematosus profunda, lymphocytic infiltration of the skin, Darier-Roussay sarcoid and strange (e.g., epoxy) contact dermatitides. (See p. 150, PCAD.)

Sources for ultraviolet treatment include fluorescent lamps, mercury-arc highway lamps and movie projector lights.

Exogenous photosensitizers include antibacterial soaps (mostly because of the halogenated salicylanilids), e.g., Zest, Safeguard, Lifebuoy, Dial, Palmolive Gold (off the market now) and Irish Spring, and cosmetics containing photosensitizers, such as bithional. Some perfumes, e.g., Shalimar, contain a furocoumarin or psoralen, which leads to marked hyperpigmentation after the erythema, as do many plants such as wild parsnip, Persian limes and, under certain circumstances, celery. Sulfonamide, anthracene, acridine derivatives and acriflavine compounds, as well as methylene blue and phenothiazine compounds, can sensitize the skin in the presence of light.

Endogenous photosensitizers include phenothiazines (Thorazine, Sparine, Compazine, Stelazine, Phenergan, Temaril and Tacaryl), griseofulvin, sulfonamides, including the antidiabetic drugs, declomycin, thiazides (Diuril, Hydrodiuril, etc.), gold, silver, stilbamadine, guanine, aminosalicylic acid, 9-aminoacridine and antihistamines, also cyclamates, furocoumarines and nalidixic acid (urinary antimicrobial).

Phototoxic reactions affect all exposed people at once. The reactions usually look like a bad sunburn and do not often itch or burn.

Photoallergy, on the other hand, has a short incubation period, looks like eczema or hives and always itches. It affects only a small percentage of exposed people.

Treatment

If there are no exogenous or endogenous photosensitizers to be eliminated, the *antimalarials* suffice, usually in twice-daily doses early in the season, tapering to twice a week through April to June or July, then stopping. A sunlamp used through the winter will often prevent the spring flare. The same is true of those who take a Caribbean vacation in February. Eye examination before and during antimalarial treatment is essential. The antimalarials are ineffective in treating solar urticaria and drug-induced light reactions. Beta-carotene (Solatene) used in one study helped about one third of photosensitive patients and most patients with erythropoietic protoporphyria.[4]

Local sunscreens are often of great assistance. The benzophenone preparations such as Uval, an oily lotion (Dome); Sol-Bar, a vanishing cream (Person and Covey); and RVP, a grease (Elder), all have wide-spectrum protection. Sunswept (Texas Pharmacal) is vanishing, and Sundare (Texas) is a washable lotion having a less wide protective spectrum but permitting some adaptive tanning. Others that have an opaque quality and block off most everything include A-Fil (Texas Pharmacal) and Solar cream (Doak). There are some others, such as Skolex, which absorb wavelengths of less than 3,200 Å, as does window glass. The atmosphere and the tilt of the earth produce less danger of sunburn before 9:30 A.M. and after 4 P.M. It is well to remember that snow reflects more than sand, which reflects more than water. Look out for white sails.

HYDROA AESTIVALE (HYDROA VACCINIFORME) HUTCHINSON'S SUMMER PRURIGO.—Children show blisters, some umbilicated, on the sun-exposed areas in summer. Puberty cures this, unless there is porphyria. Sunscreens applied locally, systemic antimalarials or estrogen, and local steroid creams usually control this. Antihistamines assist.

SOLAR URTICARIA.—Urticaria from sunlight is best treated by local sunscreens, steroid creams and antihistamines given internally (avoiding Tacaryl).

Other Sun Effects

ERYTHROPOIETIC PORPHYRIA.—Congenitally affected boys are the patients. (See p. 151, PCAD.)

HEPATIC PORPHYRIA.—There are two types: the acute intermittent and the cutanea tarda. The latter is more commonly seen, producing photosensitivity in the exposed areas, e.g., bullae on the dorsa of the hands, showing pink urine with the Woods's lamp examination. (See p. 152, PCAD.) This condition usually is seen in liver damage from barbiturates, contraceptive pills, estrogens or alcohol. The treatment is phlebotomy. Sodium bicarbonate (two 5-grain tablets taken three times a day) occasionally is helpful.

COLLOID MILIUM.—This is seen in the South and Southwest in sun-exposed fair-skinned individuals and is more or less an irreversible protein deposit.

PELLAGRA.—Pellagra is classically seen in the elderly recluse with poor nutrition and too much alcohol intake. Treatment is nicotinic acid.

XERODERMA PIGMENTOSUM.—This disease is an accelerated skin senility with extensive actinic damage going on to cancer; it can be helped with 5-FU treatment. (See p. 153, PCAD.)

SYSTEMIC LUPUS ERYTHEMATOSUS.—Antinuclear antibodies and a positive lupus erythematosus preparation, hematuria, reversal of the serum protein, leukopenia and the malar flush in a sick patient require steroids and antimalarials in combination plus other tender loving care. (See p. 143, PCAD.)

ACTINIC KERATOSES.—Five percent 5-FU in hydrophilic petrolatum, rubbed in twice a day for 3 to 4 weeks, or 1% 5-FU in propylene glycol is an effective way of controlling these things. It does a wonderful job, but has to be watched. Commercial preparations are Efudex (Roche) and Fluroplex (Herbert). (See Formulary, no. 33.) If it is used on a lip keratosis, where it is equally effective, prepare your patient for a horrendous reaction.

Seborrheic dermatitis and sun exposure coincidentally produce intensification of the response so that seasonal limitations are wise. Bowen's disease of the face *does* respond to treatment, although the condition of one patient with hand involvement failed to clear completely after many months of treatment. The duration of the treatment on the hands and forearms should be at least 6 weeks; it is worthy of trial in treating erythroplasia of Queyrat and superficial basal cell epithelioma. The iceberg effect of ending up with a more extensive response than expected should be explained ahead of time. The propylene glycol tends to dry the area, so bland emollients or steroid and emollient for nightly use are helpful. Lotion makeup to cover in the daytime helps women. Liquid nitrogen applied for 15–25 seconds is pleasanter and faster. If 0.5% triamcinolone acetonide (and presumably acetate, too) is used with the fluorouracil, the inflammatory reaction is considerably lessened and the therapeutic result is the same.[5] On occasion I have found telanglectasia to be an annoyingly persistent concomitant of this combination, however. Better to avoid the fluorinated steroids here and use plain hydrocortisone emollients.

SENILE ELASTOSIS.—This is a disease of dermal sun damage which is irreversible.

COCKAYNE'S AND BLOOM'S SYNDROME.—These congenital disorders are accompanied by increased susceptibility to rapid sunburn.

HARTNUP DISEASE.—This is a sort of congenital pellagra. Along with carcinoid, it has abnormal tryptophan metabolism leading to light eruptions.

DERMATOMYOSITIS AND SYSTEMIC LUPUS ERYTHEMATOSUS.—These often start after sun exposure. (See pp. 140–141, PCAD.)

SUNLIGHT.—Sunlight *may* act as a Koebner phenomenon, producing rapid spread in the exposed regions of lichen planus, warts, psoriasis or dermatitis herpetiformis.

REFERENCES

1. Fromer, J. L., et al.: Management of lymphoma cutis with low megavolt electron beam therapy: 9-year follow-up on 200 cases, South. Med. J. 54:769, 1961.
2. Calabresi, P., et al.: Beneficial effects of triacetyl azauridine in psoriasis and mycosis fungoides, Ann. Intern. Med. 64:352, 1966.
3. Roenigk, H. H. J., and Haserick, J. R.: Mycosis Fungoides Treated with Topical Application of Nitrogen Mustard, in Waisman, M. (ed.): *Pharmaceutical Therapeutics in Dermatology* (Springfield, Ill.: Charles C Thomas, Publisher, 1968), pp. 87–91.
4. Fitzpatrick, B., et al.: Beta carotene therapy for erythropoietic protoporphyria and other photosensitivity diseases, Arch. Dermatol. 113:1229, 1977.
5. Eaglstein, W. H., et al.: Non-inflammatory destruction of actinic keratoses by fluorouracil, Arch. Dermatol. 112:1256, 1976.

16 / Pigmentary Changes

The increase or decrease in the amount of pigmentation in the skin, especially if it is in an irregular pattern, produces problems in esthetics or social acceptance rather than ill health or discomfort. However, many people are disturbed by pigment changes and are grateful for help.

Physiologic Changes in Pigmentation

Pigmentation changes occur in suntanning or in the development of freckles (ephelides). Late in life mottled pigmentation of the face, hands and forearms appears (lentigo). In those exposed to the sun at sea, a leathery darkening of the skin occurs in the exposed areas that never really fades. Carotenosis, with yellow palms and soles in those who eat excessive amounts of carrots and squash, can occur; and postinflammatory hyperpigmentations (and occasional hypopigmentation—dyschromia) after any inflammatory dermatosis can temporarily disfigure. The mottled chloasma of pregnancy and the more geometric droplike hyperpigmentation resulting from the photosensitizing effect of perfume, e.g., Shalimar (berloque dermatitis), also are usually temporary.

Systemic Reasons for Pigment Changes

These causes include chloasma from taking birth control pills, which often disappears with change in the type of pill, Addison's disease (on the mucosa, too), hyperthyroidism, fixed drug eruption, hemochromatosis, diabetes (carotinemia or hemochromatosis), pituitary or adrenal tumors, von Recklinghausen's disease with cafe-au-lait spots, scurvy, pellagra and sprue. Heavy metal intoxication with arsenic gives freckles, with diffuse darkening of the skin of a silver or slate gray color, as does bismuth; and gold produces a lilac color. Atabrine gives a yellow color. Poikiloderma of Civatte is a reticulated pigmentation change in the neck in menopausal women. Urticaria pigmentosa, dermatitis herpetiformis and lichen planus, as well as tinea versicolor, all give blotchy pigment changes. Less common causes are Albright's syndrome with bone involvement, ochronosis, xeroderma pigmentosum, pinta, Fanconi's syndrome, phenylketonuria, leprosy, Vogt-Koyanagi syndrome, and Peutz-Jeghers syndrome (see p. 15, PCAD), with pigment spots on the lips. Acanthosis nigricans in adults is suggestive of a tumor (see p. 32, PCAD). Erythrose peribuccale pigmentaire is probably similar to Riehl's melanosis caused by sun and cream. Hypervitaminosis A has produced a darkening of the skin similar to that in Riehl's melanosis. (See Formulary, nos. 34, 35.)

Occupational and Local Causes

Riehl's melanosis, with the hyperpigmentation on the malar cheeks and forehead, usually results from long-continued use of toilet water or cologne and exposure to the sun. Local use of cosmetics containing mercury, lead, zinc or bismuth, or even plain petroleum products can cause hyperpigmentation. In persons with certain occupations, the inhalation of tar products can lead to melanodermatitis toxica lichenoides. Erythema ab igne caused by exposure to heating pads and other heat sources can lead to mottled hyperpigmentation; and pressure from bands and buttons, if continued for a long enough time, can lead to deepening of the pigment. The application of the x-ray beam similarly produces mottling years later.

Treatment

The management of many of these rather evident symptoms involves elimination of the cause, where feasible, and in other instances concealment or attempted removal by local means. Hormonal adjustment is generally disappointing, as for example in treating poikiloderma of Civatte.

Bleaching is generally used in correcting melanoderma. Eldoquin, or 2.5% hydroquinone ointment, is generally rubbed in three times a day. Eldoquin forte is 4% hydroquinone, and Eldopaque is the same with sun block. A formula for a strong depigmenting and peeling agent is:

Retin A solution 0.05%	10
Eldoquin lotion 2%	10
Aristocort cream 0.1%	
q.s. ad	30

M. Ft. Ung.
Sig. rub in three times a day until irritation occurs, then rest and later resume.

A similar preparation is as follows:

Tretinoin	0.1%
Hydroquinone	5.0%
Dexamethasone	0.1%

This should be used once or twice daily to produce peeling, then after that phase subsides, once daily. Kligman and Willis found it effective in treating melasma, ephelides, and postinflammatory hyperpigmentation, though it was not useful for senile lentigines of the hands.[1]

Mercury creams, such as are found commercially, are mild and occasionally helpful. They are usually sold as "freckle creams" (e.g., Nadinola).

Peeling can be done with carbon dioxide slush or snow, or ethyl chloride spray. Phenol painting or 25% trichloracetic acid painting is often very helpful in the management of moderate localized lesions. A small trial area should be done first, since hyperpigmentation occasionally occurs. In the case of small lentigines, it is often possible to use a very fine electrodesiccating current, mildly and superficially brushing across the lesion without anesthesia, then curetting it off. The camphor water, alcohol, bichloride and salicylic acid "freckle peeler" is useful. (See Formulary, no. 13.) The patient applies it three times a day until peeling occurs, then rests a few days and then resumes. Dermabrasion can be useful in treating diffuse severe freckling.

Sunscreens suitable for the type of sun exposure the patient endures should be designed. Eldopaque (Elder), which is a titanium dioxide sunscreen containing hydroquinone, when applied to the hyperpigmented spots of chloasma in the day and ordinary makeup is used on the normal skin, often has quite acceptable results. Ordinary makeup such as Covermark and Spotstick aid in concealing unsightly dark patches, as does a makeup sunscreen called A-Fil (Texas Pharmacal). Other sunscreens include Sol-Bar (a cream) and Uval (a lotion emulsion). Both taste bitter when they get on the lips. RVP and RVPaque are greasy and pasty, respectively, and Sunswept, the cosmetically elegant cream, is not always effective. Sundare is a greaseless liquid and washes off easily, but can be applied *under* makeup.

In managing *arsenic and gold pigmentation*, dimercaprol (British anti-Lewisite) given intramuscularly can be helpful. It is not effective in treating argyria, although possibly for mercury and bismuth pigmentation (which is rare) it would be effective.

Patchy hypopigmentation occurs in most of the conditions listed as causing hyperpigmentation, since migration of the melanocytes from one site to another is all that is needed. Albinism, kwashiorkor, pinta, alopecia areata, leprosy, canities, postinflammatory effects especially after trauma or burn, perinevoid vitiligo (leukoderma acquisitum centrifugum—Sutton's nevus), scleroderma, vitiligo, exposure to rubber antioxidants and ingestion of chloroquine can all depigment skin. Endocrine changes, heavy metal intoxication and even the use of furacin eyedrops can produce pigment loss.

Perhaps the most underdiagnosed and overtreated cause of the whole group is *pityriasis alba*. This is commonly seen in a young boy at the end of the summer and consists of small coin-sized disks of light scaly skin where the normal tan is missing, almost always on the face although occasionally on the shoulders and arms. It appears to be related to a defatting of the skin caused by the shriveling action of unremoved soap or salt water from the beach, plus overexposure to wind or sun or soap, in a skin that is only patchily maturing. A warm towel, a superfatted soap and lubrication usually clear it, although it can bedevil the most experienced therapist. Cor-Tar-Quin cream occasionally clears stubborn spots.

In the treatment of leukoderma or vitiligo, the 8-methoxypsoralens or tripsoralen tablets taken 2 hours before sun exposure daily, starting with timed short exposures and gradually increasing, are undoubtedly helpful for very cooperative patients. However, my own practice is to use diacetic acid and walnut juice paint (Owen Labs.). With skill this can keep the "white spots" completely unnoticed. This is called Dy-O-Derm and comes in various shades. Also available is Vitadye (Elder).

Sometimes repigmentation occurs spontaneously, and high doses of vitamin B enhance this tendency. In several patients this has occurred *without* treatment. Painting with phenol is certainly an excellent way of repigmenting small local areas, especially in dark skin.

Cosmetic management with Covermark, using the shading cream first (Lydia O'Leary, New York City), or simply staying out of the sun altogether so that the contrast between the untanned and vitiliginous skin is not noticeable, perhaps is the easiest way of management.

Local application of 0.1 – 1.0% of alcoholic solution of Oxsoralen followed by carefully measured and gradually increasing exposures to black light at fixed distances, and thereafter occluding sun exposure with blocking sunscreen such as Maxafil or RVPaque, is a time-consuming, but often very effective way of repigmenting small areas. (See Formulary, no. 35.) Arora and Willis found that lowering the concentration of methoxsalen and using longer ultraviolet light exposures increased tolerance.[2] A good concentration is 0.1% and the peak effect occurs at about 15 minutes after application, so expose then. Peak reaction is at about 72 hours, so treatment should be given every third day.

REFERENCES

1. Kligman, A. M., and Willis, I.: A new formula for depigmenting human skin, Arch. Dermatol. 111:40, 1975.
2. Arora, S. K., and Willis, I.: Factors influencing methoxsalen phototoxicity in vitiligenous skin, Arch. Dermatol. 112:327, 1976.

SUGGESTED READING

Fitzpatrick, T. B., et al.: *Dermatology in General Medicine* (New York: McGraw-Hill Book Co., 1971).

17 / Instrument Sterilization

Because of the existence of endemic cases of viral hepatitis (serum hepatitis) transmitted by insufficiently sterilized hypodermic needles, the use of disposable needles and syringes has become a welcome practice. However, instruments, especially sharp scissors and curettes, cannot be disposable, and these have to be sterilized in such a way as to destroy bacteria and viruses and yet maintain their sharpness. The water boiler is only moderately satisfactory for sterilization, since it is questionable whether it destroys the serum hepatitis virus.

Fig 17–1.—Autoclave.

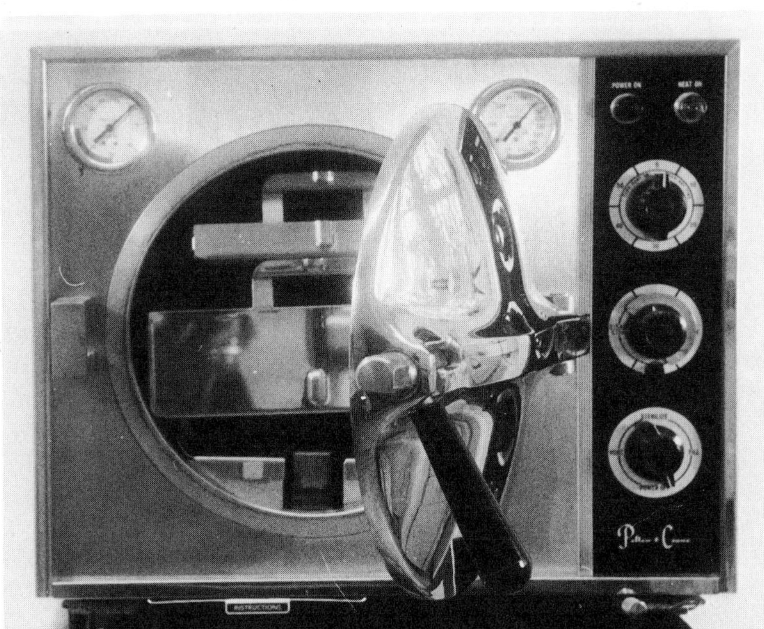

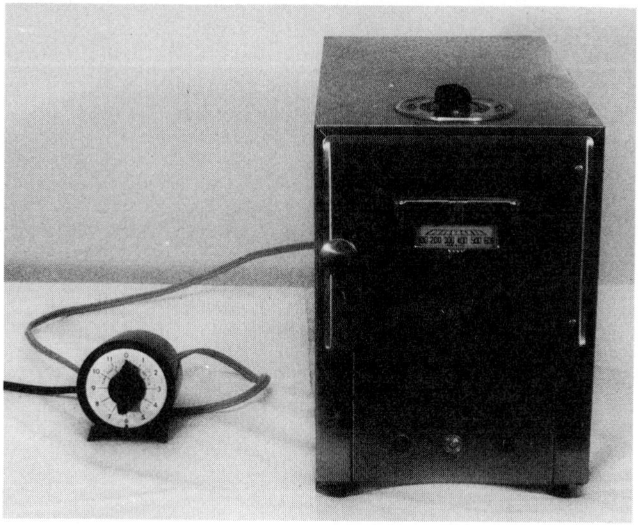

Fig 17–2. – Dry heat sterilizer.

The autoclave, while satisfactory for sterilizing gloves, drapes, towels and gauze, is hard on glassware and metalware and dulls instruments. It destroys all forms of microbial life, however (Fig 17–1).

Sterilizing with dry heat, in the form of baking in a thermostatically controlled oven, is an easy method (Fig 17–2). It does not dull sharp instruments if the lower temperature ranges are used. This can be done for longer periods (e.g., overnight) and be extremely effective. The items to be sterilized can be wrapped in aluminum foil or placed in a perforated pan, and the nurse can lock them in the dry heat sterilizer at the end of the day, set the automatic timer to shut off at, say, 5 A.M., and things are cooled off when she comes in at 8 A.M. the next day.

Table 17–1 summarizes the methods and uses of heat sterilization.

Cold Sterilization

It is our practice to wash all instruments after use with soap, hot water and nail brush and then drop them into a glass tray

TABLE 17-1.—METHODS OF HEAT STERILIZATION

STERILIZATION METHOD	TEMPERATURE	TIME	USES
Autoclave	250–254 F (120–123 C) 15–17 lb of pressure	30 min	First choice for gloves, drapes, towels and gauze Second choice for instruments, glassware and metalware
Boiling water	212 F	30 min at sea level; 5 min longer per 1,000 ft increase in elevation	Not recommended except when other methods are unavailable
Dry heat	340 F (170 C) 320 F (160 C) 300 F (150 C) 285 F (150 C) 250 F (120 C)	1 hr 2 hr 2½ hr 3 hr 6 hr (preferably overnight)	For glassware, metalware and dull instruments Use 250 F for sharp instruments and Luer-Lok syringes

containing Edisonite and tincture of green soap and let them soak. At the end of the day they are removed, washed and sterilized by whichever method is the most appropriate, usually dry heat. The following day the foil-wrapped syringes are stored in sliding racks and the needles are placed in the tray, which is put in the water boiler, an excellent storage place, being at the back of the treatment table and having a lid operated by a foot pedal. Long-handled forceps are kept standing nearby in a jar of benzalkonium chloride 1:750, in which antirust tablets can be placed. There is a form of benzalkonium chloride that comes with the antirust chemical in it. This also can be used for storage of forceps. These forceps can be used to select the small syringes and needles as required. Scissors, curettes and forceps for routine use are stored in shelves in an instrument cabinet. Scalpel handles are stored in trays containing the antirust benzalkonium chloride solution. Biopsy punches should be kept dry in wooden racks and shelves (Fig 17–3); disposable scalpel blades should be stored in the same manner, although these are usually wrapped in foil.

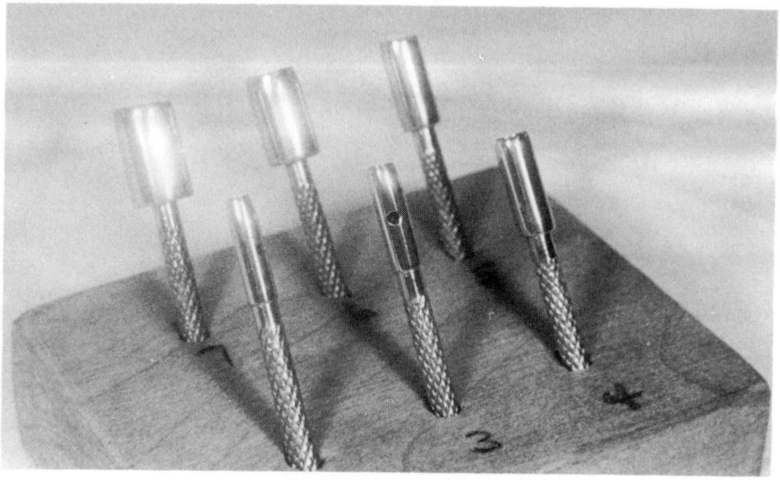

Fig 17–3. – Biopsy punches in rack.

Excision kits containing the necessary instruments, such as thumb forceps, mosquito clamps, curved kelly, needle holder, scissors, self-retaining retractor, skin hook and what is preferred, are presterilized by dry heat in foil-wrapped tin trays. By doing this, only the scalpel handle, disposable blade, gauze and suture have to be added when setting up.

Sets of Thomas towels (with the hole in them) and regular towels are also presterilized and wrapped and labeled as to size (large-medium-small), as are surgical gloves.

A small ultrasonic jewelry polisher is used to clean small instruments periodically; this is excellent for cleaning curettes and for removing oxidized debris and biologic material that occasionally cakes on.

Many of the instruments preferred by dermatologists are used in other specialties, such as otolaryngology and ophthalmology. One of these instruments, the chalazion forceps, is very useful in taking small cysts out of the lip.

Graefe's fixation forceps with their sharp teeth enables one to hold difficult tissue firmly in one hand while dissecting with the other. This is also very useful in "teasing" sebaceous cysts out through a narrow orifice. Tiny curettes, such as Meyerhoefer's chalazion curette, 1, 2 or 3 mm in diameter, are very useful for pulling the sac out of a tiny sebaceous cyst or curetting an acne cyst.

Soft rubber ear syringes are also very useful for syringing out tender external otitis ears rather than using the heavy plunger type of syringe as in removing wax.

Mosquito forceps, very tiny and very light, are far more suited to the type of dermatologic surgery usually done by the average physician in the office than are the heavy Kocher type of clamp or hemostat snap.

Needle holders should be small and light; scissors should be curved, sharp and small. Blunt-nosed scissors are useful for dissecting out the margins of sebaceous cysts and can always be used elsewhere.

Skin Surgery

Office Equipment

STERILIZER.—Dry-heat sterilizers for the instruments and autoclaves for the towels, drapes and gloves are needed. A supply of gauze squares, which the office nurse can package in foil and sterilize in the autoclave, cuts the cost of this essential item considerably.

DRAPES.—An "eye drape" (Thomas towel), made by cutting a hole in a tea towel and hemming it, plus one or two regular towels packed together in aluminum foil and sterilized in the autoclave, can be kept on hand and labeled as to size. This is largely to provide a sterile field for the suture material. Waterproof paper towels with cellophane backing on one side are useful as additional drape material underneath the sterile towels. "Scotch" brand surgical drapes and barrier towel drapes (Johnson & Johnson) and other sterile drapes (Converters Inc., Newark, N.J. and National Disposables Inc., Plainview, N.Y.) are available in the disposable line. Also, disposable rubber gloves can be obtained from most manufacturers (Pharmacy Labs., Glendale, Calif.).

OPERATING TABLES.—Expensive "electric hydraulic" tables are available, although in general a plain wooden table 76 in. long, 24 in. wide, 29½ in high, with slides or gliders on its four legs and covered by a foam rubber mattress with a sheet over this, is a very satisfactory arrangement. It is easily movable, which is a great advantage. It can be made to any height desirable to suit the operator. A large footstool (Picker X-Ray Company) is needed, and it should be untippable so that the patient can get on and off easily.

MAYO STAND (Fig 17–4).—The Mayo stand is used for instruments. The Luxor lamp, which is mounted on the wall and is flexible, plus a large ceiling installation and if possible a large window to let in daylight also help. White walls reflect light and assist the physician in visualizing difficult objects. A head mirror for examining the ear, nose and throat leaves both hands free, and the Luxor lamp can be easily placed so it is

Fig 17–4. — Mayo stand.

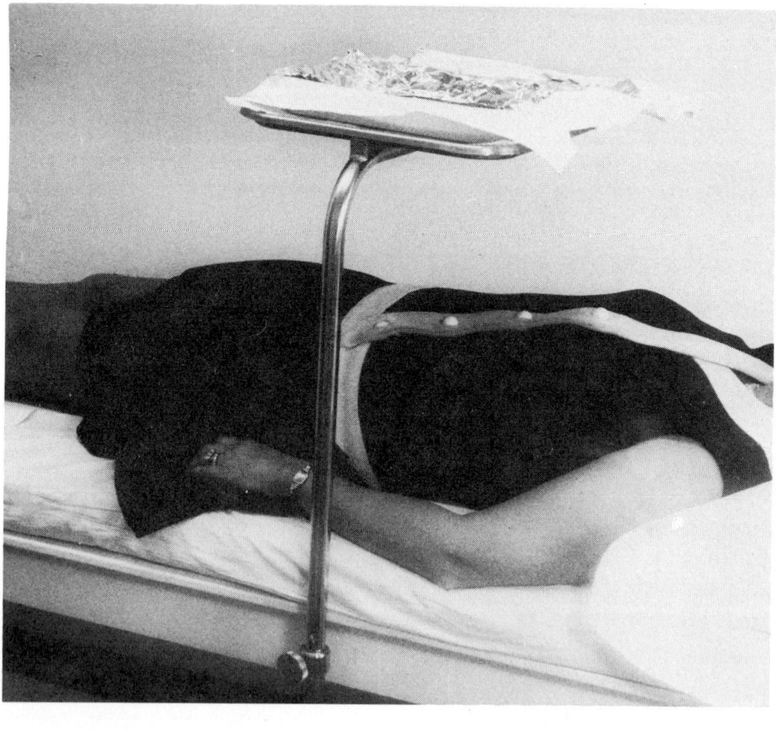

beside the patient's head while he sits on the operating table, enabling the physician to gaze easily into the recesses. In partitioned offices, through and through bolts can install a Luxor lamp swivel bracket very firmly in each of the adjoining rooms.

WALLS.—Walls should be easily wipeable, since Xylocaine and other substances constantly will have to be wiped away.

INSTRUMENT TABLES.—One or two of these equipped with cold sterilizing trays and dishes for scalpel handles, punches and other instruments should have a typed routine to follow in case of anaphylactic shock, such as that shown in Table 4–1 (p. 78).

An oxygen tank and inhaler mask should be at hand, as well as a tracheal tube of the type used in giving general anesthesia. Some offices keep an "emergency tray" handy with a tourniquet, syringe, epinephrine and "mixovials" of Cortef or Solu-Cortef, Aminophylin and other drugs.

Suture material

Dermalon (00 to 00000) is probably the most used suture material. It has a slight tendency to slip, and so knots have to be overtied. Silk sutures, usually 3-0, are best used in the oral cavity, where nylon tends to be spiky and swell too much, although silk swells too and knots must be carefully tied. Mersilene is a polyester fiber slightly stronger than nylon, but this material is almost too pliable; knots come undone quite often unless multiple square knots are tied. It has almost no tissue reaction, however. The commonly used size for small skin surgery is 0000 Mersilene.

Gut sutures actually need never be used in the skin; chromic gut should be used in abdominal surgery only. Buried sutures favor infection, and good bites with skin *retention-sutures* will close dead spaces and lead to tension-free apposition of the skin edges (with 5-0 closely applied interrupted sutures) and can be removed in 24–48 hours with little or no scarring.

All of these sutures come equipped with an atraumatic cutting needle (except gut, which is actually used more for ligature purposes, e.g., 5-0 gut), usually fully curved, which facilitates precise apposition of the wound edges. If subcuticular suturing is contemplated, a reverse cutting needle is used.

Instruments

The *Bard-Parker* handle with a #15 blade is adequate for most excisional surgery. For very fine work, a Beaver blade and handle may have some advantages, although I feel more secure with the Bard-Parker handles.

A *needle holder,* e.g., Mayo-Hegar about 5 or 6 in. long, with a good grip is needed so the instrument ties with fine sutures will not be frustratingly slippery. Other specially designed "plastic" needle holders are available, although actually a straight 5.5 in. Crile hemostat with a box lock on the finger grips is excellent.

Two or three straight or curved mosquito (Halstead) 5-in. *hemostats* with a box lock are very useful.

Fig 17–5.—Wire brushes and drills used for dermabrasion.

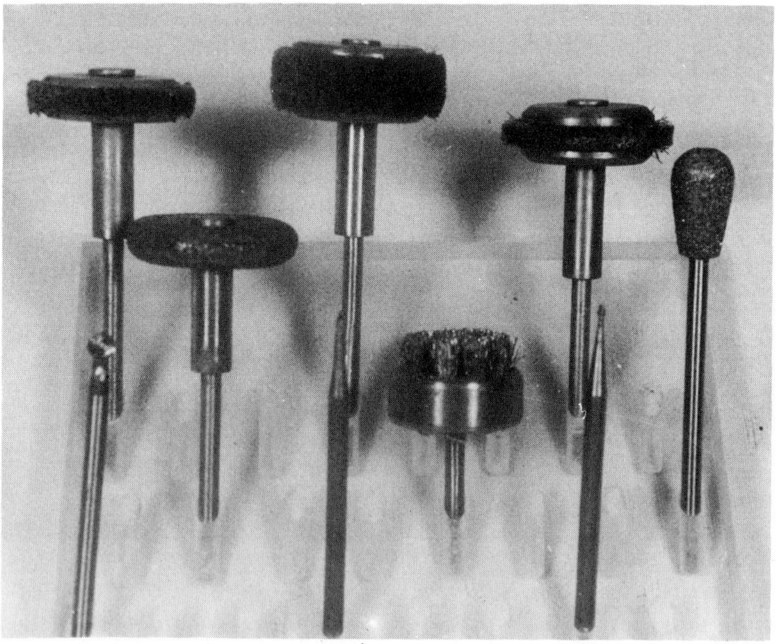

The Stille type of *tissue forceps* with the four or five teeth is superior to the "mouse-tooth," which often crosses and twists the tissue. Occasionally a long, strong pair of tissue forceps may be needed to lift up the tissue, especially when dissecting out large sebaceous cysts on the back of the neck where the skin is thick and the tissue is fibrous.

Fine curved iris *scissors* or Mayo scissors for undercutting are needed.

A *self-retracting retractor* occasionally can be very useful.

A *skin hook* is very useful to pick up and trim dog ears at the end of an excisional wound.

All of these and any other instruments desired can be prepackaged in aluminum foil and kept in rolls or trays ready for instant use (Fig 17–5). One useful practice is to enclose the foil-wrapped set in a sterile towel folded over and clipped at one side to the tray edge with a clothespin. When the towel is unfolded on the Mayo stand, it provides a sterile field where all the instruments can be used by the surgeon.

Anesthesia

Xylocaine is an effective and very safe local anesthetic which can be used without norepinephrine in electrosurgery and procedures on the digits. For facial excisional surgery, the blanching effect of the norepinephrine assists the careful work required and is to be recommended. On the palm of the hand, anesthesia is most difficult, and for local infiltration carbocaine is the preferred local anesthetic. Cyclaine can be used for questionably allergic people who are afraid of other "caines." The infraorbital and mental block are sometimes useful in performing facial surgery (Fig 17–6). Using a line drawn from the pupil to the canine tooth, the infraorbital nerve exits from the maxilla at this point on the cheek 2 cm lateral to the side of the nose. Usually the foramen can be palpated, and the needle is introduced just below and medial to the foramen so that it will slide into the foramen as it inclines upward and outward. A 22-gauge needle introduced 0.5 cm into the foramen where 1 cc of the Xylocaine is injected and another 1–2 cc is injected at the opening, gives a good block of the cheek, upper lip, side of the nose and lower eye-

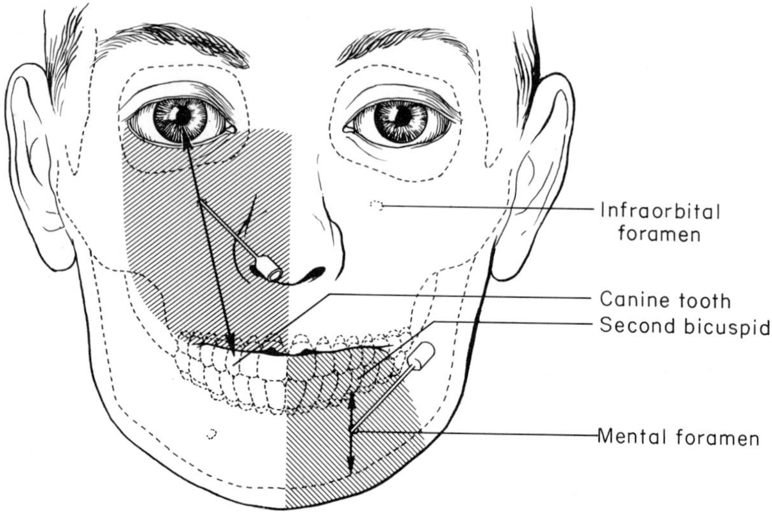

Fig 17–6.—Infraorbital and submental nerve block. (From Wise, R. A., and Baker, H. W.: *Surgery of the Head and Neck* [2d ed.; Chicago: Year Book Medical Publishers, Inc., 1962], p. 53.)

lid. In facial surgery on the inner canthus areas, it is an excellent form of anesthesia, as the distortion of the tissue is kept to a minimum.

The mental foramen lies midway between the upper and lower edges of the mandible opposite the second bicuspid tooth, although in older edentulous patients, it is closer to the upper edge. It also can usually be palpated. The needle is introduced slightly above and behind the foramen, which inclines forward and downward at an angle of 45 degrees with the skin. Skin wheals will assist in lessening the pain of probing; an injection of 1–2 cc in the canal and at the opening will anesthetize the chin and lower lip though not quite to the midline.

Most dermatologic surgery, however, is done with local infiltration either around or under (in the case of small lesions such as warts) the object of the excision. A little spray of ethyl chloride (or fluroethyl) lessens the sting of the first Xylocaine injection, and by proceeding from the edge of the numbed area, one can relatively comfortably infiltrate a large area.

Skin Preparation

Washing the area with Phisohex prior to the operation may engender a feeling of comfort in the nurse, but the antiseptic effect of hexachlorophene has to continue repetitively for at least a week to produce any reduction in skin bacteria. The cleansing powers of Phisoderm leave much to be desired. Therefore soap-and-water washing, followed by alcohol or alcohol and ether wipes before local anesthesia and again after, offers a more sensible preparation for skin surgery. (See Formulary, no. 24.)

Choosing the Line of Excision

This is probably the most important aspect of the whole procedure, since how well the resultant scar can be hidden is often the patient's chief concern and often governs his choice of a physician. Langer's lines do not always follow the wrinkle lines on the face, and where there is a conflict, it is usually wisest to follow the wrinkle lines. Wrinkle lines of excision on the face, trunk and extremities are shown in Figures 17–7, 17–8 and 17–9.

Fig 17–7.—Wrinkle lines of excision on the face. (From Kraissl, C. J., and Conway, H.: Surgery 25:592–600, 1949. Used by permission.)

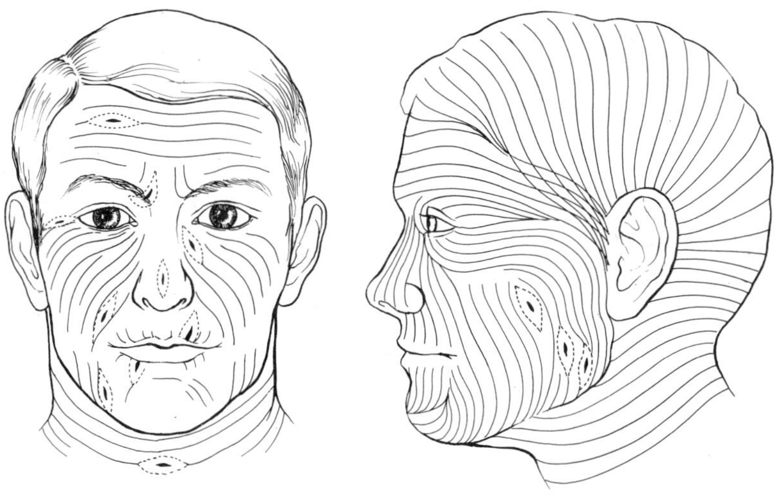

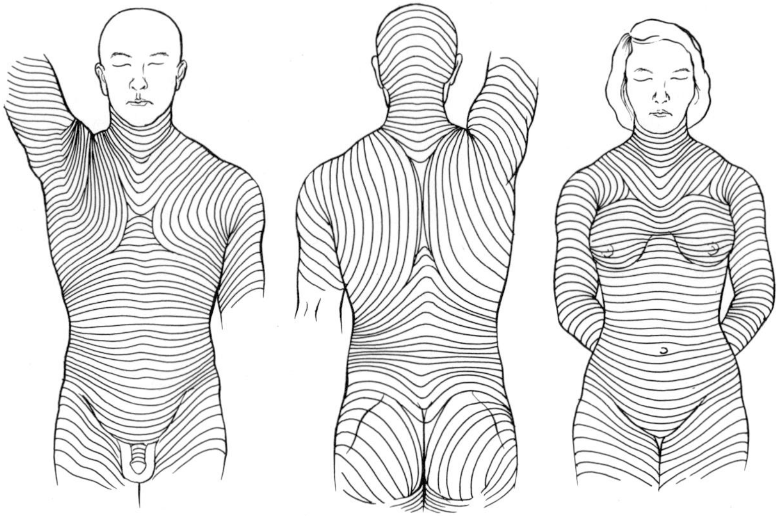

Fig 17–8.—Wrinkle lines of excision on the trunk. (From Courtiss, E., et al.: Plast. Reconstr. Surg. 31 (no. 1), January 1963. Used by permission of the publisher.)

If the shape of the lesion makes it difficult to follow the wrinkle lines, then the excisional line should follow that line that sacrifices the least tissue. Scars on the face fade beautifully, and expressive facial movements iron out most surgical scars so that in years to come they are almost invisible, no matter which way they occur.

Outlining the proposed excision line with wax pencil or laundry ink (or a sterilized ball-point cartridge) is a little self-defeating unless done *before* the local anesthetic is injected, since this always disturbs the relationship of the skin edges. One practice is to outline the beginning and end of the proposed excisional wedge with a toothpick (sterile) dipped in gentian violet (bottle held by the not-scrubbed nurse). Then mark the midpoint of the lateral margin of the proposed wedge. With the back of the scalpel, cross-hatch the skin (as in Fig 17–10, A) so that apposition will be perfect with no distortion.

Then inject the Xylocaine and clean up the skin before putting on the gloves and laying on the drapes.

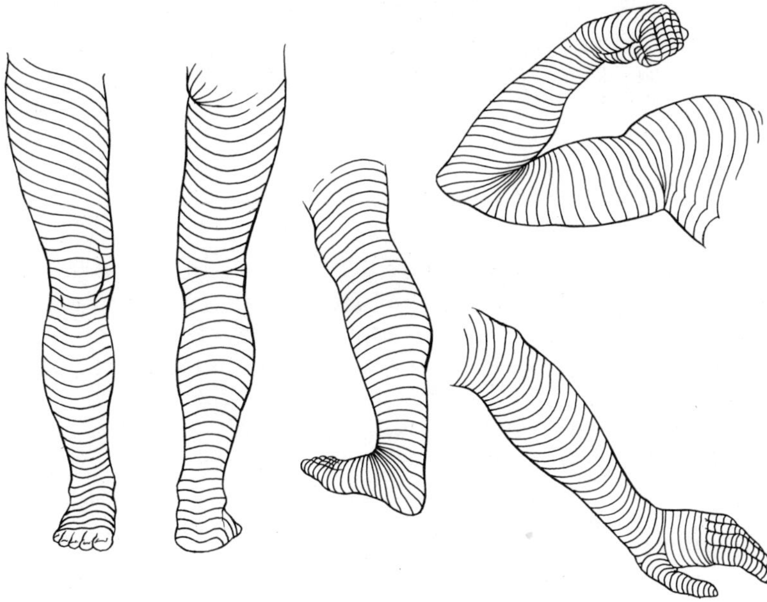

Fig 17–9.—Wrinkle lines of excision on the extremities. (From Courtiss, E., et al.: Plast. Reconstr. Surg. 31 (no. 1), January 1963. Used by permission of the publisher.)

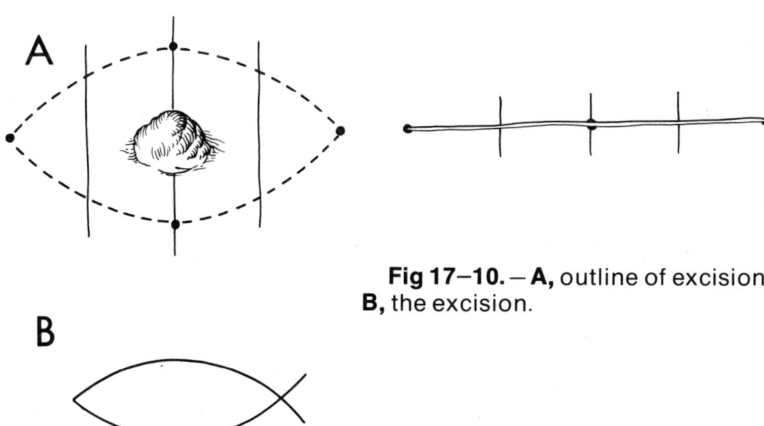

Fig 17–10.—**A,** outline of excision. **B,** the excision.

The Excision

Just as on the golf course, hackers are not appreciated. The cut must be at right angles to the skin, it must be firm, and it must start and finish at approximately the same depth. If the cut overlaps at the ends (as in Fig 17–10, B), no great harm has been done.

One end is picked up with the toothed forceps, and the elliptical block of tissue is excised by cutting toward the middle. Mosquito clamps are applied to the small bleeders and left. If there is so much tissue missing that undue tension will result from closure, then undercutting moderately deeply, preferably with flat blunt-nosed scissors such as the Mayo scissors, and spreading to find a natural cleavage level should be done now. The needle holder should be loaded, and the suturing should proceed from one end to the other. Sometimes lining up the two middle cross-hatches first assists greatly in spacing the proper number of sutures to neatly and precisely close the wound. They can be replaced later. Sometimes holding the wound edges with tissue forceps while the needle is introduced, at right angles to the skin (Fig 17–11, A), or sometimes holding it steady with the left hand is best.

Each occasion will demand its own technique. The edges of the wound should be aligned perfectly to avoid any "step" difference in level, since this will cast a shadow on the face and exaggerate the presence of the scar. If the excised tissue

Fig 17–11.—**A,** introducing the needle for closing the excision. **B,** aligning the edges of the wound.

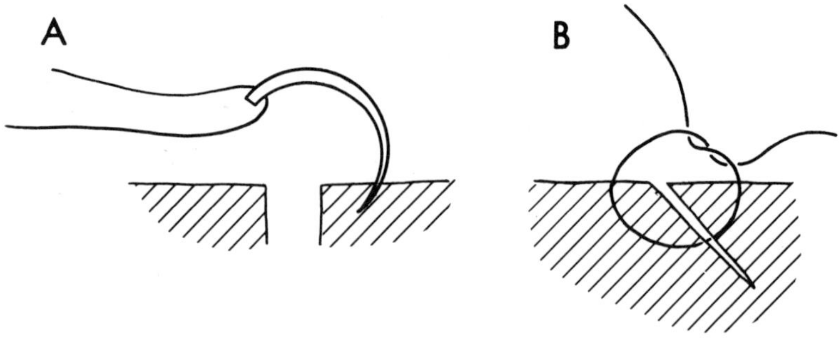

left a wound where the tissues on one side appear to be thicker than on the other, e.g., near the eyelid on the cheek where tangential "incisions" may occur, then the surgeon should take a bigger bite of the thin side, and be sure the edges are perfectly apposed (Fig 17–11, B).

If tension is a problem, there is a dead space, or pressure is needed to effect hemostasis, a retention suture, probably a big mattress suture (3-0 or 2-0), placed well out from the wound edges can be used provided it is removed in 24–48 hours. This will take the tension off the 5-0 interrupted sutures, which effect the good apposition of the edges and are now at their leisure.

In some areas, e.g., on the breast or inner thigh, where the skin edges have a strong tendency to roll in, a vertical mattress stitch may be needed to slightly evert the skin edges. Otherwise proper healing will not occur and the wound will open up when the sutures are removed. A near-far everting suture will do the same as a vertical mattress (Fig 17–12).

If dehiscence of a wound should occur, immediate resuturing is the treatment of choice.

Tying the knots is best done with forceps, tying square knots (reef knots) so they lie flat. When working alone, a surgeon's knot, which consists of two loops in the first knot, and one loop in the second knot tied in the opposite direction, will prevent slipping and is useful to pull separated edges together. Figures 17–13 through 17–20 illustrate how a knot is tied with instruments. However, one must be careful *not* to tie

Fig 17–12.—Sutures. **A** and **B,** vertical mattress. **C,** near-far everting suture.

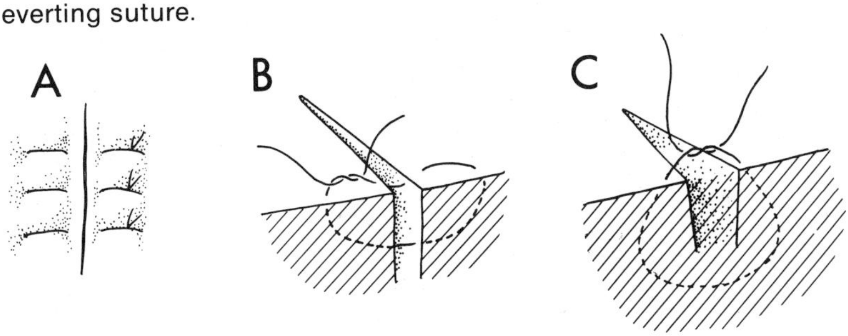

Fig 17–13

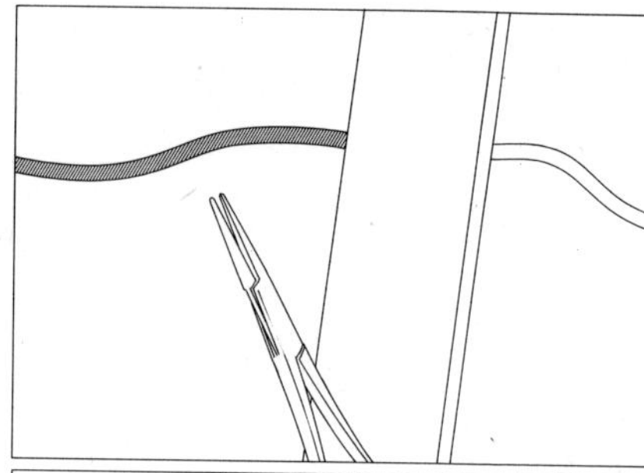

Fig 17–14

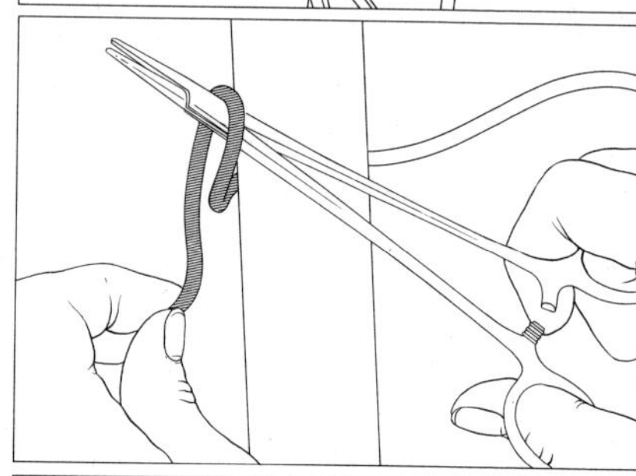

Fig 17–15

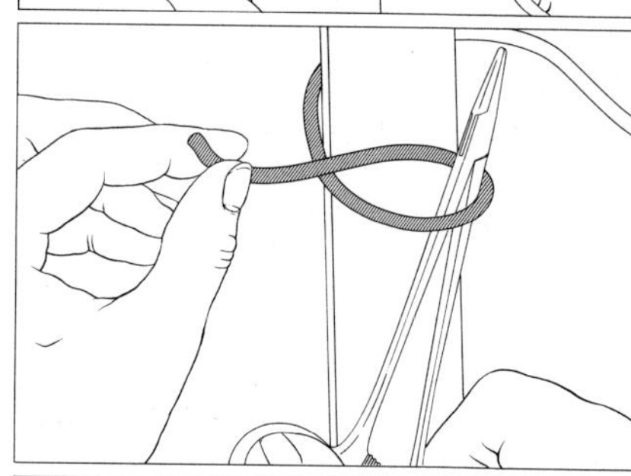

Fig 17–16

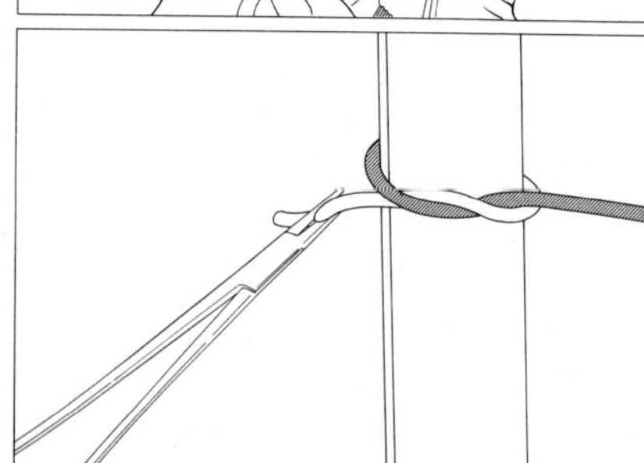

Figs 17–13 to 17–20.—Instrument ties. **Figures 17–13 to 17–16** illustrate the first half of the square knot, the overhand half-hitch.

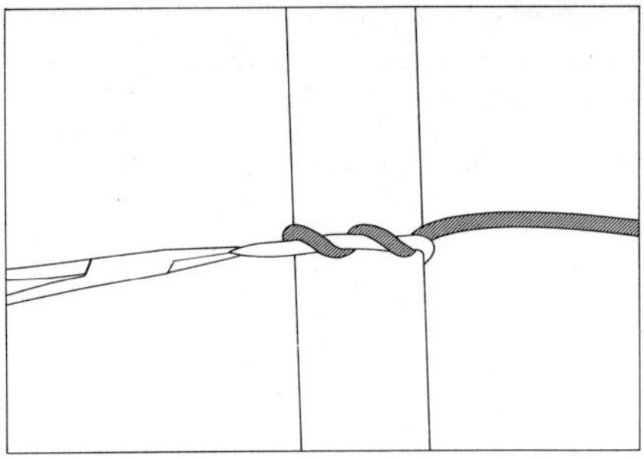

Fig 17–17

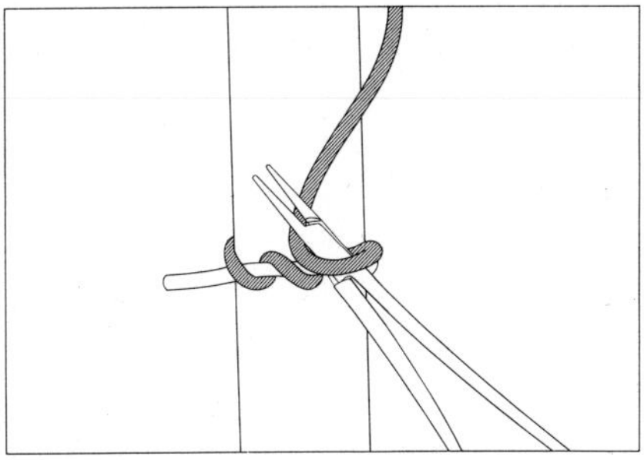

Fig 17–18

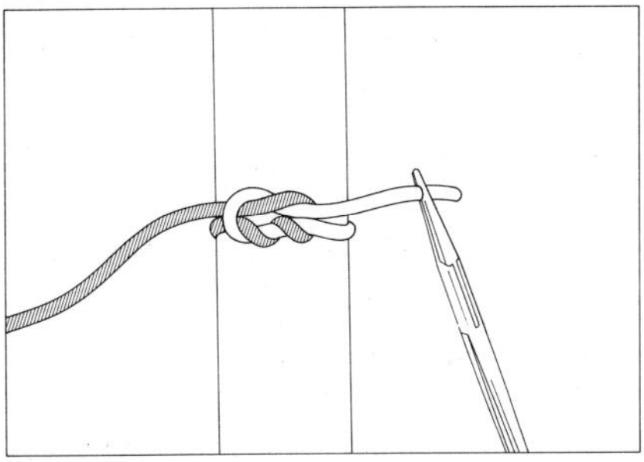

Fig 17–19

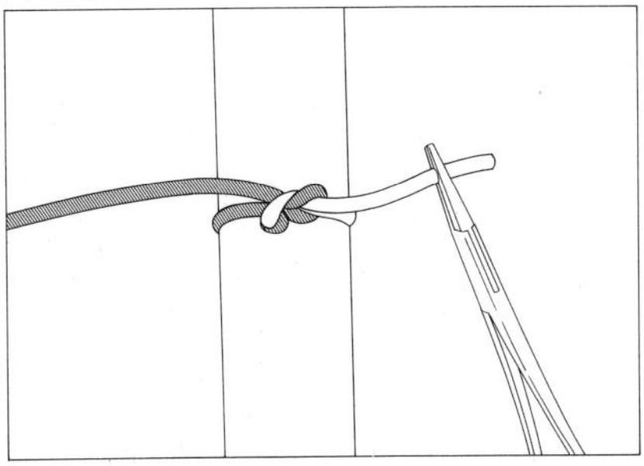

Fig 17–20

When done double twist **(Fig 17–17)** this is the "surgeon's knot." **Figure 17–18** shows the underhand knot to complete the surgeon's knot; **Figure 17–19** illustrates pulling it tight; and **Figure 17–20** shows the completed knot, pulled tight.

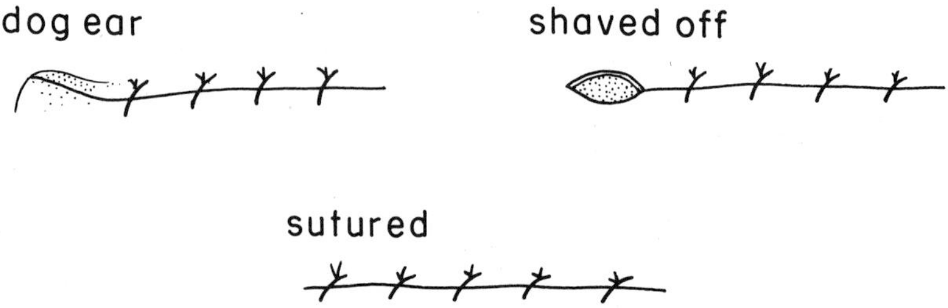

Fig 17–21.—The process of shaving off a dog ear and suturing.

them too tightly, since squeezing the tissues interferes with healing and may leave cross-hatching scars when the inevitable postoperative swelling occurs.

Dog ears, or protruding bits of skin at the end of an excision scar, look somewhat like the bow and stern of a canoe and should be removed before the final sutures are put in. If the dog ear is hooked up with a skin hook and the flat blade of the scalpel shaves it off, the resultant oval defect can be closed with one suture and will give a much smoother result (Fig 17–21).

Suture Removal

Removal depends essentially on common sense. A Little League pitcher will need at least 10 days and Elastoplast strapping for 2 to 3 weeks to prevent his wound from opening up. However, in general, removal of eyelid sutures may be done in 3 days; face 5–7 days; legs 9–10 days; and the soles 2

Fig 17–22.—Reinforcement of wound edges with crisscross overlapped adhesive tape following removal of sutures.

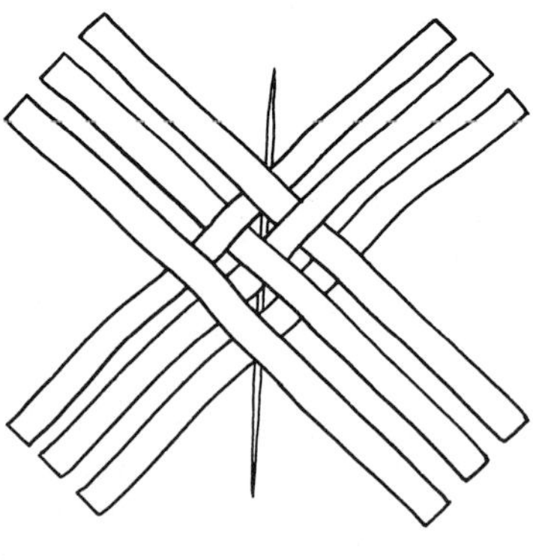

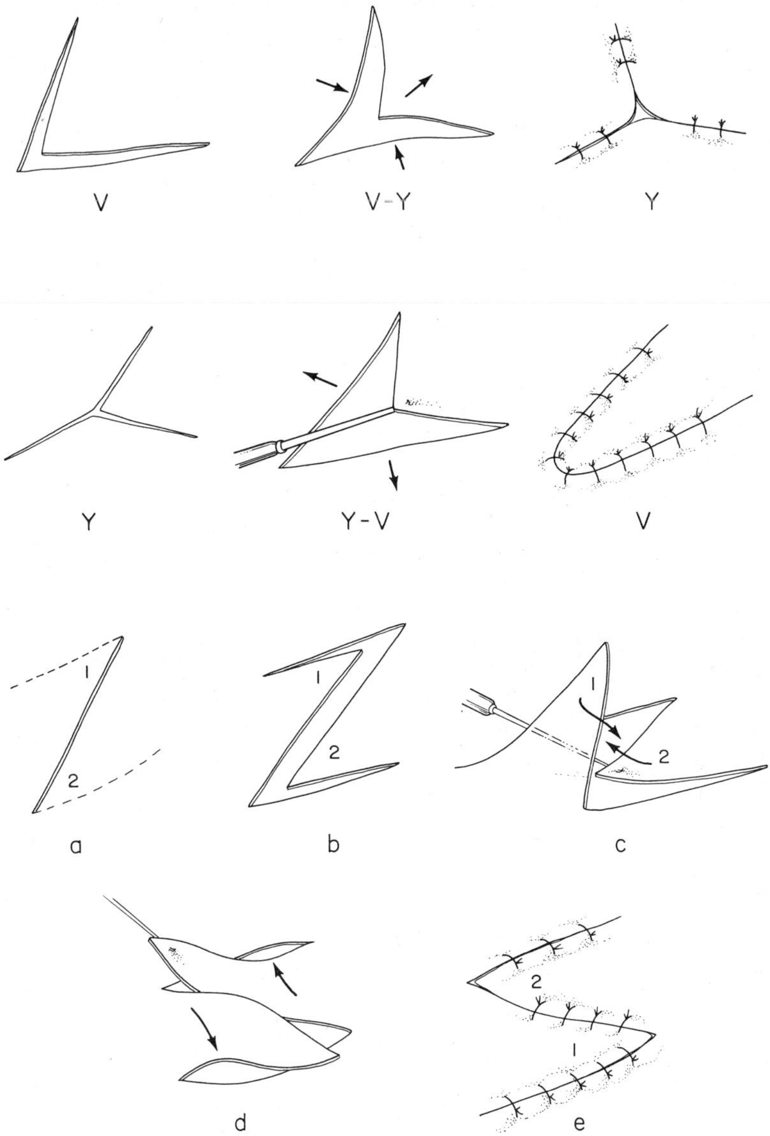

Fig 17–23.—The V-Y-, Y-V- and Z-plasties. (From Epstein, E., et al.: *Skin Surgery* [2d ed.; Philadelphia: Lea & Febiger, 1962], pp. 130–31. Used by permission of the publisher.)

weeks. Retention sutures removed in 24–48 hours is the usual practice. After removal, 3-M strips of perforated sterile adhesive will reinforce the wound edges (Fig 17-22).

Butterfly bandages in my experience do not stick, although perhaps wiping off the skin with ether first would help this.

Pressure dressings *always* help wound healing, and when possible, a *little* pressure such as that obtained with a good gauze pad over the wound, held in place by a strip of Elastoplast, is enough to increase the rate of successful "scarless" healing. In the scalp, Aeroplast can be used. All dressings should be checked 48 hours after surgery. Patients occasionally wear off or pull off the dressings and substitute inadequate ones of their own. The patient should be told not to bathe, as the wound dressing should be kept dry for 5–7 days until all the sutures are removed.

Special techniques such as the V-Y or the "Z" procedures are available for closing defects where relaxation of tissue is desirable, e.g., to prevent ectropion under the lower lid of the eye (Fig 17–23).

A Note on Tattoo Removal

Most physicians who have removed tattoos remember both the way patients beg to have tattoos removed despite the admonition that there will be a scar, and the vehemence with which the patients afterwards decry the results even if very good. Patients must be selected very carefully. The salabrasion technique first described by Crittenden[1] and more recently by Clabaugh[2] may be used successfully. The secret is not to try too hard. A gauze bandage roll with gauze wrapped around it is moistened and dipped in table salt, then rubbed briskly over the tattoo. If the epidermis is first abraded with the rotating steel brush, this is much easier. When small red spots appear, continue rubbing until a uniform redness is seen. Rinse off the salt and apply a dry dressing for 48 hours. A coagulum will form and the inflammatory reaction rejects the pigment over the next few weeks. Antibiotics may prevent sepsis if concern arises. The results are often surprisingly acceptable.

REFERENCES

1. Crittenden, F. M., Jr.: Salabrasion: Removal of tattoos by superficial abrasion with table salt, Cutis 7:295, 1971.
2. Clabaugh, W. A.: Tattoo removal by superficial dermabrasion, Plast. Reconstr. Surg. 55:401, 1975.

SUGGESTED READING

Epstein, E., et al.: *Skin Surgery* (Philadelphia: Lea & Febiger, 1962).

Wise, R. A., and Baker, H. W.: *Surgery of the Head and Neck* (Chicago: Year Book Medical Publishers, Inc., 1962).

Journal of Dermatologic Surgery

18 / Electrosurgery

Electrosurgery

Electrosurgery involves controlled and directed heat in the tissues, which results from the tissues' resistance to the passage of a high-frequency current. Electrocautery, which is used more in the West than in the East, results from the use of a hot wire (electrically heated). Electrolysis is the use of a direct current (galvanic) to release hydrogen at the negative (active) pole, e.g., in epilating hair; whereas electrodesiccation involves monoterminal current (high-voltage, low amp). Electrocoagulation uses biterminal current (low wattage, high amp), and electrocutting current is biterminal (one indifferent, usually undamped tube current) and cuts through tissue like a knife. As far as can be determined, electrocutting current is about the same as cautery.

Electrodesiccation

This is probably the most frequently used modality in the dermatologist's office. Many small growths can be removed by its use. An alternating current having a frequency of 100–10,000 kc is alternating or oscillating so rapidly that no sensation of electric shock is felt when the current is applied to living tissue, but if the current is sufficiently intense, there will be a feeling of warmth. Accordingly, anesthesia with Xylocaine is desirable. Destruction of tissue takes place from the concentration of the current at the tip of the needle, and this is referred to as diathermy or long-wave diathermy current. The corresponding wavelengths are 3,000–30 m.

Electrodesiccation uses the current from the second winding of the coil on a spark-gap machine. This provides fine control of the spark at the tip of the needle, which desiccates the lesion. By multiple insertions into the lesions and by using a heavier current, one can destroy quite large lesions. Control of bleeding is similarly achieved by sparking or actually touching bleeding points; and if curettage is used, desiccation and curettement repeated several times can achieve considerable depth of destruction. It is this method of removal that is used commonly in the treatment of keratoses and epitheliomas, particularly basal cell epitheliomas, since, from the sensation as the curette passes over the tissue, one can tell whether one has most likely achieved normal healthy structures. Spraying this spark across a tissue will gently char the surface, although a current that is strong enough to char or cause tissues to contract may lead to undue puckering of the scar with keloid formation, and adjustment of the settings of the current should, by trial and error, be arranged so that a moderate spark is achieved that does not produce undue scarring. Usually the *on* or *off* control is in a foot switch, although sometimes the switch can be mounted on the handle of the electric needle. Usually electrodesiccation either kills a cell or leaves it unharmed, and it is only an injured cell that causes pain.

Electrocoagulation is tissue coagulation by the use of a biterminal electrode, and this is not much used in dermatology. Sometimes a very low setting may be used for treating spider nevi and telangiectases, or for epilating hair.

Cutting Current

The cutting is produced by a continuous undamped oscillating bipolar current using an indifferent electrode; the feedback occurs through the air. It is an alternating current with a wavelength of 3–30 m or shorter, and is called "short-wave diathermy"—generated for the most part by vacuum tubes. It is usually between 10,000 and 100,000 kc. One may use a knife blade, a loop or a "hockey stick." This cutting current is extremely useful when shaping ala nasi after epitheliomas are removed, or in other words, for brushing away small soft fibromas or simple moles for a superior cosmetic result. Usually the cutting current will coagulate tiny vessels but causes larger vessels to bleed more, so that control of hemorrhage may be more successfully left to the desiccating current.

The postoperative follow-up for all electrosurgery is important, since there is a slightly higher incidence of keloid formation, and the natural tendency for patients is to cover their unhealed wounds with bandages and forget to remove them, leading to moist, juicy and often poorly healing wounds on many occasions, which often leads to the growth of exuberant granulation tissue. This in turn favors the later development of hypertrophic scars. If this occurs, the application of 10% silver nitrate or the occasional touching with the silver nitrate stick usually flattens granulation. The patient should be encouraged to leave the wound open to the air, daubing it with merthiolate or Zephiran only; if because of pressing esthetic considerations, a cover-up is important, the bandage should be trimmed to its narrowest to allow air in from the side. The use of bacitracin or other antibiotic ointments as dressings is occasionally necessary but may lead to moisture; consequently, dressings *must* be changed often or left off at night. Patients should be apprised of the time required for healing, that is, a minimum of 21 days, although the first scab may drop off in 6–12 days. Generally another will form, thinner and more tenacious, which when it drops off, leaves a freshly healed pink scar which is soft and flat. Wounds on the female breasts and the lower extremities take longer to heal. The deltoid and sternal areas are notorious for a very marked tendency to heal with keloidal scarring, as are other areas that receive tension and friction, such as axillary lines and the waist-band region. The patient should be seen 2 months after the surgery to assess the scar. The patient should also be advised that if the scar becomes lumpy or itchy, hard, tender and puckered, the surgeon should be notified at once, since after 7 or 8 months it is no longer easy to reverse the process.

Occasionally a patient or a physician will mistake a lumpy hypertrophic scar for a recurrence of the original lesion, so long-term follow-up is essential. Hypertrophic scars heal with age, and in the case of the occasional depressed scar resulting from electrosurgery, lots of talking, smiling, chewing and isometric facial exercises will pull the skin surface smooth and flat, and the scar will fade.

Electrosurgery is the method of choice for treating spider angiomas, discrete nodules of lymphangioma, all forms of warts, seborrheic keratoses, actinic keratoses, sebaceous adenomas and some histiocytomas. It is useful in treating condyloma acuminata, fibrous fibromas, dermal nevi and other benign lumps and bumps. Dermatofibromas and histiocytomas are better excised and sutured. Basal cell epitheliomas, squamous cell epitheliomas and keratoacanthomas respond well to removal by electrosurgery, and usually to electrodesiccation and curettage. With a good margin and careful follow-up, the cosmetic results are extremely acceptable and the 5-year cure rate is in the 98% range. Pathologic examination will differentiate the invasive and infiltrating types of basal cell epitheliomas from the "en masse" type and guide the therapist to deal very radically with the disseminated and infiltrating type.

The hair should be removed from hairy moles before the mole is removed. Deferring mole removal until all the hair is definitely out gives superior esthetic results.

Epilation

Unsightly hair between men's eyebrows or elsewhere on women's faces can be removed by waxes, depilatories, shaving, plucking and electrolysis (galvanic current) or high-frequency current epilation (spark gap). The best results are achieved by a skilled use of electrical epilation, either electrolysis or high-frequency current.

High-Frequency Current

Any spark-gap machine such as the Cameron (Fig 18–1), Bovie (Fig 18–2) or Hyfrecator (Fig 18–3) can be used. The patient should refrain from plucking hair long enough to permit the hair to grow so the operator can have an indication of the direction of the hair follicle. If the hair gets too long, the patient can clip it with scissors during this waiting period. The face should be well scrubbed and cleaned with 70% alcohol. The patient should be arranged lying down in a good light. The operator should stand or sit comfortably, so that the hand that holds the epilating needle will have easy access to the hair follicle. Anesthesia is usually not necessary, although 1 or 2% Xylocaine can be injected. A gauze square to collect the epilated hair and a well-made pair of epilating forceps should be at hand. In the case of the Bovie or Cameron

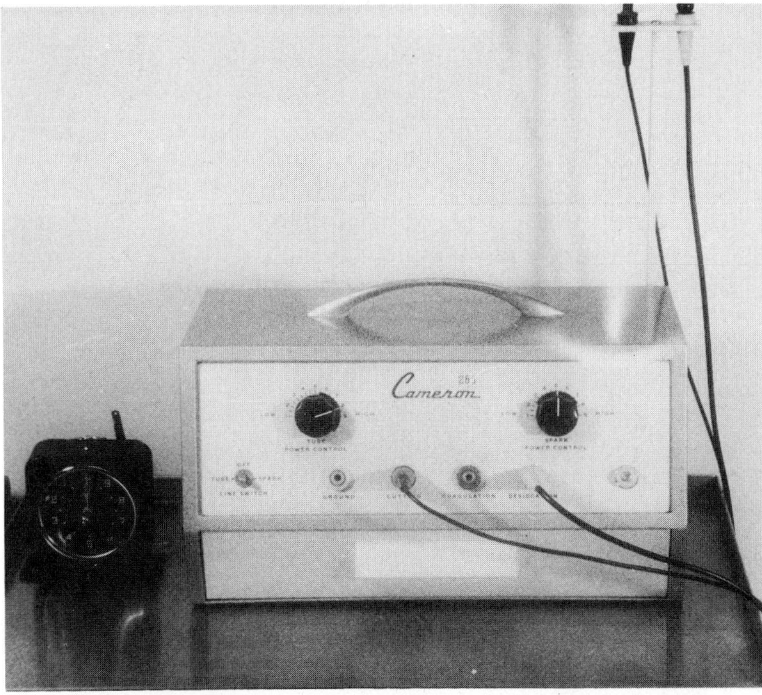

Fig 18–1. – Cameron spark-gap machine.

machine, the indifferent electrode is held by the patient and the switch is turned to "epilation."

The needle is inserted into the hair follicle gently until the bottom is reached, then the current is run for 6 – 10 seconds and the hair gently pulled out. If resistance is encountered, the hair follicle is not yet destroyed and must be retreated. With practice and experience, knowledge of the best setting (usually around 30 in the Bovie) and the length of time required can be obtained for your own machine. If the Hyfrecator is used, set the spark gap by testing against a dampened thumbnail until a minimal spark can be made to jump across. The foot switch controls the time.

Patients can minimize the tendency for the formation of a mild acneform folliculitis after the treatment if ice cubes are

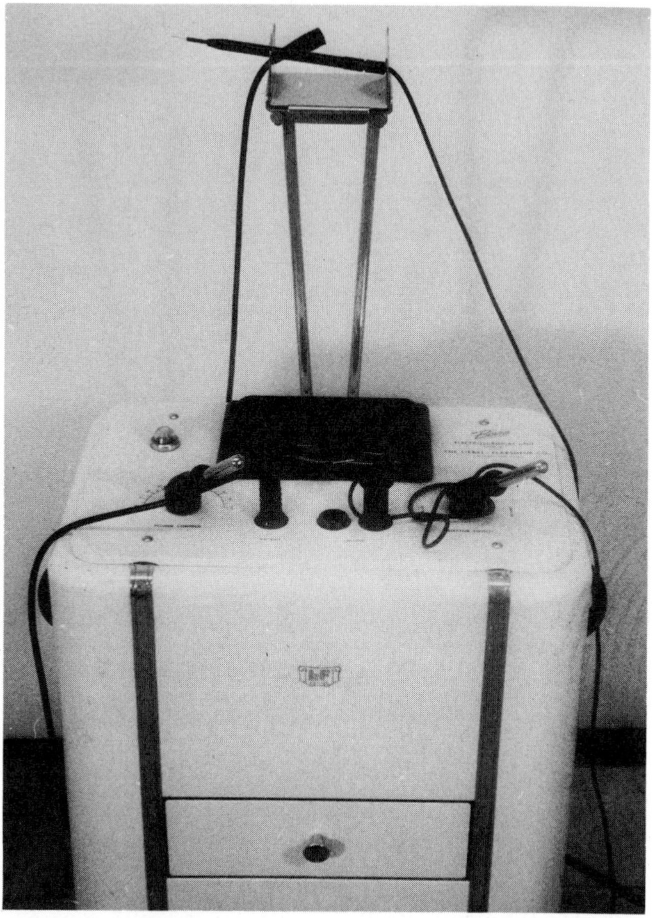

Fig 18–2. – Bovie spark-gap machine.

held against the face for a few minutes and antibiotic lotions or creams are used frequently for the first few days. Removal of hair should be spread out over as wide an area as possible, e.g., only two or three hairs per square centimeter of skin. Only about 20 to 30 hairs are done at each sitting, which can be spaced at 2-week to 2-month intervals.

Most dermatologists will refer their patients requiring

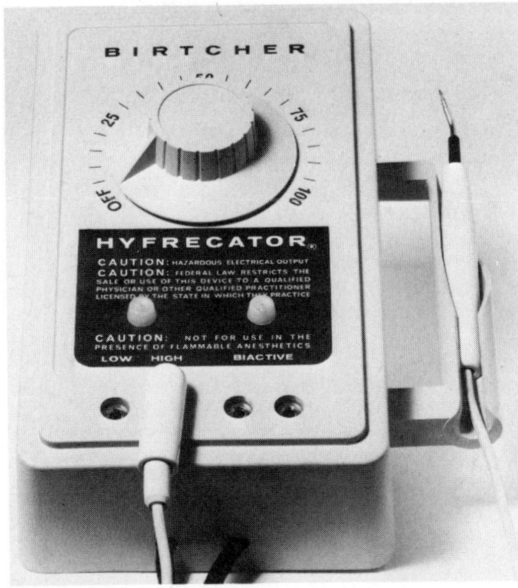

Fig 18–3. – Hyfrecator spark-gap machine.

epilating to a trained electrologist or have one in their own office to do this, but knowledge of the technique and ability to perform it are needed for the occasional hairy mole that requires epilation.

Electrolysis (galvanic)

Various machines can be purchased to convert house current (120 v AC) to direct current, e.g., the Wappler. Battery machines can be purchased or constructed by using a 22.5-v dry cell battery such as is usual with radio receiving sets. If this is hard to obtain, a 45-v battery will do. This is mounted in a wooden box with a rheostat, milliammeter and binding posts, so that the rheostat controls the strength of current. The binding posts must be marked *positive* and *negative* clearly in view of the danger of a steel needle tattooing the hair follicle. If a platinum needle is used, polarity does not matter, but if there is doubt, the negative electrode will turn red litmus paper blue or give off hydrogen peroxide in salt water.

The needle or active electrode is connected to the negative pole, and the sponge is connected to the positive pole. The patient holds the sponge and the needle is inserted as for high-frequency epilation. The current is controlled either by an assistant at the box or by a switch on the handle of the needle holder. It runs at 0.5–1.5 ma, depending on the size of the hair and the patient's pain threshold, for about 30 seconds (until a few seconds after froth appears), when the hair can generally be pulled out with forceps.

Spider angiomas can be treated with the galvanic current until blanching occurs. Usually the current is 1–2 ma, and the time required is variable with the size and depth of the vessels. Similar techniques are used in treating dilated venules and telangiectasis with multiple punctures to the various branches.

Small moles can be removed by transfixing them at the base in a wheel-spoke pattern for 30–60 seconds, and when a little foam comes out, that is usually enough.

Liquid Nitrogen Therapy

Liquid nitrogen can be obtained from companies distributing industrial gases commercially (Linde division of the Union Carbide Corporation). A cotton applicator stick, such as the kind used to apply medication, if loosely wound with cotton at the tip, can be dipped into liquid nitrogen and then applied to the lesions for anywhere from a few seconds to 30 or 40 seconds. Reactions may vary from simple redness to large bullae with various colors of blood in them. It is best to outline the area to be treated, since in the freezing process, outlines are sometimes indistinct and you may be off the target a little. Treatment is sometimes painful, since the liquid nitrogen is at −195.8 C; there is more pain in some people than in others who seem to be sensitive to cold, although generally speaking the pain subsides completely after 24–48 hours and the intense pain subsides within 15 minutes. There is actual freezing of the lesion, and blanching occurs in a small area around the application of the cotton-tipped applicator, which does not need to have pressure applied. This is an excellent form of treatment for warts, keratoses, leukoplakia, creeping eruption and picker's warts (see p. 355) on the back of the neck and scalp and can also be used for hemangiomas and various other lesions such as superficial epitheliomas. If this method of treatment is used for treating periungual warts, Xylocaine anesthesia should be used.

The applicator should be applied for 10–15 seconds for hemangioma and 15–25 seconds for flat warts, early keratoses and other lesions on thin tender skin. For warts on the dorsa of the fingers and hands, 40–60 seconds are needed, and for the palmar and plantar warts, 90–120 seconds, although some palmar warts need much less. Experience and judgment are required to estimate the right duration of freezing. With the Foster Froster (Medical Specialties, New Orleans) perhaps a little less time is needed. The treatment time is figured from when the growth turns white, remembering that it takes about as long to thaw as the time the applicator is held on the lesion. A revisit after 48–72 hours is wise, since occasionally the purple blister alarms the patient. The blister can be perforated if unduly large, although it is best if it can be left alone to scab up and dry off. In the case of plantar warts, perhaps com-

Fig 18–4.—The Foster Froster applicator for liquid nitrogen treatment.

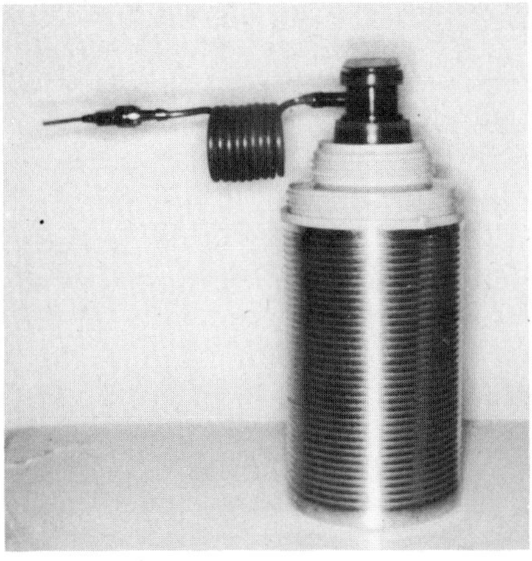

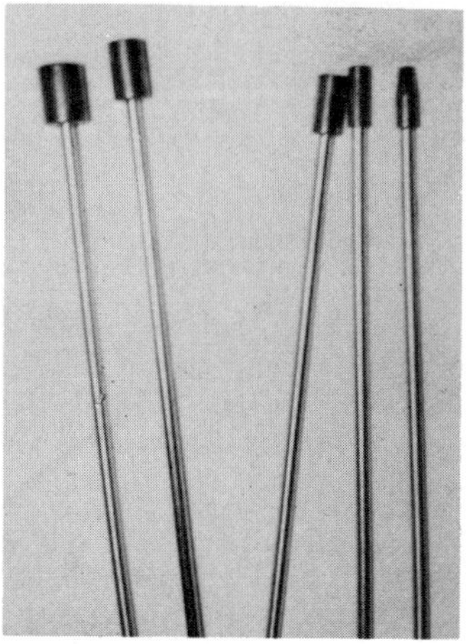

Fig 18–5.—Copper disk applicators for liquid nitrogen treatment.

fort is enhanced by a 40% salicylic acid plaster applied over the blister; this may also be done if the blister is punctured or deroofed.

Seborrheic keratoses can be treated with liquid nitrogen for 45–90 seconds, and actinic keratoses, pitted scars, keloids, especially folliculitis keloidalis and superficial leukoplakia also can be very successfully treated.

The Foster Froster (Medical Specialties, New Orleans) is a very useful hand-held and almost foolproof method of applying liquid nitrogen (Fig 18–4). The jet effect enables a number of actinic keratoses to be treated with about 15 seconds of freezing rapidly. For eyelid epitheliomas and other areas where deeper freezing is desired, the copper applicators are superior (Fig 18–5). They have to be dipped into the liquid nitrogen and should reach equilibrium in about 3 minutes. In the case of flat warts or pitted scars, a rolling or brushing technique using a large applicator often will just hit the high spots, leaving the rest alone.

Cryotherapy

Solid carbon dioxide snow (at–78.5 C) and liquid nitrogen (at –195.8 C) are the agents used by dermatologists to treat superficial lesions. The freezing produces erythema and blister formation within a few hours. Over the next 2 or 3 days, the blister breaks and a crust forms, and if undisturbed this will drop off in 2 or 3 weeks. A shave biopsy can be taken quite painlessly while the lesion is frozen. The freezing will not interfere with the fixing and staining of the tissue.

Pain is felt during the initial freezing, although it is of short duration. The pain recurs with thawing and lasts 15 minutes or so. Then it fades to a dull ache which lasts for two days. The ultimate result of destruction by freezing is usually depigmentation, although the scar is soft and flat and has good texture. Depending on the depth of the destruction and the type of aftercare, it is possible to produce a keloidal scar nevertheless.

Solid carbon dioxide snow can be obtained from ice cream companies and occasionally soda fountains. It can be stored in the refrigerator. A 1-lb cake will last all day, but it is slightly inconvenient to obtain it in this manner. A carbon dioxide cylinder or a carbon dioxide fire extinguisher will supply the gas, and it can be collected in a canvas bag or glove to solidify it. This, then, can be molded in old disposable syringes with the tips cut off to appropriate cylindrical sizes; if a point is desired, it can be shaped with a file. The Kidde apparatus is a fairly satisfactory commercially available kit complete with various sizes of applicators.

Dry ice is extremely useful in treating pigmented nevi that are flat and large. A blotting paper shield can be accurately made by outlining the lesion on the skin with ink, pressing the blotter on, and then cutting out the exact aperture. This shield will permit accurate application. Generally it will require repeated applications to blanch out the pigment. The ice should be pressed on for 6–20 seconds, rarely longer. A superficial blister may form, which will scab and peel. This can be repeated at 3- or 4-week intervals. Small painless shave biopsies can be done while the area is frozen.

For strawberry marks (simple hemangiomas), the carbon dioxide snow should be applied for from a few seconds to 20 seconds, depending upon the depth and turgidity of the hemangioma, with varying degrees of pressure. In general, pressure intensifies the depth of the reaction and has to be used on scalp hemangiomas. Thrombosis of the vessels may continue to complete involution, once started. Several treatments are generally required, however. Spontaneous disappearance is by no means invariable.

Keloids have to be treated for much longer, usually 60–70 seconds, with pressure. Discoid lupus erythematosus can be treated similarly with dry ice, although 10–15 seconds is usually enough.

Carbon Dioxide Slush Treatment

This is of great use in treating keloidal acne scars or pitted acne scars. The method is very often to take three layers of gauze and open them out so that they form a square about 8 in. wide on each side. The ice is crushed in a mortar and pestle and then dumped into this gauze, which is caught up around the edges to form a sort of small bag. (Fig 18–6). Acetone is

Fig 18–6.—Dry ice in a gauze bag.

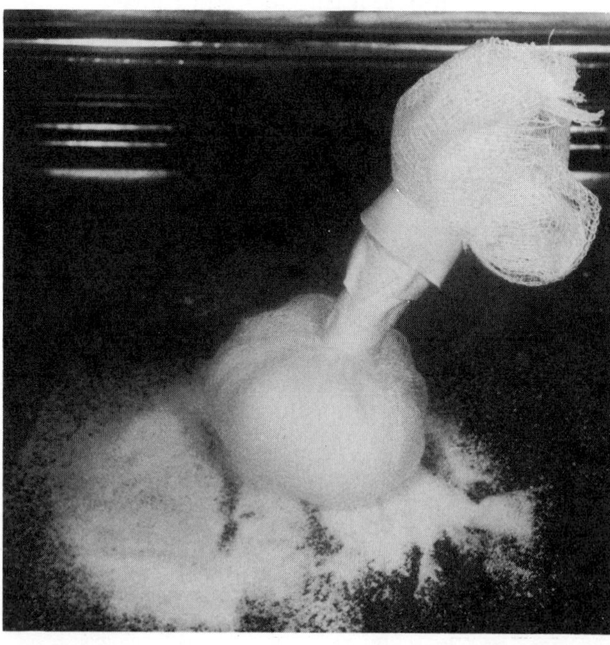

put into the cool mortar and a little sulfur precipitate is dusted in and stirred up with a tongue depressor. The bag held in a towel to protect the fingers of the operator is then dipped into the acetone and smeared across the affected area of the face, moving rapidly to produce erythema and slight peeling of the skin, which result after blanching occurs. The patient should be lying down so that the acetone does not run into his eyes. This is very useful in the treatment of acne vulgaris, rosacea and scarring, but it should be carefully done because the first treatment very often produces quite a severe edematous reaction in sensitive skins and may lead to pigmentary changes, especially in brunettes. It is our practice to do it at intervals of 2 to 3 weeks for a total of five or six treatments.

Many dermatologists have discontinued using carbon dioxide slush for acne scars, preferring dermabrasion. Unless you are doing dermabrasion fairly frequently, I believe you should refer your patients to a physician who *is* doing it all the time.

19 / Tumors of the Skin

Epidermal Tumors

VERRUCOUS NEVI.—Linear warty streaks, patches or whorls, often resembling seborrheic keratoses, are difficult to remove without scarring. Removal that is too superficial invites recurrence. Surgical excision, electrodesiccation and cryosurgery with liquid nitrogen can be used; the choice, to some extent, depends on the location of the nevus.

DERMATOSIS PAPULOSA NIGRA.—Pinhead-size black papules form on the cheeks, usually in black people. The papules respond to light electrodesiccation with surprisingly little tendency to scar.

SEBORRHEIC KERATOSES.—These greasy "stuck-on" shiny plaques on the temples, trunk and sides of the neck are best removed by electrodesiccation and curettage. (See p. 174, PCAD.) Liquid nitrogen treatment is less easy to use here because of the thickness of the lesion. In very numerous keratoses, ethyl chloride spray anesthesia (Fig 19–1) followed by quick curettage while frozen, and then hemostasis by trichloracetic acid or Monsell's solution (ferric subsulfate solution—J. T. Baker Chemical Company) are speedier.

ACTINIC KERATOSES.—Actinic skin; sailor, rancher and farmer skin; solar keratoses and senile keratoses are all the same. This is a precancerous lesion and is often found in the fair-skinned on the hands and face. One hundred percent trichloracetic acid, electrodesiccation and curettage are the methods of treatment. The 5-FU preparation rubbed in twice daily for a month produces an inflammatory reaction that leads to a scarless disappearance of these keratoses; this is a marked advance in the management of the repentant sun lover.

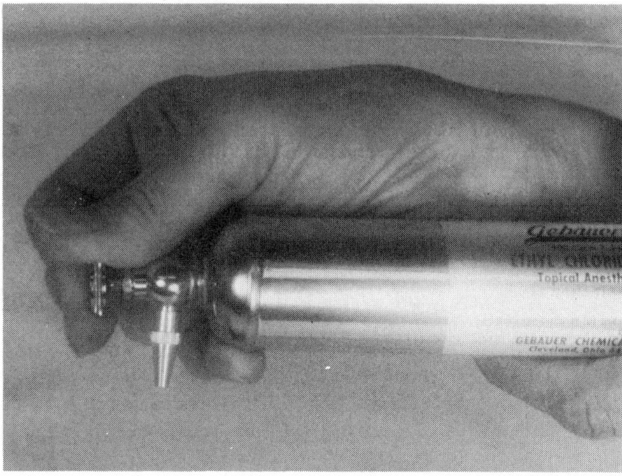

Fig 19–1.—The Gebauer metal container for ethyl chloride produces a fine spray for local freezing.

KERATOACANTHOMA.—Self-healing epithelioma of Smith is a pseudocarcinomatous hyperplasia that grows rapidly to 1–2 cm within several months and remains as a skin-colored nodule with a keratin-filled central crater. Virus-like inclusions have been demonstrated. Involution occurs spontaneously apparently, but because of the risk of error, removal by electrosurgery or surgical excision is wise. Ten percent podophyllin ointment applied under occlusion in the office daily has produced cure.

CUTANEOUS HORNS.—These occur most commonly in elderly people on the cheeks or temples. They occasionally occur in the genital region, and it is hard to say whether seborrhea or sun exposure is the major predisposing factor since both conditions seem to play a role. Occasionally changes in the base suggest squamous cell carcinoma, so they always should be quite thoroughly removed.

BASAL CELL EPITHELIOMA.—These epitheliomas are pearly nodules with rolled borders over which course telangiectases. (See pp. 175–181, PCAD.) They occur most commonly on the face in sun lovers. Uncared-for seborrheic skin seems to be predisposing, and the usual duration before seeing the dermatologist is years. The epitheliomas are usually slow-growing. They can be of several clinical types, e.g., morphealike epithelioma, which is best excised, although it is reported to respond well to radiotherapy. I have not found this to be the case.

Superficial pagetoid, button-like, pigmented and rodent ulcer and *adenoid cystic* exhibit the waxy characteristics and respond well to electrodessication and curettage, x-ray therapy or surgical excision. Pathologically all of these can be grouped as "en masse" or "infiltrative" depending on whether the tissue section shows strands of basal cells infiltrating in an invasive manner into the surrounding tissue, much like the tentacles of an octopus. This last infiltrative basal cell epithelioma is the one that produces the repeated recurrences and is a prime candidate for the controlled (repeated marked frozen sections) chemosurgical excision techniques of Mohs. If more than three recurrences develop, the patient should be referred *not* to a plastic surgeon (who may be unfamiliar with the concept of an inflltrative basal cell epithelioma), but to someone skilled in performing the Mohs technique.

Basosquamous cell epitheliomas should be treated like basal cell epitheliomas.

Intraepidermic multiple superficial basal cell epitheliomas, which often occur in patients fed arsenic as children, similarly respond well to electrodesiccation and curettage, or radiation or surgery. Sometimes one treatment of 1,200 rad at 80 kv unfiltered is enough. Routine x-ray treatment of most basal cell epitheliomas consists of lead shielding to a margin of 5–10 mm around the growth and x-rays at 100 kv unfiltered with a half-value layer of 0.9 mm aluminum, 600 rad three times a week for six treatments at a tube-skin distance of 20 cm using a glass-tipped cone. (A maximum of around 3,500 rad is average.)

SQUAMOUS CELL CARCINOMA.—Presenting as a warty fast-growing nodule on hand, lip, ear or face, this carcinoma has a base that is usually indurated and rounded and may be dusky red or purple. Crusted ulcerations may occur. If left untreated, metastases will occur sooner from tumors at mucocutaneous junctions. Anaplasia is not unknown, especially at sites of radiodermatitis, and rapid removal is imperative.

Varieties include *Paget's disease of the nipple,* which is indicative of mammary duct carcinoma and requires mastectomy. An "eczema" of the nipple requires a biopsy. *Bowen's disease,* which is intraepidermic carcinoma in situ, is often hard to differentiate from the multiple superficial basal cell epitheliomas. The "permanence" of these lesions should give rise to suspicion, although the clinical appearance in general is not hard to recognize. Electrodesiccation and curettage, excision and cryotherapy are the methods of choice.

Erythroplasia of Queyrat, a velvety erythema of the glans penis or vulva, is essentially Bowen's disease of the mucosa. The diagnosis should be pathologically confirmed since some cases of chronic balanitis can mimic the condition. The therapy of choice is 5-FU, according to W. M. Honeycutt.[1] Electrodessication is good, too. Three patients were completely cleared with topical 5-FU treatment.[2, 3]

Dermal Tumors

Angiomatous Nevi

PORT WINE STAIN.—Capillary hemangioma is best treated by Covermark (Lydia O'Leary, New York City).

HEMANGIOMA SIMPLEX.—A strawberry mark does not always appear at birth, but may appear weeks later. It involutes spontaneously in more than half the cases, but picking which ones will involute is a difficult trick. It often occurs in premature babies. (See p. 168, PCAD.) Treatment with carbon dioxide snow for 30–40 seconds in inconspicuous areas is effective.

CAVERNOUS HEMANGIOMA.—A spongy swelling with red or purple skin overlying may have varying amounts of fibrous or lymphatic tissue within. Compressibility indicates large vessels, which can be injected with 1–2 cc of sclerosing solution to produce rapid involution. Spontaneous involution occurs during a 5-year period or longer in more than half the cases. Growth may be alarming in the patient up to one year of age, when it usually ceases, while susceptibility to involution from radium lessens after one year of age. Radium or x-ray therapy in small doses produces the best clinical results. In deep cavernous angiomas that do not overlie sensitive structures (e.g., the eyelid or genitals), filtered radiation using 200 rad monthly for six times is effective. Gamma-ray therapy with radium plaques filtered with 2-mm-thick brass trays and rubber over this to cut out the characteristic radiation from the brass, applied at contact, is excellent therapy. However, fear of sequelae on the part of the general public and the highly specialized skills and knowledge required make the use of gamma-ray therapy much less common than formerly. In problem cases, the risks of future late sequelae (e.g., thyroid tumor) must be frankly and thoroughly discussed with informed parents. Radium therapy should be done only by those well trained in its use. It is being used less and less.

Surgical excision can exsanguinate a child if the angioma is large. However, surgical excision can be of great assistance in areas where the abundant stretchable skin of the infant permits rapid closure. Short courses of steroid treatment are reputed to be effective in inducing resolution, though most of the recent reports of this technique in the German literature concern liver hemangioma.[4]

SPIDER NEVUS.—Telangiectasia and stellar nevus are most often seen in old people and babies, in pregnant women and in persons with alcoholic cirrhosis and other liver diseases. These nevi are best blipped with a low spark and fine needle, or negative pole of the galvanic electrolysis apparatus. However, the central vessel must be destroyed since the angioma will blanch from the edema of a near-miss and recur a few days later. Retreatment should be planned therefore approximately 6 weeks later.

SENILE ANGIOMAS.—Ruby spots are usually on the trunk. These are of no significance other than a minor cosmetic one. Electrosurgical destruction is the treatment of choice.

VENOUS ANGIOMAS.—These are usually on the lip in older people. They can mimic a melanoma, though are easily destroyed by electrodesiccation. They bleed profusely when pricked.

ANGIOKERATOMA.—All varieties respond well to either cryosurgery or electrodesiccation.

Lymphatic Nevi

LYMPHANGIOMA CIRCUMSCRIPTUM.—Grouped deep-seated vesicles ("frog spawn") in the groin, axilla and tongue secrete lymph if pricked. Excision or deep electrodesiccation can cure them.

Vascular Tumors

GLOMUS TUMORS.—These are very painful and require complete excision.

KAPOSI'S MULTIPLE IDIOPATHIC HEMORRHAGIC SARCOMA.—Typically, violaceous plaques and nodules on the foot and ankle initiate the disease, which appears to consist of multiple new growths rather than metastases. Telangiectatic cystic lesions occur on and around the lesions. (See p. 184, PCAD.) Edema from lymphatic infiltration may occur. Involvement of viscera occurs as a late manifestation, and the disease may eventually end as a lymphoblastoma or a reticulum cell sarcoma. Meanwhile it appears to be exquisitely chronic and radioresponsive to small doses of radiation given by experts. *Sun*bathing helps. Vinblastine is helpful in treating those with visceral involvement, using 0.1 mg/kg given piggyback intravenously weekly (watch for leukopenia).[5]

Fibromas

HISTIOCYTOMA.—Also called fibroma durum, noduli cutanei, nodular subepidermal fibrosis, dermatofibroma lenticulari and sclerosing hemangioma, a histiocytoma is a single round or ovoid purplish nodule which feels larger and deeper than it looks. It is firmly attached to its overlying skin, which may have a slight central dell. It occurs mostly on the shaved legs of women and is probably the result of some granulomatous change resulting from either an insect bite or a shaving folliculitis long since forgotten. It never seems to grow larger than 1.5 cm in diameter, and it never becomes malignant. Occasional mild itching is the only symptom. Histiocytomas are better left alone, but if removal is attempted, it must be wide surgical excision since recurrence with scarring is not uncommon. Cryotherapy with 60–90 seconds of liquid nitrogen treatment often clears these, although it leaves a white spot occasionally.

FIBROMA MOLLE.—The soft dome-shaped tumors of normal skin color appearing on the faces of middle-aged women (and men) are benign, unsightly growths, usually removed with elegance by electrocutting current, smoothing them down to blend with the surrounding skin. They are of no importance.

KELOIDS.—Hypertrophic scars (fibrotic scars) follow burns, scalds, electrosurgery on the chest, trauma and tension on any scar. They are occasionally very tender and always unsightly. Blacks seem to develop them most easily. Treatment of choice is carbon dioxide snow block applied through a blotting paper shield cut to surround the keloid for 60–90 seconds with pressure. Anything shorter than 60 seconds is just teasing it. Liquid nitrogen application with copper disks is also effective. Xylocaine applied underneath may be needed if the treatment hurts too much. The pain is worse when thawing occurs, and Empirin with codeine (Empirin compound Tabs #3, Burroughs & Wellcome, containing one-half grain of codeine each) may be prescribed. Intralesional injection of Kenalog suspension mixed with Wydase (hyaluronidase—Wyeth) is effective if a dental syringe with finger grips is used and it is carefully and thoroughly done (with or without fluoroethyl spray). Immediate postoperative treatment of known keloid-formers with a 6- to 8-week oral steroid regimen will often prevent keloids, e.g., in gallbladder scars. If plastic excision of keloids is attempted, steroid and x-ray treatment 1 week before and 1 week (and later) after the operation is the preferred treatment.

SKIN TAGS OF THE NECK (ACROCHORDON).—Pinhead or larger in size, these tags are often pedunculated fibromas occurring at the sides of the neck in women. They are also seen in the axillae and around the eyelids. Occasionally flat warts and seborrheic keratoses will occur in this distribution. Clipping and blipping are the treatment of choice, using Xylocaine anesthesia.

SUBUNGUAL FIBROMAS.—Fibromas appear beside the nail in fingers and toes as small pinkish growths. Usually unilateral and solitary, if allowed to progress they will displace the nail upward and backward and become bony hard; pressure from the shoe produces pain. Scooping them out with a small sharp strong curette or surgical excision is the method of choice.

CHONDRODERMATITIS NODULARIS CHRONICA HELICIS.—This is probably a form of delayed reaction to frostbite or other injury, e.g., sunburn. It consists of a cornlike cartilaginous spur on the inner rim of the ear in men, which is exquisitely tender and often interferes with sleep and using the telephone. Cure is by careful excision, being sure to take the wedge of cartilage and make the edges of the remaining cartilage *very* smooth to prevent the development of a new nodule at the excision margin.

Lipoma

Fatty tissue, usually lobulated and encapsulated with connective tissue strands, forms subcutaneously, most commonly on the trunk, as small discrete moveable lumps. Movement of the skin over them often produces a traction dimple. They must be considered benign and usually are easily excised. They are not to be confused with Dercum's disease in large-hipped women (adiposis dolorosa).

Adnexal Tumors

Syringoma, steatocystoma multiplex, eccrine poroma, spiradenoma, hidradenoma, myoepithelioma, and adenoacanthoma of sweat glands. These are all benign and often diagnosed only on biopsy. However, there are several disorders of real importance, such as carcinoma of sweat glands, which regularly metastasize. Carcinoma of sweat glands often looks like a basal cell epithelioma, although it can proliferate, and resembles dermatofibroma sarcoma protuberans when occurring in the groin or axilla. Wide excision is the treatment of choice. *Adenocarcinomas of sebaceous glands* occur chiefly in the lids, and these too metastasize. Other adnexal tumors of moderate importance are cylindromas (turban tumors), which occur in women and are rubbery, lobulated, numerous and familial. They can be fairly easily cured by excision with either scalpel or electrosurgery. *Trichoepithelioma* looks like syringocystadenoma clinically and occurs around the eyelids. It is easily cured by electrosurgery using a fine needle and a low current. Basal cell nevi are simply basal cell epitheliomas, though curious, and must be treated similarly.

Metastatic Tumors

On many occasions an unexplained lump in the skin, when biopsied, gives the first clue to a hitherto unknown internal malignancy. This may be true of malignant melanoma, hypernephroma and adenocarcinoma of the gut, prostate, lung, kidney and stomach. The most common metastases in the skin (often the scalp) result from mammary carcinoma. The histology is typical of breast malignancy. Leathery infiltration of the skin of the postoperative mastectomy area is another form of metastatic carcinoma which progresses to "cancer en cuirasse." Rarely does an "erysipeloid" hot erythematous infiltration result from invasion of the subpapillary lymphatics.

Treatment of Skin Tumors

In weather-beaten sailors and farmers exhibiting much actinic damage, the easiest way to handle their periodic basal cell epitheliomas (or squamous cell carcinomas) is by desiccation and curettage. However, in areas such as the neck, midcheek, bridge of the nose, midforehead and preauricular region, there are times when scalpel excision and suture give a superior final result. In elderly patients, radiotherapy gives quite satisfactory results and may be the method of choice in areas where excision without grafting is impractical, e.g., on the tip of the nose and the inner canthus of the eye. A shrewd assessment of the depth of the tumor should be made, and the appropriate hardness of radiation selected. The power to penetrate varies with the kilovoltage, and the filter will filter out the soft rays, selecting harder-quality radiation. The further the tube is from the skin, the more parallel the rays become, and the higher the percentage of rays that will penetrate. At a greater distance, surface irregularities mean less and dosage variation is less, too.

It is not good practice to generalize about x-ray dosage, but it is our practice to use 20 cm tube–skin distance with glass-tipped cones and 100 kv, 5 ma unfiltered (half-value layer of approximately 1 mm aluminum) radiation for the treatment of all basal cell epitheliomas. The dose is between 650 and 750 rad, given three times a week for a total of six doses (3,900–4,500 rad total). The shielding is to within 1 cm of the margin in tumors larger than 1.0 cm in diameter and about half the diameter of the tumor, or a minimum of 5 mm when smaller. This shielding is a little on the narrow side and should not be too rigidly adhered to, but it suffices as a guide. The dosage used is a good deal lower than that recommended by many textbooks, but it is my feeling that if this amount of radiation fails to eradicate an epithelioma, 8,000–10,000 rad probably will not do it either and the patient requires *other* means of therapy. The sequelae over 20 years with this dosage are inconsequential, whereas higher dosages may lead to late difficulties and even atrophic changes if applied over cartilage, e.g., on the tip of the nose.

Simple surgical excision and suture of most skin cancers give a satisfactory cosmetic result if attention is paid to the lines of tension in the facial skin. Cross-hatching, with the point of the Xylocaine needle making two or three transverse scratches across the proposed excision lines, will enable proper apposition of the wound edges to be made when closing. The excised wedge of tissue should be about four times as long as it is wide, and undercutting will facilitate closure. If tension is a problem, 000 retention sutures removed in 48 hours will take the strain off the 00000 (5-0) sutures used to approximate the edges. If dog ears occur at the ends of the wound, clip them off with either a flat blade or a straight sharp scissors, and suture or leave them to granulate, but do it at the time.

Electrosurgery with electrodesiccation and curettage, the chief method, should be done repeatedly over the tumor-bearing area until the texture of the curetted skin indicates healthy tissue. A sharp curette will pick up tumor-bearing areas with great accuracy. If the location of the scar requires consideration for cosmetic elegance (e.g., the ala nasi), then a little sculpturing with the electrocutting current is advisable to produce an inconspicuous scar.

Pigmented Moles

There are essentially five kinds of pigmented nevi: (1) the epidermal nevus or lentigo, (2) the junction nevus at the epidermodermal junction, (3) the dermal nevus in the dermis,(4) the compound nevus, with dermal and junctional elements, with or without hair, and (5) the blue nevus, which is made up of spindle-shaped melanoblasts deep in the dermis and which is usually of such a distinct slatelike color that diagnosis is easy.

There is a sixth type of pigmented mole, the protuberant polypoid papilloma, which is usually flaccid with a narrow stalk and most often located in the axilla and groin. Often actually a fibroma, this occasionally contains nevus cells and so should be classified with the moles. Clip and blip is the proper removal technique.

The decision as to which moles should be excised completely, which should be removed with a superficial cosmetically acceptable result, which should be left alone and which should have a small excision biopsy can be made by physicians only after many years of experience looking at moles and their microscopic tissue. In general, when in doubt, perform a biopsy. If the patient is concerned and if he or she is having *any* symptoms from a mole, the tissue must be examined microscopically. Trust your clinical judgment; in general it is reliable.

From the therapeutic viewpoint, the pigmented moles that are subject to irritation by friction of clothing, or in other ways, can degenerate and become malignant. This is much more apt to occur with junction nevi. It has been the impression of numerous observers that sudden severe sun exposure (e.g., northern people vacationing in the Caribbean in February) may initiate malignant melanomas at the site of *no* preexisting junction nevi. This probably accounts for about 25% of all malignant melanomas. The late Doctor McNeer used to say "hazel eyes" predispose;[6] and I agree.

JUNCTION NEVI.—These can arise at birth or later; pigmented nevi located on the genitals, palms and soles are usually junction nevi. If the nevus is smooth, hairless, flat or only slightly raised and light to dark brown, with a "superficial" look to it, it is probably a junction nevus. If it is enlarging, especially in a pregnant woman, it should be excised. If it shows any of the usual signs of increased activity, such as growth, increase in depth of pigment, change of shape, crusting or flaking on its surface, itching or repeated easy irritation, it should be excised. If the junction nevus is inactive or is a cosmetic hazard, it may be removed by any of the usual methods of cryotherapy with liquid nitrogen; carbon dioxide snow pencil applied for 10–30 seconds, depending on the apparent thickness; electrosurgery (cutting current has a slight tendency to stimulate the return of pigment in the scar, and patients should be warned); or scissors or scalpel excision. In choosing the method of removal, tempering justice with mercy, in a woman especially, the physician should consider the cosmetic result. Lentigo or freckle-like nevi can be treated similarly, cryotherapy having much less tendency to permit pigment return later and less tendency to form keloids. A nice way to excise a superficial junction nevus is to balloon it up with Xylocaine, hold it with the fingers of the left hand and snip it off with sharp curved scissors. This is sufficient for a pathology exam, and the tiny scar is most acceptable.

COMPOUND OR DERMAL NEVI.—These nevi can be excised with scalpel or punch, though often this later-spreading excision scar is a poor cosmetic exchange. Treatment with cutting current in a mature patient gives satisfactory cosmetic results, though since occasionally a bit of the mole is left behind to grow again, this may have to be revised a few months or years later and smoothed down again. Keloids form with greater frequency in patients between the ages of 11 and 18, so removal of such moles is better postponed until after age 19 unless pressing reasons, such as daily shaving, make an earlier removal desirable. If the mole is hairy, hair should be removed by electrolysis epilation every 2 months until sure that all hairs are out, then the cutting current (or galvanic electrolysis transfixion) may be performed. After removal, the scar will be especially sun-sensitive for a few months, and sunscreens should be used.

BLUE NEVI.—These should be excised or left alone. Malignant change is rare, but can occur.

JUVENILE MELANOMA ("SPINDLE CELL NEVUS").—Characteristically these nevi consist of sudden rapid growth of a mole in an adolescent or a child approaching adolescence, with many of the features of malignant change both clinically and microscopically. (See p. 167, PCAD.) Single wide local excision suffices to cure them. Melanomas can occur in babies and in adults well past adolescence, and their correct assessment may test the pathologist's skill. A consensus is usually wise.

MALIGNANT MELANOMA.—These usually arise from junction nevi, but may also less commonly arise from intradermal and compound nevi or from apparently normal skin. They are one of the most malignant of all tumors and require wide and extensive surgical intervention by skilled surgeons. Recognition is not difficult for the physician, who often sees the patient for the first time when dissemination has already occurred. The superficial spreading melanoma may be recognized by the disorderliness of the outline, color and surface texture, particularly multiple colors (blue, gray, brown, red, black, white). (See pp. 182–183, PCAD.) Regression, leaving white areas, is suspicious, especially when a white halo forms.[7] The cardinal signs of a nonhealing sore, deepening of pigment, enlargement often with pseudopod-like projections at the margin, bleeding and ulceration, and finally satellite lesions, with regional lymph gland enlargement, give the show away. If a biopsy is taken, it should be all-inclusive with scalpel excision and suture.

Any woman who has had surgery for a malignant melanoma should never become pregnant. Malignant melanomas seem to run in families, and if there is a family history, the index of suspicion should be high.

Clark's levels II to V classification has made prognosis of malignant melanoma according to depth of infiltrate much more accurate than formerly. Recently a more objective histologic system has been introduced, using an ocular micrometer in the microscope eyepiece and measuring from the granular layer to the deepest extent of the tumor. A width greater than 0.75 mm carries a more grave prognosis.

Direct injection of pox virus into the metastases of malignant melanoma has resulted in temporary remission according to Malcolm M. Lane Brown of Sydney, Australia.[9]

LENTIGO MALIGNA.—Hutchinson's malignant freckle is usually a slowly enlarging dark brown or black freckle on the cheek of an elderly patient, which microscopically is malignant melanoma, but which clinically runs an essentially benign course for years (up to 25) until eventually real malignant melanoma supervenes. It can be cured by complete though superficial removal by any satisfactory method, including electrodesiccation.

SUBUNGUAL MELANOMA.—Such a melanoma should be biopsied and diagnosed early, since cure by amputation of the finger is a favorable outcome in most cases. Sometimes it is mistaken for a fungus infection. It usually starts as a light brown spot on the lateral nail fold.

BATHING-TRUNK NEVI.—In large hairy moles that have extensive dark pigment with a blackish tint, the danger of the patient experiencing malignant degeneration even before puberty is great. Excision and flap or graft by a good plastic surgeon is the method of choice. Andrews has used cryotherapy successfully for inoperable cases.[8]

MONGOLIAN SPOT.—This is a blue nevus over the sacrum in dark-skinned newborns. It usually fades.

REFERENCES

1. Honeycutt, W. M.: 5-FU in treatment of erythroplasia of Queyrat, Derm. News (no. 7), 1969.
2. Goette, D. K., Elgart, M., and DeVillez, R. L.: : Erythroplasia of Queyrat treatment with topically applied fluorouracil, J.A.M.A. 232:934, 1975.
3. Goette, D. K.: Erythroplasia of Queyrat treatment with topically applied fluorouracil, Arch. Dermatol. 110:271, 1974.
4. Zarem, H. A., and Edgerton, M. T.: Induced resolution of cavernous hemangioma following prednisolone therapy, Plast. Reconstr. Surg. 39:76, 1967.
5. Tucker, S. B., and Winkelman, R. K.: Treatment of Kaposi sarcoma with vinblastine, Arch. Dermatol. 112:958, 1976.
6. McNeer, G., and Das Gupta, J.: Prognosis in malignant melanoma, Surgery 56:512, 1964.
7. Clark, W. H., Jr., and Mihm, M. C., Jr.: Lentigo maligna and lentigo-maligna melanomas, Am. J. Path. 55:39, 1969.
8. Domonkos, A. N.: *Andrews' Diseases of the Skin* (6th ed.; Philadelphia: W. B. Saunders Co., 1971), p. 815.
9. Brown, M. M. L., and Milton, G. W.: The limited role of attenuated smallpox virus in the management of advanced malignant melanoma, N. Z. J. Surg. 35:286, 1966.

20 / X-ray Treatment

Electrons are released from the filament in a vacuum tube, and these negatively charged particles are driven with great force (when a high voltage is applied across the tube) across to the anode target disk. The electrons smash against this target and bounce off as x-rays (Fig 20–1). The current or rate of flow of electrons is controlled by the milliamperage, usually 5 ma in x-rays used in dermatology. The force with which the electrons hit the target and bounce off is determined by the kilovoltage (similar to the water pressure behind a tap), which will produce "harder" (that is, more penetrating) rays when there is a higher kilovoltage. The inverse square law holds true for all radiation, assuming it to come from a point source; that is, the intensity varies inversely with the square of the distance. (If you cut the distance in half, you quadruple the intensity.) So the distance must be measured accurately. The further the tube is from the target, the more parallel the rays will become and possibly a little harder and therefore more penetrating. By inserting filters, the soft rays can be blocked, allowing only the harder rays to penetrate, though at a slower rate.

X-ray Treatment

The x-rays hitting tissue will set up secondary radiation or back scatter, which may enhance the "air-dose" by 20–30% (usually). If the tube is close to the skin, say 15 cm, the peripheral margins of the treated field (unshielded, that is) may receive only 50% of the dose the center gets. However, if the tube–skin distance (TSD) is 30 cm, the margins get 80% of the dose or so. So in treating large fields, either overlap or increased TSD is usually needed to produce even dosage.

The depth of the lesion is important, especially when treating epitheliomas, where it is important to reach the deep cells

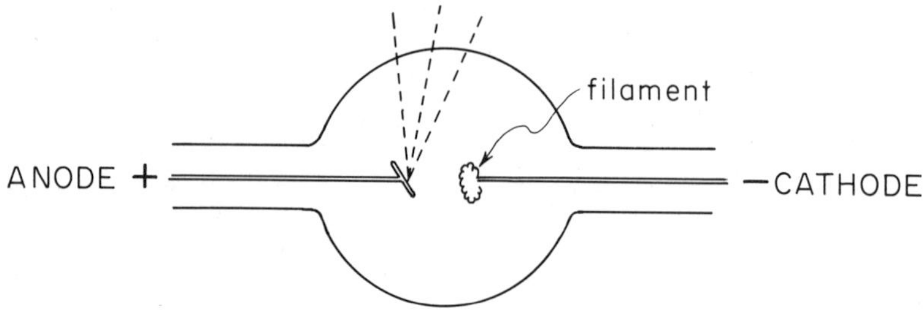

Fig 20–1.—Formation of x-rays in a vacuum tube.

as well as those on the surface. Therefore the quality or penetrability of the beam has to be expressed in some convenient manner to build knowledge of the "ideal" combination of factors. The half-value layer does this. The half-value layer is that thickness of aluminum in a filter that is required to reduce the original exposure by 50%. Filtration adds to the homogeneity of the beam, which aids even absorption of the remaining radiation through all thicknesses of the target tissue. In other words, each layer in depth absorbs the same percent of the remaining radiation. For most average basal cell epitheliomas, a kilovoltage of 100 with a half-value layer of 0.9 or 1.0 mm aluminum is adequate to ensure successful treatment, i.e., successful depth dose. It is best to have two or three techniques and learn them well!

For tumors in the skin of the face, 100 kv, 5 ma, 20 cm TSD producing 600–650 rad every other day for six treatments, shielding with a margin of 6–10 mm to the tumor edge and a total dose of around 3,600 rad will be adequate for cure without late radiation sequelae or telangiectases and hyperpigmentation. At times a higher dosage may be needed, e.g., 1,000 rad for four treatments and 750 rad for two treatments, to give a total of 5,500 rad. For very superficial lesions, 80 kv is adequate with 5 ma, 20 cm TSD, and perhaps a slightly higher total dose, e.g., 750 rad for six treatments to equal 4,500 rad. Generally speaking, when a lesion is large, e.g., 2.5 cm in diameter, 500 rad for six treatments will suffice, that is to say, the air dose can be smaller; whereas if the lesion is very small,

650 – 750 rad, or even a few doses up to 1,000 rad may be needed to destroy it.

When treating any skin area, an effort should be made to get the part to be treated in a perfectly flat position that can be comfortably maintained for the duration of the treatment. Sandbags, pillows and lead cut-out shields should be taped in place. A special glass-tipped cone will assist visibility of the lesion during treatment (from the lead-lined booth where the operator watches through lead glass).

Genitals should be shielded at all times, and pregnant women should never be treated with radiation, at least partly because of the extreme apprehension so generated.

Special locations such as eyelids can be treated with brass shields inserted under the eyelids. Pontocaine drops and castor oil may be used to lubricate first, or Xylocaine may be injected into eyelid and chin and then the lid sutured away from the eyeball; coning, with a small glass cone directing the beam away from the eyeball, is also advised. This has been an extremely satisfactory method in many instances. In elderly patients, fear of late sequelae is not realistic. Calibration of the x-ray tubes (and the grenz-ray tubes) should be done by a radiation physicist yearly.

Grenz Radiation

Ostensibly on the borderline between ultraviolet and x-ray, this very soft radiation is usually given at a distance of 20 cm and 10 kv and 12 ma. Since it is supersoft, penetrating rays are almost inconsequential, the vast majority of emissions being absorbed in the epidermis. Therefore in chronic diseases subject to frequent remissions, where retreatment is probably going to be required, grenz rays are safer. Grenz rays are also more suitable for treating the eyelids and gonad skin and they have a strangely beneficial effect in psoriasis. The air absorption of the grenz rays is a more important factor since the rays are so soft, and the TSD is therefore rather important. The patient should be cautioned to be still. The usual dose for treating benign conditions, e.g., psoriasis, is 200 rad grenz weekly for 4 to 6 weeks.

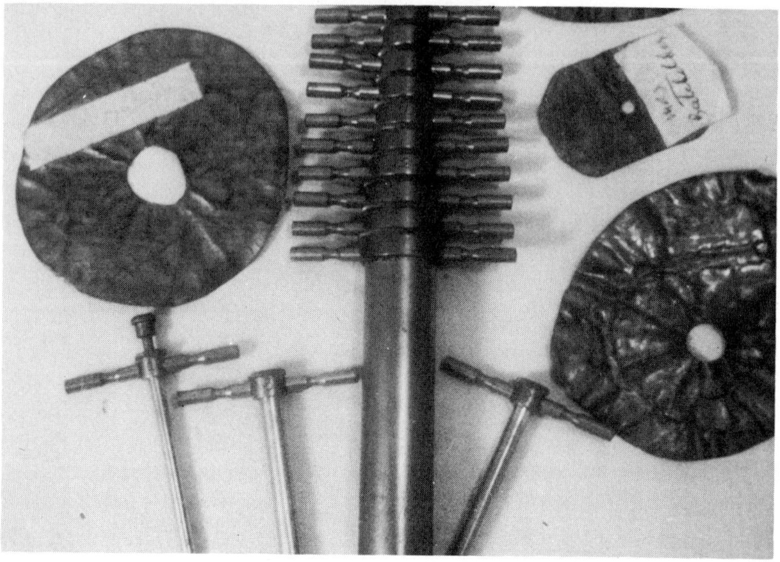

Fig 20–2.—Cork borers of various sizes for cutting lead shields.

Grenz radiation will produce hyperpigmentation with great regularity. Tars should *not* be used coincidentally with radiation.

Shielding

Lead shields can be made with cut-outs of varying sizes and shapes by outlining the field on the skin with a ball-point pen and pressing on blotting paper to pick up the ink outline. Then this can be transferred to lead. Cork borers can be used to produce various diameters of small holes which can later be altered to fit the lesions more accurately (Fig 20–2). Lead and rubber shields for under the chin and covering the hairline, eyelids and other sensitive areas can be cut out. Figure 20–3 shows paper-covered lead eye shields.

Controversies

The use of x-rays and grenz rays in dermatology has never been without controversy. It is a very useful modality, but of

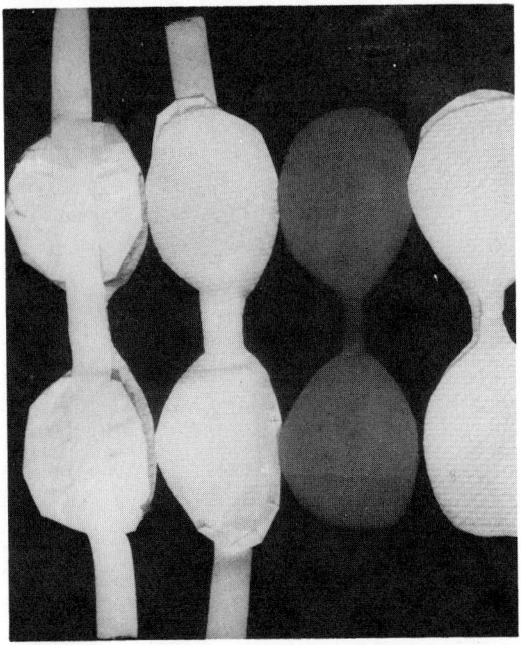

Fig 20–3. – Paper-covered lead eye shields.

course, through negligence, can cause grave harm. Almost all skin cancers developing in x-irradiated skin result from *overdosage*. The examples we have seen of skin damaged by quacks using x-rays to epilate superfluous hair on the face serve to accentuate this point. This was gross, negligent overtreatment. The operator must know his machine, it must be calibrated by a physicist annually, and it must have an automatic timer. X-rays should never be used as an easy way out of a difficult problem in therapy, and yet they are most helpful in treating cases like a 65-year-old patient with dermatitis herpetiformis who has compressed fractures of the spine from steroids and glucose 6-phosphate dehydrogenase deficiency, so that sulfones produce a hemoglobin value of 4 gm in nothing flat! To decry the use of x-rays through ignorance is unpardonable as well as unscientific. It must be admitted, however, that in the minds of the general public (and a great many surgeons as well) radiation is evil. It *can* be dangerous and must be reserved for intractable problems or for well-selected malignancies.

A recent HEW report[1] surveying the use of radiation treatment summarizes the situation:

"While the survey confirms the belief that the use of ionizing radiation in dermatology has decreased, it also shows that radiation therapy is still a regularly used integral modality in dermatologic therapy. . . . Our survey showed that 55.5% of the dermatologic offices are equipped with superficial x-ray machines and/or grenz ray units and that 44.3% of dermatologists use superficial x-ray or grenz rays regularly. Even if one assumes that all dermatologists who did not respond to the questionnaire are not using radiotherapy, the survey would undeniably prove that at least 22.5% of all dermatologists use radiotherapy; the real percentage is probably higher. . . . The replies also confirm that dermatologists are well aware of the cumulative effects of small radiation exposures. The overwhelming majority of dermatologists limit their total doses in benign disorders to radiation quantities that are considered safe and unlikely to lead even to mild cosmetic radiation sequelae."

REFERENCE

1. *A Review of the Use of Ionizing Radiation for the Treatment of Benign Diseases* (HEW Publication [FDA] 78-8043) (Washington, D.C.: HEW, 1977), pp. 25–26.

21 / Contact Dermatitis

The diagnosis of contact dermatitis is usually made by the clear-cut delineation of the dermatitis to a site recognizable as being in contact with the potential source of the dermatitis, e.g., a watch band, brassiere strap or earrings. Figures 21–1 through 21–6 show the common sites and causes of contact dermatitides. (See pp. 39–41, PCAD.)

Primary Irritant Type

This is generally found in men who clean grease off their hands, using either methylated spirit or a detergent or trichloroethylene parts cleaner, in mechanics who use other strong primary irritant chemicals, and in housewives who use detergents. (See Formulary, nos. 22, 36, 37.)

Sensitizer Type

An allergic eczematous contact dermatitis is produced, and the causes of this are usually fabric finishes, dyes, oils, tars, rubber, soap, cosmetics and perfume, insecticides, wood resins, plants, paints, plastics, glues, fiber glass, metals, polishes, ointments (home remedies) and occupational hazards (e.g., lithographers).

The sensitization type of allergic eczematous contact dermatitis usually occurs anywhere from 5 to 7 days and occasionally as long as 20 days after the initial or sensitizing contact, *at the site of contact*. There are no circulatory or otherwise detectable antibodies produced, although there is local tissue allergy. This condition is usually, though not invariably lifelong. The most common sensitizers are plants, paraphenylenediamine, nickel, rubber components and the dichromates.[1]

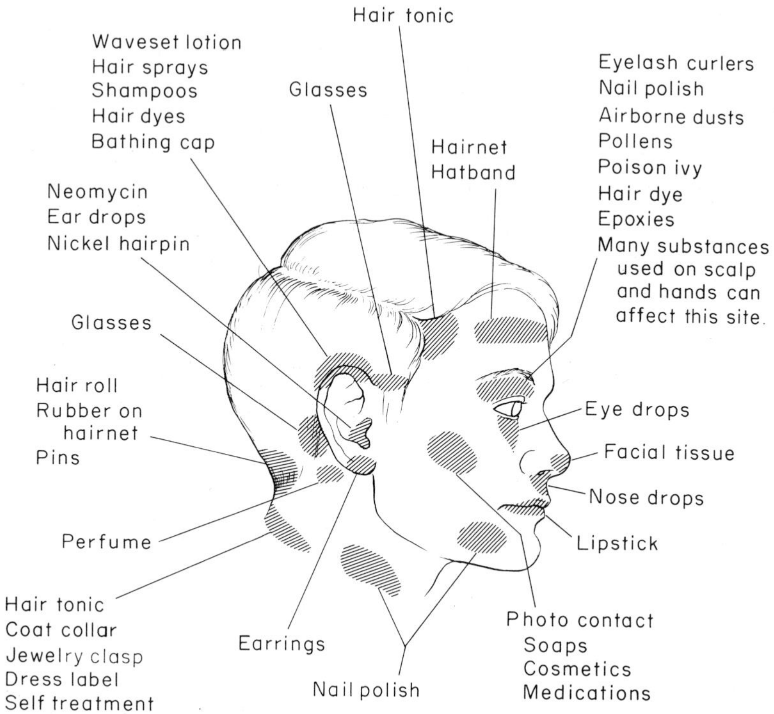

Fig 21–1.—Sites and causes of contact dermatitis on the face (women).

Atopy is a distinct entity, separate from contact dermatitis and eczema (epidermal skin lesions), and separate from the urticaria-hay fever-asthma group that produces wheal reactions with intracutaneous testing. In children contact dermatitis *can* occur in such other groups, which accounts for the occasional help from intracutaneous testing if the allergen is the same in each instance.

Causes

Elucidation of the cause can be difficult, and if the eczematous contact dermatitis goes on and on, the "broadening of the base," spoken of by Stokes,[2] occurs, and new allergic reactions may enter the picture, not uncommonly induced by overtreat-

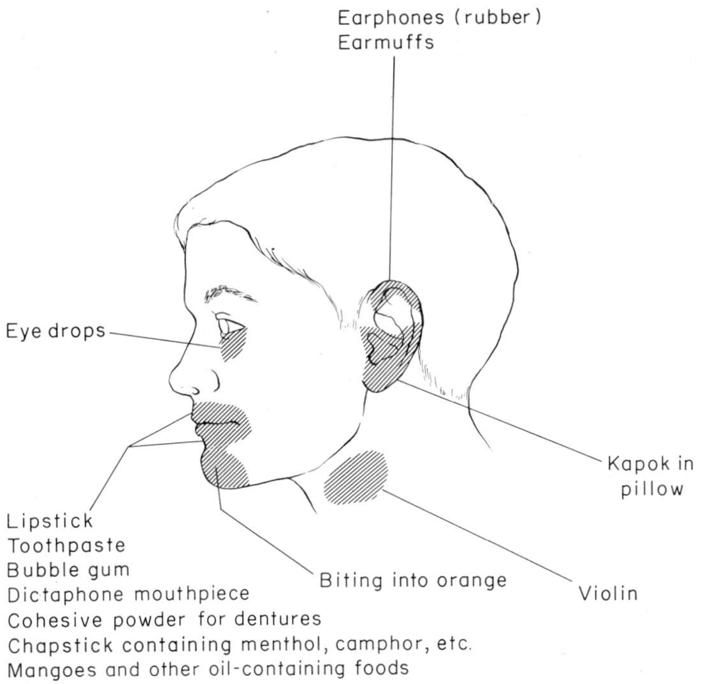

Fig 21 – 2. – Sites and causes of contact dermatitis on the face (men).

ment with anesthetic medications (as for example, the "caines," antihistamines such as pyribenzamine, or antibiotics such as neomycin or furacin, or penicillin, or sulfa). Hypersusceptibility to otherwise comparatively inert substances may occur, with ultimately a complex situation where many factors prolong the eczema. Not the least of these is apprehension on the part of the patient that there is no cure.

Plants

Allergic dermatitis from poison ivy, oak, sumac, Japanese lacquer tree, cashew nut and Indian marking nut (all varieties of catechols) usually results in intense edema, erythema and vesicles or bullae, and intense itching in the areas of contact. After 2 hours the plant oil is irretrievably fixed in epidermal union and cannot be washed away, and the "irreversible" re-

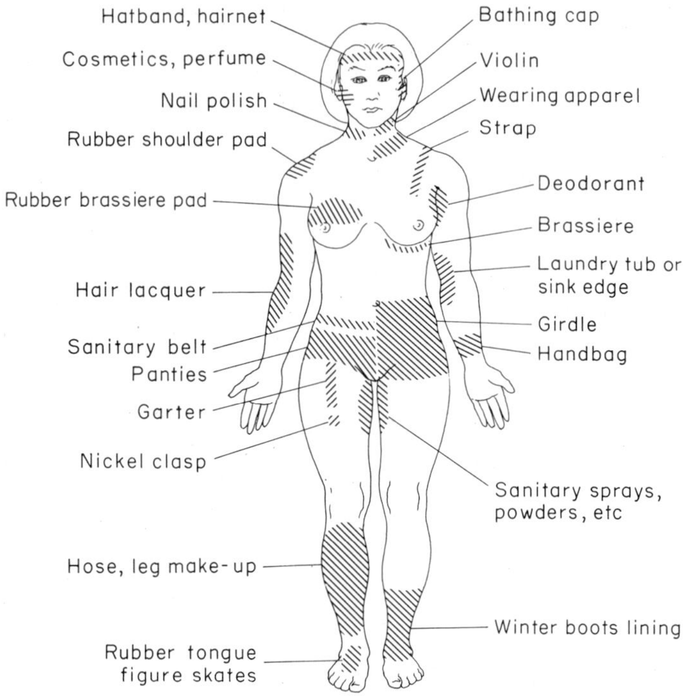

Fig 21–3.—Sites and causes of contact dermatitis in women (front view).

action commences. It is usually clinically evident after 8–48 hours and goes on for a few weeks. Dermatitis develops from contact with dead leaves, roots, branches, as well as contaminated fur, golf balls, shoes and garden utensils.

The appearance of new lesions several days after exposure is due to more dilute amounts of the oil being distributed during the 2 hours after exposure; the longer time taken to develop clinically evident lesions is perhaps explainable by (1) the dilution of substances reaching the secondary contact areas, and (2) the gradually increasing reactions as the allergy runs its course. Linear streaks of vesicles are characteristic.

Other varieties of plant dermatitis include those caused by

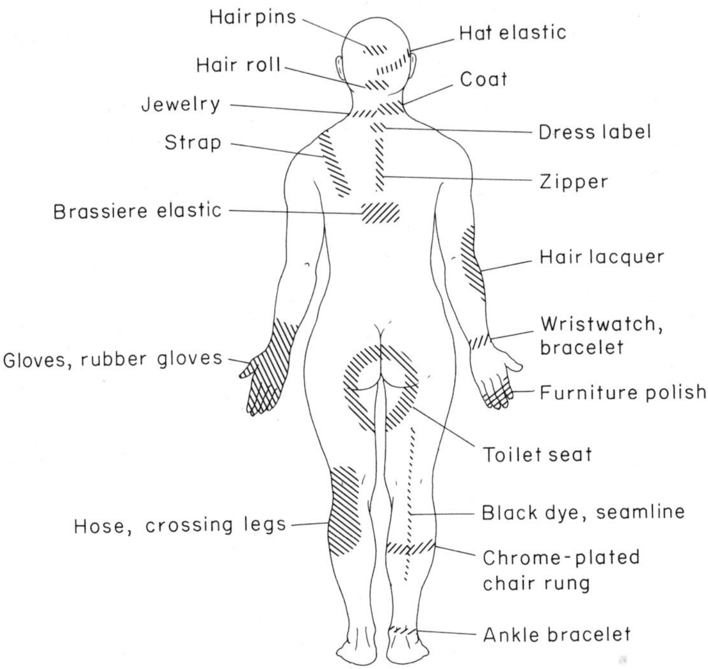

Fig 21–4.—Sites and causes of contact dermatitis in women (rear view).

primrose and African violet, seaweed and algae getting under bathing trunks, and ragweed pollen in the air producing dermatitis on the exposed skin of gravediggers, track walkers and others. Shelmire lists 56 different plants for patch testing.[3]

Some plants and their juices contain a proteolytic enzyme which can produce irritation of the skin. Pineapple juice is one of these. Chewing buttercups occasionally releases an enzyme that produces blisters around the lips. Some members of the daisy family produce blisters if crushed on the skin.

Plants containing furocoumarins, e.g., wild parsnips, gas plant, fig and mustard, will, if the "juice" gets on the skin and then if there is subsequent strong *sunlight*, produce a crop of striated criss-cross blisters that heal with hyperpigmentation.

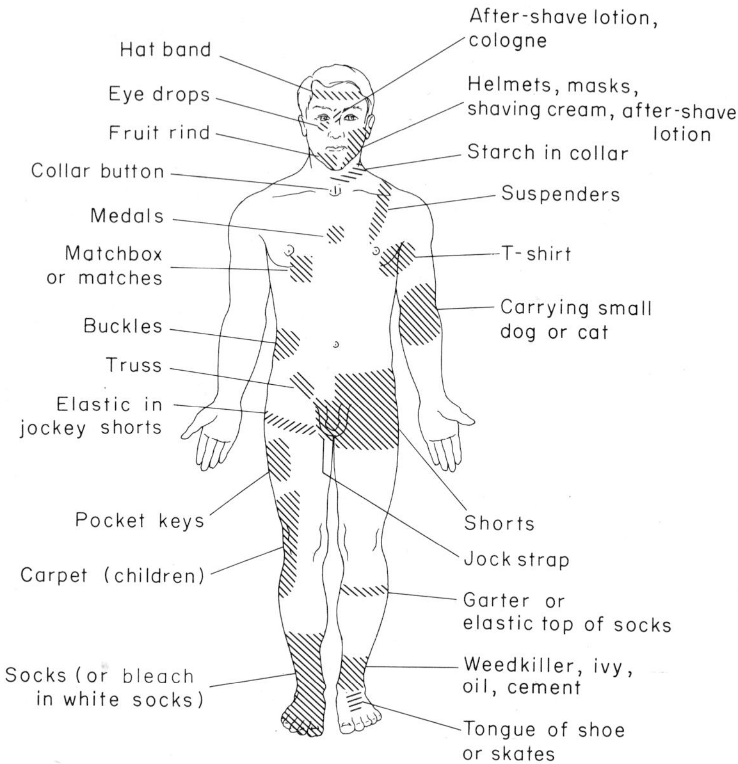

Fig 21–5.—Sites and causes of contact dermatitis in men (front view).

These appear 12–24 hours after contact. (Celery-picker's dermatitis is due to a "rust" which causes photosensitizing eruptions.)

Onions and garlic can show cross reaction with tulips and hyacinths, and split and fissured fingers may result in those who handle them.

Gardeners often are sensitive to primrose. *Florists* find chrysanthemum to be the most frequent sensitizer (late fall). *Foresters* are occasionally sensitive to birch, beech, pine, spruce and other evergreens. *Farmers* mostly become sensitized to ragweed. Other occupational groups such as nursery-

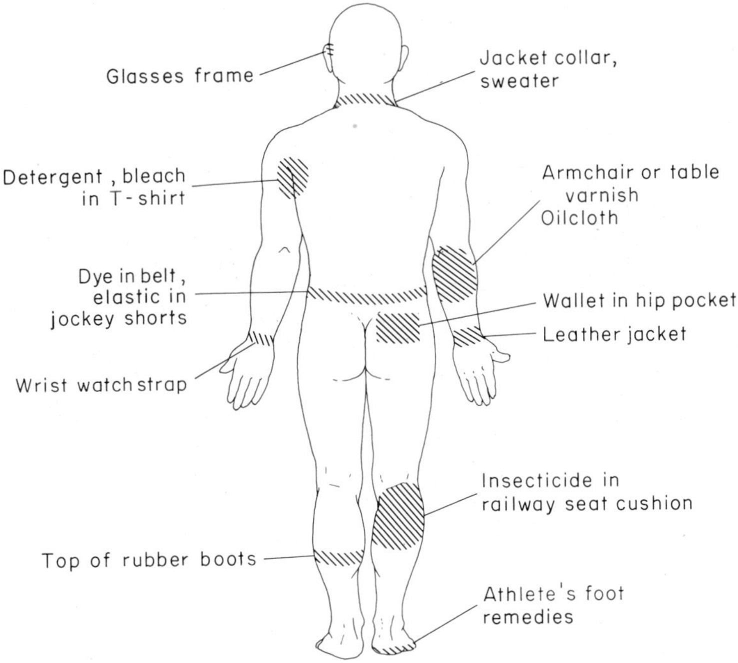

Fig 21–6.—Sites and causes of contact dermatitis in men (rear view).

men, carpenters, boat builders, lumberyard workers and furniture makers may develop sensitivity to teak or California sequoia (ship builders), silver spruce (airplane factory workers), mahogany (cabinet makers), cocus wood (flute players) and cocobolo wood (from knife handles).

The mango (catechol) dermatitis is a classic in red-lipped persons recently arrived from Florida. Eugenol (a substituted catechol) is used in dentistry and is present in oil of cinnamon, oil of cloves, and in some soaps and in bay rum.

Pollen dermatitis is probably missed more of the time than it is diagnosed.

Memorial Day, May 30, heralds June grass; July 4, timothy; Easter, trees; and Labor Day, ragweed. Often the onset of the seasonal flare of the dermatitis coincides.

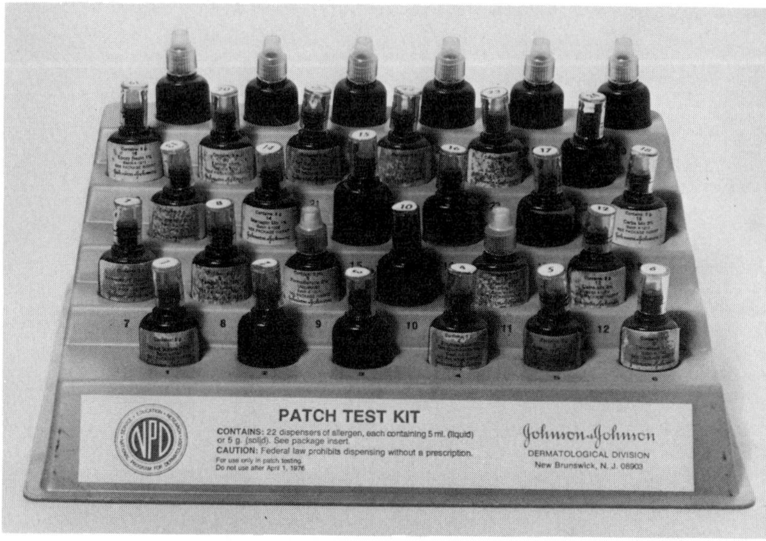

Fig 21–7.—Patch test kit available through the Academy of Dermatology.

Elucidation of the cause in a susceptible case of plant dermatitis involves a careful history of any seasonal or occupational variation, and patch testing (Fig 21–7) to either the slice of carrot or tulip, as the case may be, or to prepared oleoresins (Hollister-Stier Labs.)

Treatment

Oral desensitization with plant oleoresins (Graham Labs.) is practical and should be commenced *after* the season ends.

Acute poison ivy usually responds best to an intramuscular injection of Kenalog, though a schedule of tapering steroid doses in oral form is adequate if continued over a *planned* dosage schedule (never mind how cured the patient feels) to prevent the rebound relapse. In treating mild cases, cool soaks, antihistamines and shake lotions are enough. Sometimes Decadron spray or hydrocortisone lotion 1% help, as does Periactin at night.

Specific hyposensitization is worthwhile if started in February, and if oral, continued through the summer in very sensitive patients.

Cosmetics

Dermatitis most commonly occurs from hair dyes, nail polishes, perfumes, lipsticks and sunscreen agents. The chief site of the eruption is the eyelid area, with ears and neck next.

Eye makeup, such as mascara, eye shadow and eye pencil, seldom causes dermatitis (although eyeliner often does) whereas nail polish, while seldom causing trouble around the fingernails, affects the eyelids first. Lower eyelid dermatitis is often from wetting solutions or eyedrops. Various formaldehyde resins are used in nail lacquers and nail hardeners, as are sulfonamide derivatives, both of which can sensitize.

Lipsticks contain waxes and fats (occasionally cocoa butter sensitizes), perfumes (occasionally sensitize), and dyes (especially tetrabromofluorescein), which may occasionally dry the lips and produce photosensitivity. Special lipsticks are available that contain neither fluorescein dyes nor perfumes, like, for example, Almay (Texas Pharmacal) or Ar-Ex.

Deodorants and antiperspirants may contain neomycin, zirconium, formaldehyde and antibacterial agents, such as hexachlorophene, which can sensitize, as well as aluminum salts. Deodorant soaps containing salicylanilide derivatives or hexachlorophene analogs can photosensitize (Dial, Zest, Lifebuoy, Safeguard, Palmolive Gold, Irish Spring, Coast).

Sunscreen preparations containing PABA (para-aminobenzoic acid), hydroquinone or digalloyl trioleate can sensitize, and in some cases, photosensitize. Bleaching creams are sensitizers too, either mercury or hydroquinone being the culprit.

Toothpaste and mouthwashes can cause dermatitis from oils, cinnamon or other flavoring, or antiseptics.

Hair dyes are mostly of the permanent or "oxidation" type, containing para-phenylene diamine (PPDA), soap, ammonia and other modifiers which penetrate and color the hair when mixed with 20 volumes of peroxide. This type of dye accepts shampoos and cold waves and sensitizes most commonly. The azo and aniline dyes produce a semipermanent coloring which is tolerated well in most PPDA-sensitive patients, but lasts through only a few washings. Metallic hair dyes (Romans used a lead comb dipped in vinegar to darken gray hair) are also referred to as hair "restorers" and are mostly still based on lead and do not sensitize. Vegetable rinses are usually made from henna, which is nonsensitizing, although some pyrogallol combinations *are* sensitizing. Methylene PPDA *can* cross-react with PABA in sunscreens, local anesthetics and sulfonamides—thiazides (Diuril), tolbutamide (Orinase), chlorpropamide (Diabinase) and saccharin.

Permanent-wave solutions, usually thioglycolates, are alkaline reducing agents which make the hair malleable; the hair is "waved" on rollers and then "fixed" with an oxidizer (hydrogen peroxide, perborate, bromates of citric acid). Thioglycolates rarely sensitize, but do occasionally cause primary irritation if not carefully mopped up, and can split and break the hair.

The adhesive used to attach toupees and false eyelashes occasionally causes dermatitis, in which case Duo Surgical Adhesive (Johnson & Johnson) sometimes is tolerated well. Bleaching or freckle creams usually contain mercury or quinones, and all can sensitize; Benoquin (Elder) is a very potent sensitizer. Face powders and rouge rarely cause dermatitis. Sunscreens, at least those made of PABA (Pre-Sun, Sundown, PABA gel, Sunbrella, etc.) or digalloyl trioleate (Sundare, Sunswept and A-Fil), can sensitize and photosensitize. The benzophenones, e.g., Solbar or Uval, seem promising, although there have been sensitizing cases. Sundare, RVPaque, RVP, Almay Sunburn Preventive, Liquid Sunshine (H. Rubenstein), Sun-Proof Cream (Ardena), Sun-Tan Gelee (Rexall) and Sun Bath (Revlon) are generally acceptable.

Patients should be advised to apply perfume to their clothes if possible rather than to their skin and certainly should avoid using photosensitizing perfumes (e.g., Shalimar) on their skin in bright sun.

Hypoallergenic cosmetics are manufactured by several companies, two of the best being the Almay division of Schieffelin & Company and the Texas Pharmacal Company.

Soaps and Detergents

Those whose occupations involve extensive soaping of the skin, such as dishwashers, housewives, laundresses and surgeons, clinically show dehydration or shriveling of the keratin layers, which leads to irritation of the "primary irritant" type. Patch tests with 2% soap solution theoretically can pick up a true allergy, but I am unconvinced. Perhaps coconut-oil-containing soaps are worse than others. Neutral soaps, such as Lowila, Basis, Oilatum, Hazeline or Dermaphyllic, are much less drying. Many of the stronger antibacterial soaps, such as Dial, Zest, Lifebuoy, Safeguard and Palmolive Gold, are sensitizing as well as drying, and may be photosensitizing.

Contact with clothing washed in strong soaps or detergents (e.g., sheets used by bed patients) can lead to dermatitis. This is especially true if bleach or whitener is used. The great offenders in this regard are Axion, Bold, Ajax Detergent, Cold Power, Salvo Tabs, Coldwater All, Amway, Arm & Hammer, Era and Dynamo.

Fair-skinned, sensitive or elderly people who bathe a lot in hot showers or tubs can develop an asteatotic eczema that can be extremely intractable. Remembering that the skin's pH is acidic, around 5.0, and all water is slightly alkaline, especially if there are many calcium and magnesium salts in it, it is easy to see how this happens. Cessation of bathing and showering for a while is necessary to clear the skin of these unfortunate patients. An alkaline skin is increasingly susceptible to the irritant effects of water alone, and the hyperirritability of the skin can be protracted; it takes 3 months for a fracture to heal, similarly with the skin. The skin must be put at rest and allowed lubrication for that length of time before it recovers.

The usual result of continuous and excessive exposure of the skin to soaps and detergents is impaired alkaline neutralization with drying, fissuring and defatting of the keratin layer leading to increased permeability of the horny layer (in both directions). The loss of water-holding capacity and the increased penetrability of comparatively innocuous substances (e.g., vegetable juices) can lead to sensitization with resultant allergic contact dermatitis subsequent to the original primary irritant effect. It can be almost self-sustaining, and many laundry soaps contain chemical additives which are the actual irritants (e.g., sodium silicate, sodium phosphate, sodium carbonate). Hand cleaner soaps contain small harsh particles to assist in grease removal, such as pumice, talc, borax, corn meal or wood flour. These are sometimes irritating. Some yellow laundry soaps contain "rosin" to make the bar more soluble, which is also a sensitizer.

Clothing

Natural fiber clothing, made from wool, cotton, linen and mohair, have never in themselves been shown to be sensitizers. Sizing and stiffening cotton with starch or rosin may produce dermatitis.

Synthetic fibers include polyester (Dacron), rayon, rubber, saran and spandex. With the exception of rubber, saran and other vinyl plastics (vinyl plastic tablecloths, elastiglass wristwatch bands), we encounter a dermatitis only from spandex. This may be due to the mercaptobenzothiazole contained in some spandex or to a rubber edge in the garment.[1] Fisher says spandex garments manufactured by Vanity Fair and Warner Slimwear lingerie are rubber-free and safe.

CLOTHING DYES.—Dermatitis may be induced more easily by dark clothing. Heavy perspiration, especially in oily-skinned individuals, enhances bleeding of the dye (e.g., widow's dermatitis).

FABRIC FINISHES.—These are used to increase durability, to soften or stiffen a fabric, or to impart waterproofing, fireproofing, crease resistance or other properties to the fabric. The use of formaldehyde or its resins in clothing is widespread, but the incidence of resulting dermatitis is comparatively low. These are used to make fabrics crease resistant, water repellent and shrink resistant. Dermatitis occurs mostly in obese women who demonstrate a dermatitis starting in the axilla and later affecting the sides of the neck, the antecubitals and the inguinals. In men, it is usually in the inner thighs, gluteal folds and back of the knees.

Stoddard solvent or other dry-cleaning solutions will occasionally produce a clothing-oriented dermatitis, as will moth crystals. Airing the clothes for a few days before wearing them will usually prevent this.

Management of clothing dermatitis involves the use of Decadron spray, which contains isopropyl myristate, a film or "spray-on-shield" (Kleinert) which suppresses sweat and may protect the fabric and acts as a deodorant. Weight loss in obese women sometimes seems to help, as does avoidance of panty girdles.

Those who are sensitive to formaldehyde must avoid wash-and-dry or wash-and-wear and drip-dry clothing.

Footwear

The chief causes here are the thermoplastic or rubber-boxed toes, and the cements and dichromates used in tanning. Dyes, anti-mildew agents, formaldehyde and nickel eyelets or nickel in arch supports also can cause dermatitis. A waterproofing silicone spray externally applied has also been the cause. The dermatitis usually begins on the dorsa of the big toe and spreads to the dorsa of the foot. Atopic children will often show a similar dermatitis which, however, will have negative results on patch-tests to shoe ingredients. Sox washed in Bold or bleached with a strong whitener can also cause dermatitis.

Safe sneakers are Converse (Official Boy Scout—Sears), although you must rip out the rubber insole and replace it with the "Vy-Foam" (urethane foam) insole (Dr. Scholl). Weejuns (Bass) have no accelerator in them.

While a patient with a shoe dermatitis is being evaluated, he should wear sandals or unlined cloth or plastic shoes, which are inexpensive and generally safe. Unlined moccasins also are usually fairly safe (L.L. Bean deerhide). If the rubber-box toe is the cause, the Celastic box toe (Celastic Box Toe Company, Kearney, N.J.) may be the answer. Otherwise for *men*, Johnson & Murphy, French Shriner & Urner and Stacey Adams make excellent shoes. For boys and girls, Gerberich-Payne shoes contain the Celastic box toe, and "Little Yankee" makes a nice shoe for boys.

Weejuns (Bass) are tanned with chromate though often successfully worn. Dermapedic shoes are all vegetable tanned, and their glues are vegetable based. They make men's and boys' boots and shoes. Plastic-molded sandals for women may be obtained from Sandak. Kinney plastic shoes are available in the Northeast. The Musebeck-Foot-So-Port Shoe Co. (Oconomowoc, Wisconsin) makes a kit and has a catalog which they will send to any physician requesting it.

Occasionally wearing down the heel pad or lining will expose adhesive which will cause dermatitis. A felt insole and use of fish glue will assist this. Doctor Fisher says Celastic box toe shoes do not contain any phenolic or rubber adhesive.[1]

Formaldehyde is used in the tanning of white leather shoes in "elk," "white kid" and "new bucks." Tannins obtained from trees are used to tan leather (vegetable tanning) and do not cause dermatitis. However, if the shoe is made of vegetable-tanned leather, the lining should not be chrome-tanned.

Dyes are not often the cause of footwear dermatitis unless the shoe has been redyed.[4]

MANAGEMENT OF HYPERHIDROSIS.—Sweat leaches out chromates from leather, so controlling perspiration is essential. Zeasorb Powder (Stiefel) and Dr. Scholl's foot granules in a soap are excellent for reducing some of this. Wearing Surgitube under the sock and then throwing it away is helpful, too, and the old-fashioned foot soaking in a teaspoon of formaldehyde in a pint of water occasionally helps. The astringency of Burow's solution soaks is also helpful.

Metals and Their Salts

NICKEL.—Nickel sensitivity is probably the most common of all contact dermatitides. Mercury and chromates are the other two important sensitizing metals, and occasionally but rarely does sensitivity arise from cobalt (masons, tile setters, dentists, printers, mechanics and machinists).

Nickel is usually the sensitizer in dermatitis caused by chrome-plated jewelry because the plating leaves "pores" or pinholes through which the heavier nickel leaks to contact the skin. Garter clasps, zippers and costume jewelry are usually nickel plated, and nickel in hairpins can sensitize the scalp. Plastic clasps and clips (Dux Company or Delrin Trolley Garter Grips) should be substituted. In the case of earrings, spraying with Decadron spray (isopropyl myristate, a "synthetic beeswax" and dexamethasone) often permits them to be worn for a few hours. Scotch-tape covering is messy and not recommended. Most gold rings contain nickel in varying percentages, which is most commonly the sensitizer. Plastic sleeves are available to cover nickel eyeglass frames, although plastic eyeglass frames of cellulose acetate almost never sensitize.

CHROMIUM.—Nonindustrial exposure to chromates occurs from contact with leather articles, glues, matches, paints, detergents and bleaches, e.g., Javelle water. Chromate sensitivity can be detected by patch testing with 0.25% aqueous solution of potassium dichromate. Certain occupational groups, particularly those who work with cement, such as masons and tile setters, are apt to develop a disabling chromate sensitivity because of the "alkali-itch" effect of the cement, which enhances the development of allergy to the chromates. Other similar groups include acetylene workers, blueprint makers, electroplaters, lithographers, photoengravers, Diesel engine mechanics, or railroad or trucking company employees, tannery employees and welders. Extreme care in avoiding contact appears to be the only successful management technique. This has saved a few lithographers, but so far no tile setters or masons, in my experience. The chrome-sensitive employee almost never loses his sensitivity.

MERCURY.—Mercury is found in preservatives and medications and in industry. Merthiolate (thimerosal), Mercurochrome (merbromin), ammoniated mercury and bichloride of mercury all produce dermatitis. Merthiolate is often used as a preservative in a variety of ointments and may cause contact dermatitis. Phenylmercuric salts used in weed killers and fungicides on golf courses can produce an ankle dermatitis. They are also used as preservatives and in contraceptive jellies.

Cinnabar used for red in tattoos, chromium oxide for green, and cobalt blue for blue all can suddenly be "rejected" with an allergic reaction of itching, edema and either eczematous or granulomatous changes in the tattooed skin. Cadmium sulfide, which is the yellow, can produce a phototoxic reaction to sunlight; similarly it can cause itching and swelling. Zirconium, silicone and beryllium can also produce granulomatous reactions in the skin.

Rubber

Natural rubber latex almost never sensitizes, whereas synthetic rubber frequently *does* sensitize. Fully finished and polymerized plastics seldom cause an allergic contact dermatitis, whereas fully "cured" rubber articles do so quite frequently. Of the antioxidants used to prolong the life of the rubber, monobenzyl ether of hydroquinone (which can depigment skin) and phenyl-beta-naphthylamine are the most common sensitizers. The accelerators, mercaptobenzothiazole, tetramethyl thiuram monosulfide and diphenylguanidine, and the peptizer, thio-beta naphthal, are the chemicals causing most of the dermatitides attributable to rubber. Two other accelerators, disulfuram (Antabuse) and thiuram, will produce itching, erythema and urticaria in those exposed who ingest alcohol. Thiuram is also used as a lawn fungicide (Tersan). Occasionally bleach will activate a rubber accelerator, zinc dibenzyl dithiocarbamate (ZDC) to become highly allergenic.[5]

Rubber-glove dermatitis can be a trial for surgeons who should switch to "eudermic" surgical gloves (B.F. Goodrich Industrial Products Company), Nuprene gloves (Pioneer Rubber Company) or latex or plastic gloves. Parke-Davis will send samples of eudermic gloves on request. Other sources of gloves for surgeons are The Original Brown Mill Gloves (Seamless) and Elastyren gloves (V. K. Gloves) made in Denmark.

Warner's or Vanity Fair Spandex garments (without rubber or accelerator) are safe for use. If rubber dress-shield dermatitis is the problem, Kleinert's nonrubber dress shields are available. Elastic in hair nets may cause dermatitis, and ribbons or wrap-around hair nets may have to be substituted. Where an eruption is due to a rubber condom, Fourex (Schmidt) fish-skins can be substituted.

Adhesive tape can cause a miliaria-like occlusion of poral openings, although true allergic contact dermatitis spreads beyond the margin of the contact with the tape. If this occurs, Dermicel tape (Johnson & Johnson), Steristrips or Micropore Surgical Tape (3M) can be substituted, or spray-on "Bandaid."

For toupees and ileostomy stoma irritated by other rubber cements, Duo brand surgical adhesive (Johnson & Johnson) is well tolerated by many.

Latex cements are used in the shoe and textile trade. Vulcanizing solutions come in two solutions which, when mixed, seal punctures. It takes a few hours to cure, and sensitization can occur from the various chemicals. Nonvulcanizing rubber solutions are used in the shoe industry and automobile trimmings and can cause dermatitis.

Nonrubber Adhesives

These are chiefly synthetic resin adhesives which can sensitize, although fish glues generally do not. Glues made from cotton (e.g., cellulose acetate) are not sensitizers, and neither is collodion. Vegetable gums such as karaya, acacia and tragacanth are sensitizers.

Plastics and Synthetic Resins

Usually solid, these are used for making knobs, gears, dishes, dentures, clothing, plastic panels and ornaments, glasses, eyeglass frames, adhesive plaster and many other things that come in contact with the skin. Resins are formed by fusing a large number of monomers into a larger polymer, often in the presence of a catalyst or activator. Once polymerized, plastics are usually inert allergenically. However, incompletely "cured" resins, or monomers, or catalysts may be irritants or sensitizers. Phenols, aldehydes, allyl alcohol, styrene, acrylonitrile and vinyl monomers are examples.

Epoxy Resins

These are widely used in enclosing transformers, insulating cables, adhesive purposes in aircraft and other industries, tool and die casting, as well as household adhesive purposes. These are extremely sensitizing, and even sawing or grinding of the completely polymerized resin can sensitize, e.g., boat builders under a laminated deck being ground smooth develop quite a dermatitis of the eyelids. The household glues generally consist of two tubes, A and B, one of which is an aliphatic amine "hardener." When the two are mixed, polymerization rapidly occurs. These amines are usually dimethylene triamine or triethylene tetramine (patch tests with 0.1% aqueous). Another epoxy component, "biphenol A," is a potent sensitizer, too.

In handling epoxies, great care *must* be exercised, and a "no-touch" or glove and paper benchcover technique should be used. If accidental skin contamination occurs, the epoxy chemical should be *instantly* removed. Fastidious workers last longer.

Fiberglass (glass wool)

In its finished state, fiberglass is considered to be nonallergenic, although the wide disparity in reaction between individuals exposed to comparable "doses" suggests more than mere mechanical irritation by broken-off spicules. Clothing contamination in workers or contamination by washing machines and curtains can lead to "mysterious" eruptions.

In all branches of the plastics industry, sensitization is a potent hazard and is best prevented, since it can almost never be cured except by removal from the environment. Scrupulous technique and cleanliness, not only of the person but also of the workbench area is essential. Sloppy or "fast" workers should be transferred and every effort made to provide washing and other cleaning facilities close at hand. Clean uniforms and frequent changes along with protective aprons, sleeves and gloves for those requiring them, are of great help in controlling sensitivity development.

State health departments are of great assistance in advising manufacturers how to make the necessary changes, as are insurance company safety inspectors.

As for the consuming general public, completely cured plastics are usually safe. One occasionally sees sensitivity to elastiglass wristwatch straps, to methyl methacrylate dentures and to melamine dentures, but I have never seen a plastic steering wheel produce a hand rash. The boating enthusiast who does his own repairs with epoxy glues is likely to develop a dermatitis. Usually the eyelids are the site of the most intense edema and vesiculation with erythema.

Diaper Rash

Usually the cause of diaper rash is ammonia produced by stool bacteria harbored by the diaper fermenting the urea in the urine. Occasionally antiseptics in diapers provided by diaper services will be the cause, and then a parent will have to boil the diapers for 10 minutes, soak them in vinegar or Diaparinc tablets, or use disposable diapers. Pedameth capsules (S.F. Durst Co.) or sodium-acid phosphate (sodium biphosphate NF) in the infant's milk will acidify the urine (10 grains three times a day for those over 6 months of age and 15 grains twice a day for those over 12 months of age). For local treatment, 1% hydrocortisone in equal parts of bacitracin and zinc oxide ointment is a very satisfactory treatment, using mineral oil to cleanse.

Toilet seat dermatitis in older children is usually from antiseptics (e.g., C.N.) or strong detergents applied to the toilet seat. It has a horseshoe shape. Incontinent adults will develop a similar eruption, perhaps more extensive and more localized if they are hemiplegic or paraplegic. Erosive lesions and moniliasis may be part of the picture. Breakdown of the skin with the formation of decubitus ulcers is to be avoided; and good nursing care with disposable bedpads, sheepskins, frequent movement, linen changes and plenty of powder, tightly drawn sheets and oral sodium acid phosphate (20 grains three times a day) to reduce a buildup of ammonia all help. If all else fails, a retention catheter in a special "incontinence bed" may be needed. In debilitated patients, antibiotics administered locally or systemically either with or without enzymatic debridement, plus transfusion and gamma globulin may assist in forestalling impending bed sores. Rubbing with lotions and painting with compound tincture of benzoin or dilute Castellani's paint also are helpful.

Care of Stoma in Ileostomies and Colostomies

Dermatitis around stoma usually occurs because of the irritant nature of right-sided intestinal secretions, which are liquid and tend to seep under an ill-fitting or loose appliance disk. Karaya gum comes in powder form, in "disks" or in sheets made of karaya and glycerine. It can be applied to raw peristomal skin and have an appliance cemented over it, while healthy skin grows under it. Karaya gum is not quickly washed away by ileal discharge, urine or feces and is protective. The disk or "washer" fits snugly around the stoma, leaving no skin exposed to corrosive wastes. Generally karaya is not an allergen, and ileostomy cement will stick to it.

Neokaraya is a combination of karaya and aluminum hydroxide gel (e.g., Amphogel, which can be used, too). If karaya seems to be irritating, then Orabase (Squibb) can be used in its place, either with or without Kenalog. Sometimes a thin roll of absorbent cotton will assist in making the base of the stoma watertight.

For odor, bismuth subcarbonate, 0.6 gm given three times a day with meals, will reduce the odor from both the feces and the bag, often with striking effect.[6]

A. A. Fisher believes solvent should not be used to remove the appliance face plate, which should be *gently* peeled off the skin.[1] However, cleanliness is essential, and if too much cement film collects, the use of a medicine dropper to apply solvent one drop at a time may make it safer and easier to use.

When severe irritation occurs, Lassar's paste with 1% hydrocortisone and covering with Saran Wrap can be used under the appliance ring.

Other Irritations of Contact Origin

GRANULOMAS FROM ZIRCONIUM.—Beryllium used in fluorescent lighting tubes, if allowed to enter through an abrasion in the skin, can produce a nodular granuloma not unlike a sarcoid. Similar granulomas have been reported to occur from contact with deodorant sticks containing zirconium, used in the underarm area and producing persistent firm purplish nodules that eventually disappear spontaneously. Zirconium salts used in poison ivy remedies have reportedly caused similar nodules elsewhere. Swimming pool granulomas similarly occur in abrasions, although here the cause is considered to be bacterial.

LICHEN PLANUS-LIKE ERUPTIONS FROM COLOR DEVELOPER. —Certain 8-mm color movies require development in a bath containing a modified paraphenylenediamine developer known as CD-2. The necessity for quickly grabbing a broken film leads to unprotected exposure, and the dermatitis develops with great regularity in those exposed.

PURPURA.—Purpura from fiber glass-contaminated clothing is occasionally seen, as is telangiectatic urticaria at the site of contact.

CHLORACNE.—Industrially acquired follicular plugs and acneform eruptions caused by chlorinated hydrocarbons, oils and waxes in contact with the forearms and thighs usually necessitate a change of job. This is peculiarly stubborn to treat while exposure continues. See #4 Formulary.

URTICARIA.—Water (so-called aquagenic urticaria) or ice, certain exotic woods or epoxy fumes, or chromate fumes in Diesel engine coolants can produce this.

SOLVENTS.—Petroleum solvents, such as gasoline and benzine, defat the skin and dehydrate and shrivel it, as do coal tar solvents, such as benzol, toluol and xylol, which can be absorbed through the skin to produce systemic toxic effects. Turpentine produces dryness and fissuring on the basis of its primary irritant effect. It is a sensitizer, too, however. Trichloroethylene and carbon tetrachloride, used to degrease machinery parts, are primary irritants that produce drying and fissuring. Ketones, glycols and alcohols are generally mild skin irritants.

CUTTING OILS.—Cutting oils, used on machining metal to keep the cutting edge cool and sharp, are essentially of two types: (1) the insoluble oil, which almost never causes dermatitis, although occasionally an oil folliculitis will result; and (2) the soluble oil, which is emulsified with water, is milky and alkaline, may contain antirust chemicals or wetting agents and occasionally will cause dermatitis.

RUST-INHIBITING GREASES.—The grease used to pack ball

bearings and other metals is occasionally a cause of dermatitis.

PHOTOSENSITIZERS.—Photosensitizers, such as the halogenated salicylanilides, are found in antiseptic soaps such as Safeguard and Lifebuoy. Bithional (Actamar or Bisphenol) in cosmetics, shampoos, medicated soaps and creams also has a photosensitizing effect, although it has largely been removed from these items now. Blancophores, or "whiter than white" chemicals, can photosensitize and are found in soaps, detergents and textiles as well as cosmetics (stilbenes). Certain dyes, e.g., eosin in lipstick, certain sunscreen preparations, especially PABA and trigalloyl trioleate, and antimildew agents (chlorosalicylanilide) as well as locally applied phenergan ointment (a phenothiazine) and sulfa ointments can photosensitize. The oleoresin of ragweed is a photosensitizer as well as a sensitizer, and nurses who handle phenothiazine medications (e.g., Thorazine, Stelazine, Compazine and Phenergan) and excretion products of patients on high doses can become sensitive and photosensitive. Similarly, phenothiazine insecticides, coal tar products, and psoralens (furocoumarin) in fruits, vegetables and perfumes can lead to light eruptions (berloque dermatitis) with hyperpigmentation. The yellow pigment in tattoos (cadmium sulfide) and occasionally the red (cinnabar) will selectively sunburn at times, displaying unusual sensitivity to light. Internal medications with thiazides, sulfas and Declomycin lead to photosensitivity reactions, too, although these are really not part of a contact exposure. For patch testing, the ordinary Wood's lamp treatment takes about 30 minutes at 6 in. to produce an erythema, so 5 minutes at 6 in. can be used as a photo patch test, applying the light to the site 24 hours after the patch is applied (cleansing with acetone before ultraviolet light treatment).

Sunlight is reflected with the greatest intensity from snow, with less intensity from sand, and still less from water. It has its peak effect at around noon. Usually window glass filters out the burning waves (below 3,200 Å or 320 nanometers). Sunscreens such as RVP (Elder), RVPaque (Elder), which contains zinc oxide plus a cinnamate, Solbar and Uval, which contain a benzophenone, Skolex (glycol paraminobenzoate),

Sunswept (digalloyl trioleate), A-Fil (menthyl anthranilate), Skol (PABA) and Solar Cream (PABA and titanium dioxide) are available. Opaque fabrics, preferably reddish, used in covering clothing, worn with wide-brimmed hats, dark glasses and gloves, do assist in keeping the sun away.

Repeated short sun exposures may eventually produce enough tanning (with or without psoralens given 2 hours before) to afford protection in sun reactors. Antimalarials and Actifed also help (Actifed is an antihistamine made by Burroughs & Wellcome). Once the eruption has occurred, antihistamines, to minimize or prevent eruptions in persistent light reactors, or steroids may be needed, in addition to maintaining a darkened environment.

Summary

In general, a knowledge of some of the occupational hazards of patients is essential for the successful management of contact dermatitis. The patient will not be able to tell the cause, although he can run through the mechanical aspects of his job quite easily. A phone call to the foreman or supervisor quite often turns up information essential to a proper assessment of the situation. In the case of professional people, such as nurses, physicians, artists and photoengravers, an intelligent discussion of the hazards of their work often leads the patient to quickly discern and pinpoint the cause. Removal of the cause, removal of the patient from exposure or, which is often more difficult, the substitution of something else, such as neoprene for rubber or spandex for playtex, is curative. Women *can* get earrings that sit *on* the ear rather than hang from it, thus avoiding the nickel rash on the lobes. In every city there will be one shoe shop where you will be able to get shoes made of untanned or chrome-free leather.

There is nothing more fascinating or more frustrating than the Sherlock Holmes style of tracing the cause of a contact dermatitis. Often the answer is so simple when you have found it, it is humbling. This is good for the soul and good for the patient.

In *acute oozing dermatitis*, treatment should include wet

dressings of boric-acid or Burow's solution, suitably diluted. Treatment should not be continuous; more commonly dressings should be applied for an hour every 4 hours or so, with shake lotions in between and steroids administered by mouth or injection (I prefer 60 mg Kenalog given intramuscularly for ivy rash, for example, which gives 90% remission in short order). Antihistamines should be prescribed to allay the itching, with steroid spray or cream lotion at night, as things subside.

In *chronic mystery dermatitis,* physicians should not give up. They may shift to Vioform, tar, paste, protection; often a change from 1% hydrocortisone lotion or cream to triamcinolone cream will work wonders. The steroid percentage may be increased up to 2% (in the case of hydrocortisone) or even more. For example, Aristocort Cream 0.5%, 5 gm in aquaphor and water, equal parts, q.s. to 15, makes a suitable strength. Or one can simply put 300 mg of hydrocortisone powder in 0.5 oz of USP hydrophilic ointment. A short course of steroids, e.g., one tablet given three times a day for 3 days, may get the patient out of a slump. Try to avoid Phisohex and stymie well-meaning friends who "had the same thing once." It should be remembered that Mycolog cream contains an ethylenediamine which is also found in aminophyllin. Patch-tests for this can be in 1% concentration.

Barrier creams are often a help in treating hand dermatitis (we will deal with this more in the chapter on hand eczemas). For wet work, Kerodex 71, and for dry or oily work, Kerodex 51 are good protective creams (Ayerst). Silicote cream (Arnar—Stone) and Covicone cream (Abbott) are two varieties of silicone protectives that are well tolerated and effective. Dupont puts out Protek, and there are "Ply" protective creams, with numbers from 1 to 9 indicating the special protective design. For housewives' hands, Keri and Shepard hand creams are well-tolerated effective emollients.

REFERENCES

1. Fisher, A. A.: *Contact Dermatitis* (Philadelphia: Lea & Febiger, 1967).
2. Stokes, J. H.: *Fundamentals of Medical Dermatology* (7th ed.;

Philadelphia: University of Pennsylvania, Department of Dermatology Book Fund, 1942), pp. 115, 134, 419.
3. Shelmire, B.: The etiology of eczema, South. Med. J. 17:297, 1933.
4. Fisher, A. A. Management of shoe dermatitis, Cutis 21:450, 1978.
5. Jordan, W. P., Jr., and Bourlas, M. C.: Allergic contact dermatitis to underwear elastic, Arch. Dermatol. 111:593, 1975.
6. Rowbotham, J. L.: Stomal care, N. Engl. J. Med. 279:90, 1968.

SUGGESTED READING

Cutis
Archives of Dermatology.

22 / Hand Eczemas

Hand "eczemas" include pustular psoriasis, drug eruptions, systemic toxic eruptions, infectious eczematoid dermatitis (including nummular eczema), streptococcal dermatitis (those that follow trauma, including erysipeloid from fish), dermatitis repens (which is often actually a *Pseudomonas* infection), psoriasis, pustular bacterid, dermatophytosis, dermatophytids, pompholyx, disseminated neurodermatitis or atopic eczema, dermatitis venenata and monilial paronychia. (Keratoderma palmare et plantare really does not belong in this group.)(See Formulary, nos. 6, 36, 37.)

Generally speaking, contact dermatitis involves the dorsa of the hands; psoriasis or fungus involves the palms. Ids are vesicular and involve the sides of the fingers, and if the webs are involved, gloves or liquids may be the causes.

Many vesicular eruptions of the hands defy diagnosis and can be classified best as "mystery hands" or varieties of either *dermatitis repens,* which responds as a bacterial infection with an allergic host response (*Pseudomonas* or other bacteria), or Hutchison's *cheiropompholyx,* which may be dyshidrotic, mycotic, idlike, toxic or even contact if followed until a definitive diagnosis can be reached. The relationship of emotion to cheiropompholyx is striking.

In any event, except in *occupational* cases, where protection with barrier creams, gloves, avoidance techniques or moving away from exposure may be necessary, the patient is not really interested in the diagnosis. He wants successful treatment.

In the case of toxic erythemas, drug eruptions and psoriasis the diagnosis is moderately straightforward, as it is in dermatophytosis. Severe ids, however, can be annoying, and internal steroid treatment may be needed to control the severity of the disease on the hands while clearing the foot fungus infection. Locally a 1% hydrocortisone lotion controls itching; and if severe vesiculation occurs, Burow's soaks or ice-cold boric acid will help.

Pustular Psoriasis and Pustular Bacterid

Pustular bacterid is the diagnosis when there is not enough psoriasis elsewhere to be sure. Often a focal infection can be unearthed by a willing dentist if x-rays of the *roots* of the teeth are taken with a view to finding root granulomas rather than cavities. In the event that no focus can be found, sulfa or other antibiotics taken internally along with steroid-antibiotic creams locally, grenz or (rarely) x-ray therapy, and occasionally tar or mercury in modest percentages will help. Occasionally Vioform, such as Ze-Tar-Quin 0.5%, or Vioform hydrocortisone cream 1% will be effective. Treatment here is perhaps related to the immunosuppressive effect of the sulfa, more so than to its antibacterial effect.

Dermatitis Repens

Often two Gantrisin tablets a day plus Vioform hydrocortisone cream and some clipping and filing of ragged nails lead to control. Treatment has to be *protracted*, and avoidance of sweat-provoking footgear, such as Cordovan shoes, and in the case of the fingers, cessation of hangnail biting and chewing are helpful measures. Children who allow their fingers and toes to get "messy" seem prone to this. I suspect that causative organisms can range through a wide spectrum, the responding characteristics of the skin being more closely linked to the patient's constitutional proclivities than to anything else.

Atopic Eczema

This eczema usually clears in summer, and is worse in winter: There is often a family history of asthma, eczema, hay fever, and Dennie's line under the lower lids. The eczema flares with emotional strain, fatigue, and soap and wool exposure, and it fits no contact dermatitis pattern. It responds to Periactin at bedtime, Atarax – 10 mg given three times a day, 1% hydrocortisone lotion or Aristocort formula locally, *plus* protection and avoidance of exposure to repeated irritation. It tends to involve the wrists, so clothing should be checked at that area. Generally, using bath oils to wash hands or at least using superfatted soaps and drying with a warm towel is helpful in management. (See Formulary, no. 31.)

Streptococcus Dermatitis

This is an acute cellulitis with or without lymphangitis. An acute hot, red swelling, it is responsive to penicillin. The subcuticular streptococcal infections that occur around the nail respond to simple deroofing of the blister, soaks and local antibiotic creams. The erysipeloid (Rosenbach) seen in fish handlers responds dramatically to penicillin treatment.

Infectious Eczematoid Dermatitis and Nummular Eczema

These diseases are more prevalent in dark skin. They do not seem to be related to defatting exposures, but they itch extremely and consist of small coin-sized plaques of "dirty vesicles" that crust and scab and slowly enlarge unless treated. Effective remedies are 2% hydrocortisone in Terramycin ointment, or 1% crude coal tar in Aristocort cream 0.5%. The disease occurs mostly on the extremities. Tar paste (Doak Company) is helpful. Either triamcinolone 5 mg/cc intralesionally or 60 mg intramuscularly clears these attacks. The Decadron gel that Merck introduced experimentally a few years ago had phenomenal success; it is now available as Decaderm in estergel. Lidex ointment is often very affective. Some remedies used years ago consisted of the following ingredients:

Pine tar unguentum	1 part
Vioform unguentum	2 parts
Acid mantle cream or Lassar's paste	3 parts (to make an ointment)

Monilial Paronychia and Dermatitis

If a toothpick glides under the nail fold, which looks a little raised and sore, and there is no lunula at the nail, this is probably the diagnosis, which is easily confirmed by culture. Twenty percent aqueous sodium caprylate solution and the avoidance of water are often helpful. In stubborn cases x-ray treatment may be required. Other treatments consist of 3% Chrysarobin in chloroform and 1% gentian violet, both of which are colored treatments. Mycostatin cream is disappointing as a cure, but it may be helpful to withstand the excessive drying of the sodium caprylate and perhaps does help when rubbed in at night. Lotrimin lotion is good. (See Formulary, no. 25.)

Pompholyx

So called dyshidrosis occurs with acute large deep vesicobullous lesions on the palms and soles, often without a reasonable explanation though just as often after a severe emotional strain. Sometimes it recurs every few months. X-ray treatment is remarkably effective, and may have to be resorted to in difficult cases; so are steroids (80 mg Kenalog given intramuscularly) though the blister roof should be checked for mycelia. Sometimes mycelia appears *after* the acute phase has passed. Soaks, antihistamines, cooling soothing local measures and systemic sedation such as Atarax, 25 mg given three times a day, can work wonders. Steroid lotion locally helps, though the plastic-glove technique usually does *not*. The idea that this is some sort of paradoxical sweat-retention syndrome persists, though many studies tend to refute this. Probanthine does not seem to help, but 5% salicylic acid in alcohol occasionally does help. Shriveling soaks of Burow's solution are helpful.

Contact Dermatitis

Fifty percent of the hand eczemas fall into this category, with "housewives' hands" being the leading group. Many are of the primary irritant type with constant repeated exposure to alkaline bleaches or detergents and cleansers. Lack of time to recoup leads to a chronic fissuring and dry itchy skin often on the thenar or hypothenar areas of the palm. Patients give a history of seeing many physicians, having many treatments and having their hand dermatitis persist. Repeated explanation and encouragement are the only hope for this group. They all admit to slipping up on their protective technique. Commonly this is heard: "I love to soak in the bathtub after the kids are asleep" (often with bubble bath and Dial soap!). Other offenses are: peeling vegetables without gloves; drying dishes without gloves; frequent shampooing without gloves; handling clothes and putting them on the line without gloves; and rushing around the kitchen without gloves. (See Formulary, nos. 22, 36, 37.)

A fracture takes at least 3 months to heal. The cast has to stay on that long no matter how comfortable the leg feels. Similarly, a housewife has to apply the missing protective film to her hand skin *externally* for 3 months no matter how well her hands feel. Shepard and Keri hand creams, applied every hour on the hour, are very helpful. Wearing cotton lining under rubber gloves, or liner gloves, which should not be worn for more than 15 minutes at a time and not in very hot water, all assist in recovery. Steroids taken internally are a quick remedy but it is too easy for many patients, who will then rely on this instead of common-sense care and will fail to completely cure. Aristocort 0.5% in acid mantle or aquaphor and water, or USP hydrophilic or Keri hand cream can be manipulated to fit appropriate needs. Tar or Vioform can be added for treating stubborn fissures or lichenified areas. If *very* stubborn, x-ray therapy is a last resort. Bath oil or superfatted soap for washing lessens the drying effects of all soap.

Allergic contact dermatitis from specific things such as the cocobolo-wood handles of knives in the kitchen and from musical instruments, leather golf-club handles, turpentine, varnish, polishes, plastics, oilcloth, various vegetables (especially onions, garlic, lettuce, carrots, oranges and tomatoes), insecticides, mothballs, horseradish, plants, paints, epoxy glue, and rubber can sometimes be deduced by the pattern on the hands. Dermatitis from a small bar, like a golf club, is usually on the fingers; a large bar is on the palms. A large ball causes dermatitis on the fingers and palms, and so on.

Another prescription that we use a great deal is 1% hydrocortisone in bacitracin ointment. Aristocort 0.5% cream can be mixed with equal parts of Chloromycetin 1% cream. Or a capsule of Chloromycetin 250 mg may be dumped into 1 oz of steroid cream, thereby rendering it reasonably antibacterial, at the same time not using neomycin, which occasionally can be a sensitizer.

A variety of formulas can be extemporized in hand treatment. Cade oil seems to have marked benefits in treating the atopic. Antibacterial agents seem to assist greatly in the management of nummular eczema. Sometimes a paradoxical response will occur, and nummular eczema will respond much better to 0.01% Synalar than it will to 0.025% Synalar. Experience is the best teacher in the management of hand eczema.

Ten percent urea in Valisone cream can occasionally rescue an "impossible" problem. Excellent lubricating and mildly protective and inexpensive hand creams are Shepard hand cream (Dome) and Keri hand cream (Westwood). Equal parts of unguentum aqua rosae and zinc oxide ointment make a soft soothing cream.

One of the most frustrating and annoying problems the practitioner faces is a chronic hand dermatitis in a highly skilled mechanic who has to work bare-handed and simply will not or cannot take time off or switch occupations. A lucky choice of a protective cream may save the day.

The West Company (Long Island City, N.Y.) manufactures creams designed specifically for use against special categories of irritants, e.g., *311 West Cream* protects against water-base paints, acids and alkalies; *211 West Cream* protects against inks, stains, dust, grime and fiber glass; and *411 West Cream* protects against most other things, e.g., solvents and cleaners.

Kerodex 71 (Ayerst) protects against soaps, shampoos, detergents, coolants, emulsified cutting oils, plating solutions, acids and alkalis (water-soluble agents). *Kerodex 51* protects against furniture polish, insoluble cutting oils, paints, enamels, solvents, cleaning fluids and poison ivy (water-insoluble agents).

Silicote ointment (Arnar-Stone), 30% silicone, is almost too greasy. *Silicote cream,* 20% silicone, is better.

23 / Foot Conditions

Excessive sweating of the feet often leads to problems when the chemicals in the sock or shoe go into solutions and produce irritation (as in Clorox-soaked socks) or allergic dermatitis from rubber cement or chromate-tanned leather.

Soaking in a dilute solution of formaldehyde (one teaspoon per pint) for 15 minutes at night and the use of Dr. Scholl's Granulated Foot Soap every night to cleanse the skin and empty the sweat ducts where bacteria may reside are effective methods of reducing the sweatiness. A lotion of 5% tannic acid in 70% alcohol applied in the morning and evening is a time-honored remedy. Burow's solution 1:40 for foot soaks is a little milder than the formaldehyde soak, though moderately astringent. A twice-daily change of socks and avoidance of Desert Shoes, Cordovans and rubber-soled shoes as routine footwear also are helpful measures. Zeasorb powder (Stiefel) and Bromhidrosis powder (Dr. Scholl) are commonly available.

Stronger effects can be obtained by the following dusting powder:

Tannic acid powder	
Boric acid powder	$\overline{aa}$
Zinc oxide powder	

Hyperhidrosis

A helpful treatment is 10–25% aluminum chloride in distilled water painted on the feet at bedtime and following with talcum powder. This method may also be used to treat axillary hydrosis, although aluminum chloride should not touch fabric, since this rots it and may cause stains. A wedge resection of the central one-third of the axilla, as advocated by Shelley,[1] is good treatment. Drysol (Person & Covey) is commercially available.

Corns (Clavi)

These circumscribed hard conical thickenings of the keratin often overlie the middle interphalangeal joint of the fifth toe and result from sliding pressure and friction. Once established they are difficult to cure. The pain they produce can be severe and disabling. The spike of hard translucent horny tissue presses inward on joints or sensory nerves with each step. Corns can also occur on the tip of the second or third toe, especially if hammer toe is present or if the shoes are very pointed. They also can occur on the soles of the foot, either in the center of a larger callus or, without much surrounding callus formation, usually at the site of pressure on the ball of the foot. They often will occur at the head of the third metatarsal in women who have broken down the anterior transverse (metatarsal) arch and who wear high heels that throw their weight forward on the heads of the metatarsal bones. When pared, corns are translucent with a yellowish clarity and contain no black dots or ruptured capillaries as do plantar warts, from which they *must* be differentiated. Plantar corns recur after removal with disappointing regularity, whereas plantar warts are cured 85% of the time by removal. Plantar corns are due to mechanical failure and undue pressure of a bone on the skin, plantar warts are due to a virus infection at a site of cutaneous susceptibility.

Corns on the Dorsa of the Toes

Unless there is an underlying bursa or inclusion cyst, corns should be pared and padded to protect them from pressure. One hundred percent silver nitrate applied every 3 weeks after paring will sometimes cure, if protection is continued. Well-fitting shoes that bend at the great toe joint and do not rub the fifth toe are essential. Padding can be lifesaver-shaped, small felt doughnuts, adhesive on one side, or moleskin with or without a central opening for the corn. Various corn paints consisting of salicylic acid, lactic acid and glacial acetic acid, 10% of each in collodion flex, can be used for home treatments. If excision by a good orthopedic surgeon is refused or difficult, and if the patient is elderly, the pain is severe, and all else fails, x-ray therapy, shielding the area with lead, using a dose of 300–600 rad at 100 kv unfiltered, 20 cm tube–skin distance at intervals of 2 weeks for a maximum of three treatments, may palliate successfully for long periods. Electrosurgery usually produces a scar that is no better than a corn, though I have on occasion had successful results with this method. Dilute intralesional triamcinolone may give relief.

Corns on the Sole

The measurement of the foot for an arch support to raise up the metatarsal heads and create a more normal division of weight-bearing points is perhaps the most effective single measure. A plaster cast of the foot (Gypsona Plaster Roll—Curity, 4 in. wide) can be used, which requires some skill, since the foot must be perfectly positioned while the cast hardens, marking the corn with wax pencil or lipstick. From this cast a Mayer-type arch support can be made to raise the metatarsal heads and make an anterior transverse arch. H & W Orthopedic Arch. Supports Inc. (Brooklyn, N.Y.) will supply the therapist with yellow paper sheets on which the patient can stand; the outline of the foot is then traced with a pencil. The site of the corn can be marked with wax pencil or ink and the technician will devise a pad notched at the site of the corn, with the lift behind this to take the weight off the corn. The lifts can be of any desired height, from 1/8 in. to 1/4 in. or more, made of soft or hard rubber, leather-covered and can be inserted inside the normal shoe to make a very comfortable, inexpensive arch support. The form submitted provides for listing the height of lift and the size of shoe, as well as the height, weight, sex and age of the patient and what sort of heel is worn.

Various types of insoles are available, and if the problem is complicated by a congenitally short first metatarsal bone (Morton's toe), a pad can be incorporated to raise the head of the first metatarsal (Morton's pad). If the longitudinal arch is flat, a scaphoid pad can be incorporated, or the Mayer-Schaefer arch support (more rigid) can be ordered. They are very inexpensive.

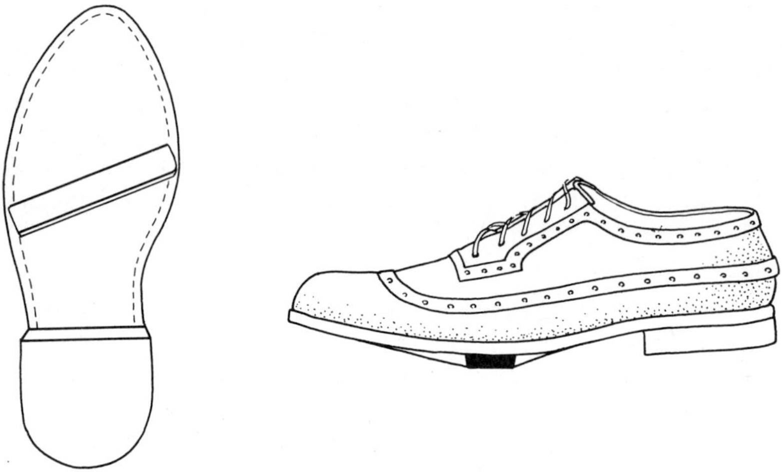

Fig 23–1.— Metatarsal bar on the outside of the sole.

Metatarsal bars on the outside of the sole of the shoe also can be used to take weight off the painful metatarsal heads. They should be ¼ in. thick and about ½ in. to ¾ in. wide or wider and be *behind* the metatarsal heads (Fig 23–1). A rocker bar has a similar effect and consists of a new outer sole, which is thicker over the metatarsal heads and thinner in front and behind. Sponge rubber can be put in the center of the cushion.

Electrosurgery is contraindicated in treating plantar corns; recurrence is almost invariable. Cryotherapy with liquid nitrogen for 90 seconds often will produce resolution. A painful blister may have to be pared later.

Corns on the Tips of the Toes

These corns are often due to cramping flexion of the toe because of pointed or open-toe shoes. As Dr. Royal Montgomery has pointed out,[2] a sling made of ⅜ in.-thick felt, with a cylinder long enough to go under the middle three toes, can be inserted into ½-in. (size #1) Surgitube, making a loop that can be adjusted on the patient's foot with the felt under the toes until just right. The sling is then removed and fixed in this shape with adhesive tape, then replaced. When the patient wears shoes with the sling, pressure will be removed from the toe tips while walking, and often the corn will disappear. A longer shoe should be worn to accommodate the slightly "lengthened" toes.

Hammer Toes

These can similarly be helped by a padded sling, the pad being about the same thickness, but wider, like a class ring, and worn with the pad over the dorsal aspect of the proximal phalanges of the middle toes.

Soft Corns

Soft corns occur in the toe webs, usually the fourth web, probably because of pressure from adjacent condyles (one metatarsal head against the proximal phalangeal condyle of the adjacent toe). They are often soggy and macerated before paring, and hard, shiny and translucent after paring. A sinus may result with extreme pain and even osteomyelitis. Treatment of early cases may be merely a matter of protection and dryness. Tincture of merthiolate with 5% salicylic acid in it applied three times a day has cleared a few cases though more often a small sponge-rubber pad shaped to keep the toes separated helps more (Fig 23–2). (See Formulary, no. 19 for urea-cordran lotion.)

Simple lamb's wool loop winding also protects; inserting sponge rubber in the inner space between the toes is very effective. On occasion the "duck bill" recommended by Royal Montgomery separates the metatarsal heads more efficiently.[2] This consists of a thin felt pad trimmed into the shape of a

Fig 23–2. – A sponge-rubber pad to separate the toes.

duck's head and bill. The narrow part is brought between the toes, and the main body of the pad is placed under the metatarsal heads.

If soft corns continue to persist, removal of the condyles or removal of the toe surgically usually provides a cure. The dread of the deformity causes most patients to postpone this solution to their problem, which usually is very satisfactory.

Plantar Warts

Solitary warts on bony prominences; mother-daughter warts, consisting of one or two large warts with multiple small satellites surrounding them; and mosaic warts, which are a collection of coalescent small warty cores fitted together like a mosaic, usually painless and of years' duration, are all included here. Mosaic warts are resistant to radiation and most other forms of therapy, including electrosurgery. The other warts can be treated with *one* course of radiation therapy (650 rad every 2 weeks) for a total of three doses, 1,000 rad at a crack, once, electrosurgery carefully done, acid or any of the other acknowledged wart treatments. The patient should have a knowledge of the natural course of infection with the wart virus and expect a recurrence. He should guard against walking barefoot in areas subject to trauma. For example, a dog hair or a thumb tack stuck in the sole often leads to a wart later.[3]

Mosaic Warts

Royal Montgomery cured 90% of 109 cases over a 5-year period in an average of 11.2 visits each, using a chemosurgical technique with either 100% silver nitrate or a saturated solution of trichloracetic acid followed by 40% salicylic acid plasters.[2] In more keratinized lesions, he augmented this treatment with 60% salicylic acid in white ointment USP or 100% monochloracetic acid rubbed in, and on occasion he used acid nitrate of mercury. (Acid nitrate of mercury is made by fuming nitric acid 45 cc, adding distilled water 15 cc, mixing and *then* adding red oxide of mercury 40 cc.

The wart is pared and the appropriate chemical applied with a toothpick, wearing finger cots to protect the fingers. Tattooing with a sharp pointed "World's Fair" toothpick helps. A 40% salicylic acid plaster (Beiersdorff) is cut to size and held in place with moleskin, which is covered with Elastoplast. The foot is kept dry for a week and the patient is given Empirin, codeine or Darvon for pain. On a return visit, the macerated tissue is pared and treatment repeated. If a sterile abscess results from the chemical destruction, it is deroofed. When the area thins, 100% silver nitrate only is used. (See Formulary, no. 21 for additional treatments.)

Plantar Radiodermatitis

Typical signs of telangiectasia, atrophy, erythema and hyperkeratosis, ulceration and occasionally pain are present. When pared, the area often gives the appearance of soggy or honeycombed small sinuses. The border is diffuse and blends in with surrounding tissue. If the lesion is ulcerated, there may be typical areas of radiodermatitis surrounding the ulcer, and there may be deep fibrosis and adherence to underlying structures. Treatment is with antibiotic ointment and perhaps systemic antibiotics and protective padding. In stubborn cases, bed rest in addition is indicated. If all else fails, proper plastic surgery is required. These unfortunate disasters are few and far between. They usually result from accidental overdosage—leaving the filter out, leaving the machine unattended, etc. Be careful! Several of my patients were not treated by dermatologists. I have not seen any malignancies, although some of them concealed their previous radiation.

Keratoderma Plantaris

Whether keratoderma plantaris is from psoriasis, climate or just plain obesity, if the heels are involved, translucent plastic heel cups supplied in various sizes (Mayflower Podiatry Supply Co., Brooklyn, N.Y.) are extremely helpful. These can be worn inside the stocking and are not noticeable. They serve to protect the heel from friction of the shoe as well as to hydrate the keratin to lessen dry fissuring. They also keep medication in contact with the heel, e.g., 40–60% salicylic acid in white ointment for mosaic plantar warts.

Plain Elastoplast, using the 3-in. variety, can be applied to fissured heels, with or without tar, and left on for three or four days with marked improvement.

Keratoderma climactericum often responds dramatically to systemic estrogen treatment. In three of my patients, when postmenopausal vaginal bleeding was induced by the estrogen, a dilation and curettage done to rule out uterine malignancy apparently was instrumental in permanently clearing the keratoderma. Some gynecologists say there may be uterine hormones secreted from postmenopausal endometrium.

Occlusion with Saran Wrap and various steroid creams is useful treatment of psoriasis of the feet. Keralyt (Westwood) is helpful (6% salicylic acid gel).

Keloids and Scars

These are often the result of a lesion on the dorsa of the foot which is constantly rubbed in the instep by shoe laces or the tongue of the shoe. Kenalog parenteral (10 mg/cc) injected intracutaneously with a 50% dilution of sterile water is very helpful treatment. Liquid nitrogen destruction is effective.

Subungual Fibroma and Exostosis

For these conditions, removal by *deep* curettement under Novocain or Xylocaine anesthesia with partial nail plate removal with or without electrodesiccation is the best treatment.

Onychomycosis

Direct examination often shows the mycelium when cultures grow nothing. Debridement after maceration with 40% salicylic acid plaster and an electric hand drill of the inexpensive variety is a safe and effective method of treatment. Griseofulvin administered for 12–14 months is required. (See Formulary, no. 25.) Micatin cream applied locally has curiously helpful results. One percent 5-FU in propylene glycol is also helpful.

Ingrown Toenails

The nail should be cut straight across. A cotton pad or Celastic (United Shoe Machine Company) should be put under the ingrown corner to raise the sharp nail from cutting into the toe fold. Tincture of merthiolate helps to dry these areas, and the patient should use soaks and mild antiseptic treatment of various kinds. Sometimes removal of the proud flesh by electrosurgery, using Xylocaine, is very helpful.

Glomus Tumor

This is bluish and very painful on pressure. The treatment, of course, is excision.

REFERENCES

1. Hurley, H. J., and Shelley, W. B.: A simple surgical approach to the management of axillary hyperidrosis, J.A.M.A. 186:109, 1963.
2. Montgomery, R. M., and Locascio, W. V.: Padding and devices for foot comfort, Arch. Dermatol. 93:739, 1966.
3. Pipkin, J. L., et al.: The treatment of plantar warts by single dose method of roentgen ray, South. Med. J. 42:52, 93, 1949.

24 / Diseases of the Blood Vessels

Vasomotor Conditions

Varieties of constrictive or obstructive vessel disease produce cyanosis or blanching of the tips of the fingers and toes. These include Raynaud's disease, acrocyanosis, acrosclerosis, as well as cryoglobulinemia, which may result from other diseases or be without any discoverable cause. Management of these diseases revolves around measures to protect and warm the parts, as well as vasodilating measures such as massage and treatment with Priscoline, niacin or alcohol. Investigation to rule out a diagnosis of anemia, focal infection and serum protein abnormalities are important. Occasionally blotching erythema of the ankles will occur in women for no good reason. Recurrent small ulcerations may accompany this. This condition is livedo reticularis. Treatment is purely symptomatic unless abnormal serum globulins or hypertension underlie this. Sympathectomy may be partially successful. (See p. 122, PCAD.)

Purpuras

This symptom results from extravasation of blood into the skin or mucous membrane. This can be petechial, ecchymotic or a hematoma. (See p. 14, PCAD.) It can be the result of *infectious disease* (tuberculosis, rheumatic fever, subacute bacterial endocarditis, Rocky Mountain spotted fever, meningitis, typhus, measles, spotted fever, smallpox, malaria, influenza, herpes zoster, anthrax) *allergic disease* (chocolate, nuts, fish, belladona, phenobarb, iodides, quinine, gold, arsenic, penicillin, mesentoin) or *thrombocytopenic* (which may be due to a drug, or idiopathic, e.g., Dilantin, quinidine). Purpuras may also result from:

1. *Defects in the fibrin clotting mechanism*—Vitamin K deficiency, hypothrombinemia induced by dicumarol or other drugs.

2. *Serum deficiencies*—hemophilia, afibrinogenemia or hypofibrinogenemic states—hemolytic anemias.

3. *Fragile vessels*—scurvy or hereditary hemorrhagic telangiectasia.

4. *Abnormal serum proteins*—Waldenstrom's, various globulin changes, cryoglobulinemias, systemic lupus erythematosus, multiple myelomas, lymphomas.

5. *Senility*—usually because of lessened connective tissue support for the vessels, small amounts of shearing strain will rupture the small vessels in older persons. Treatment involves slower movements and sleeve protection.

6. *Circulatory obstruction*—caused by tight clothing, tumors, asthma, cardiac failure, whooping cough.

7. *Allergic vasculitis*—see p. 123, PCAD.

Treatment

Depending on the cause, treatment should include elimination of foods or drugs, addition of vitamin C or K, antihistamines and on occasion steroids. The assistance of an internist is advisable.

Allergic Vasculitis

This term includes benign local reactions and disseminated fatal diseases. There is a tendency for the number of gamma globulins to be increased, as well as for a reaction in and around the small blood vessels compatible with sensitization. This can vary from proliferative to necrotizing in type. Those primarily in the skin include erythema nodosum (see p. 10, PCAD)(in the shins), nodular dermal allergy of Gougerot (buttocks and extremities), allergic arteriolitis of Ruiter, dermatitis nodularis necrotica of Werther (buttocks and extremities—with polymorphism), necrotizing angiitis with granulomas (Churg-Strauss), also known as allergic granulomatosis as well as periarteritis nodosa cutanea, the allergic microbids of

Miescher, erythema elevatum diutinum (Hutchinson type) and acute parapsoriasis. (See p. 27, PCAD.)

More serious forms include papulosis atrophicans maligna (Degos' disease), lethal midline granuloma of the face (McBride), Wegener's granulomatosis, which has more widespread manifestations, and of course periarteritis nodosa. (See p. 122, PCAD.) Pyoderma gangrenosum may occur with ulcerative colitis and is probably an autoimmune disease. Solitary chancriform angiitis is a highly fatal vasculitis, produced by drugs or serum, and usually begins as a dermatitis with fever and gradually worsens. It is similar to Lyell's epidermal necrolysis. (See p. 11, PCAD.)

Sulfonamides, streptomycin, para-aminosalicylic acid bacterial extract injections, weed sprays and petroleum products, as well as the rheumatoid factor, appear to be implicated as causes in many cases of allergic vasculitis.

In Winkelmann and Ditto's study of 38 cases of vasculitis, 19 patients gave a definite history of some sort of preexisting allergy; in 20 cases, drugs or chemicals were implicated in the onset; and in several, there had been injections of bacterial extracts.[1] In six of 15 idiopathic cases, the rheumatoid factor seemed to be implicated. The onset was preceded by flu-like symptoms. Table 24–1 lists the forms of cutaneous and systemic necrotizing vasculitis.

Investigation should include a careful study of the patient's history to discover drug or other toxic products encountered in work or hobby. Anti-streptolysin titer, erythrocyte sedimentation rate, serum protein electrophoresis, the rheumatoid factor and biopsy of the skin, as well as routine blood and urine studies should be done.

Treatment

Treatment is based on the avoidance of exposure to drugs and chemicals; in mild cases, rest plus elevation of the legs, patience and antihistamines may be all that is needed.

In treating acute cases, short courses of steroids, perhaps repeated, and in severe cases, steroids in large doses appear to be the only course. Autoimmune mechanisms must be a factor in many of the cases, and Winkelmann and Ditto used sulfapyradine treatment for two patients with gratifying results.

TABLE 24-1.—FORMS OF CUTANEOUS AND SYSTEMIC NECROTIZING VASCULITIS*

PRIMARILY CUTANEOUS	PRIMARILY VISCERAL	CUTANEOUS AND VISCERAL
Arteriolitis allergica (Ruiter), often drug	Allergic granulomatosis (Strauss, Churg and Zak) with asthma	Allergic angiitis
Dermatitis nodularis necrotica (Werther)	Anaphylactoid purpura (Glanzmann)	Leukocytoclastic angiitis
Erythema elevatum diutinum (Hutchinson type)	Henoch-Schoenlein purpura (abdominal pain)	
Facial granuloma with eosinophilia	Hypersensitivity angiitis (Zeek), drug or serum	
Hemorrhagic microbids (Miescher)	Hypersensitivity type of periarteritis nodosa skin in one-fourth cases	
Idiopathic lethal granulomas of the midline facial tissues (McBride)	Necrotizing angiitis (Zeek)	
Monosymptom, bisymptom, trisymptom and pentasymptom complexes (Gougerot)	Noninfectious necrotizing granulomas	
Nodular dermal allergids (Gougerot and Duperrat)	Pathergic granulomatosis (Feinberg)	
	Peliosis rheumatica	
Pyoderma gangrenosum	Purpura rheumatica	
Acute parapsoriasis	Wegener's granulomatosis glomerulitis, fever, granulomas all over beginning in upper respiratory tract	

*From Winkelmann, R. K., and Ditto, W. B.: Cutaneous and Visceral syndromes of necrotizing or "allergic" angiitis: A study of 38 cases, Medicine 43:59, 1964; Reprinted with permission of the Williams & Wilkins Co. and Doctor Winkelmann.

The effect of this drug in treating dermatitis repens and pyoderma gangrenosum has been known for some time. In treating acute parapsoriasis, it has been shown that methotrexate is remarkably effective, while in many cases of pyoderma gangrenosum, debridement, either surgical or enzymatic, is helpful. Lamprene has been found effective in Sweden.[2] A patient with Wegener's granulomatosis treated with Imuran (azathioprine) and steroid responded well.[3]

In the days when Meleney's symbiotic gangrene was considered more often in the differential diagnosis, zinc peroxide paste was considered very helpful treatment. Its manufacture now seems to be a lost art. One wonders if this might be useful in managing many cases of so-called midline granuloma of the face (McBride). Certainly the use of systemic antibiotics and steroids with local antibiotics (powders or ointments) and either 1% neomycin solution, wet dressings or hot saline compresses, plus peroxide irrigations can be of benefit. Supportive therapy and search for any debilitating disease and its correction are part of the attack. The similarity of vegetative pyodermas to perifolliculitis capitis abscedens et suffodiens is more than coincidental.

Poikiloderma Atrophicans Vasculare (Jacobi)

A widespread superficial diffuse telangiectasia with small capillary hemorrhages and atrophy suggesting "x-ray skin" often appears after sunburn or exposure to cold. There is no successful treatment. Possibly some cases progress to mycosis fungoides or lymphoblastoma. Poststeroid flushing can generally be differentiated easily.

Pigmented Purpuric Eruptions

These involve the lower extremities. These appear to be relatively benign conditions which may be related to drug eruptions, especially aspirin, and appear to be self-limited. Perhaps overindulgence in hot baths or showers plays a greater part in their development than is generally acknowledged. Purpuric pigmented lichenoid dermatitis (Gougerot and Blum's disease), purpura annularis telangiectodes (Majocchi's disease) and progressive pigmentary dermatoses (Schamberg's disease) are the varieties commonly seen. (See p. 13, PCAD.)

Treatment involves the use of steroid emulsions and lubrication with elimination of drugs or foods suspected of being implicated with the onset. Avoidance of strong soap and long hot, frequent baths and moderate elevation of the feet when possible, plus vitamin C taken orally, usually suffice.

Angioma Serpiginosum

This angioma consists of minute angiomatous puncta occurring in groups in which proliferation and involution go on more or less simultaneously to produce small ringlike or serpiginous patterns. They are a curiosity, no etiology or treatment being known.

Telangiectasia

The appearance of tiny clusters of superficial capillaries with a central red point leads to the term *spider angioma*. These angiomas are commonly seen on the face and hands of fair-skinned children who are in the sun a lot, as well as in pregnant women. Sailors and farmers who are exposed to the elements, as well as the more sheltered martini drinkers, may exhibit spider angiomas in the central portion of the face, the so-called expensive complexion! Treatment is by galvanic electrolysis or diathermy spark. Correction of dietary indiscretions usually is not quite enough.

Small red capillary angiomas on the trunk of people over 40 years of age are referred to as DeMorgan's spots or senile ectasia. These can be destroyed by electrodesiccation.

Hereditary hemorrhagic telangiectasia (Osler-Rendu-Weber) results in nose bleeds, development of angiomas and spiders on the lips, tongue and floor of the mouth, and other symptoms, which gradually increase in number with the passage of time. Estrogen is reported to help these people, who may have frightening hemorrhages from time to time. Bleeding areas can be cauterized or injected with sclerosing solution (Sylnasol – Searle).

Extensive telangiectasia may occur in persons with subacute lupus erythematosus, dermatomyositis, scleroderma and rheumatoid arthritis, commonly on the terminal phalanges. After one of the exanthemas, a generalized telangiectasia may occur, as can happen in pregnancy. This can occur also after radiodermatitis, adenoma sebaceum, cirrhosis of the liver, heart disease and nephritis.

Widespread telangiectasia of the legs of middle-aged women (also men) with or without arborescent venules can be a disfiguring condition which on occasion can be helped by electrolysis or injection of sclerosing solution *foam* (shake the bottle up and use only the foam) using a #30 needle and great magnification. If the foam gets outside the venule, a brown stain may result, or there may even be a small slough. It is exasperating work, and the patients are often equally exasperating in their demands for perfection. Twenty percent saline with a small amount of heparin in it is a better technique, using a #30 needle and pushing about 1.0 cc of air ahead of the solution to blanch out the vein.[4]

Telangiectasia may be a part of several congenital conditions, such as Thomsen's disease (congenital cutaneous dystrophy), Rothmund's syndrome, or Bloom's syndrome, when dwarfs look as if they have lupus erythematosus. Telangiectasia of the cheeks occasionally occurs in patients with the tetralogy of Fallot.

Sickle Cell Anemia

In this disease there is a punched-out ulcer, usually on the ankle for years before any other symptoms occur. It is common in blacks and is familial. Diagnosis is by blood examination, and treatment with steroids is temporarily curative. Other leg ulcers can occur with pernicious anemia, Cooley's anemia, congenital hemolytic anemia and polycythemia, as well as ulcerative colitis.

Thromboangiitis Obliterans

Vascular occlusion of the vessels of the legs leading to pain, gangrene and amputation characterize this condition. (See p.

123, PCAD.) It is almost exclusively found in young middle-aged men, and often in cigarette smokers. Sympathectomy helps for a while.

Arteriosclerotic Leg Ulcer

This type of ulcer is most often on the medial aspect of the lower third of the leg like a varicose ulcer. However, usually there are no varicose veins, and there is often a history of intermittent claudication. The arteries can usually be felt. Treatment is by measures designed to improve the circulation, e.g., bed rest, elevation or supporting bandages, as well as antibiotics. Sympathectomy is disappointing, but sometimes vascular surgeons can be very helpful and should be consulted.

Varicose Veins and Varicose Ulcers

Usually stasis eczema results from seepage of serum proteins into the skin. Pigmentation may occur from leakage of red blood cells and resultant hemosiderin deposition. Edema

Fig 24–1.—The zinc paste bandage is applied directly on the skin. There should be no wrinkles or folds.

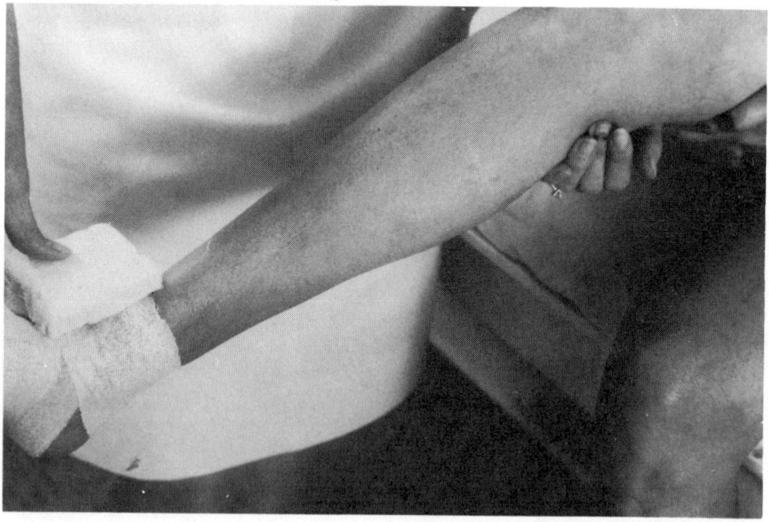

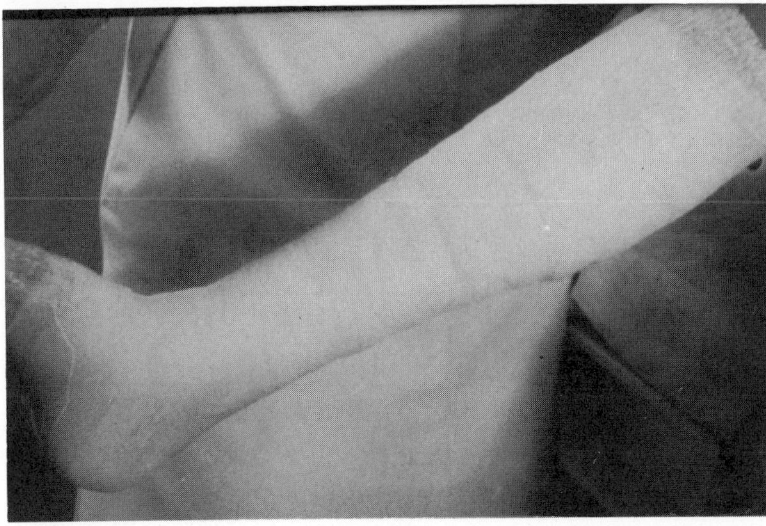

Fig 24–2.—The zinc paste bandage completely wrapped from toe to knee. It is smoothed on like a cast.

Fig 24–3.—Elastoplast is applied over the zinc paste bandage. Here the toe is too pointed.

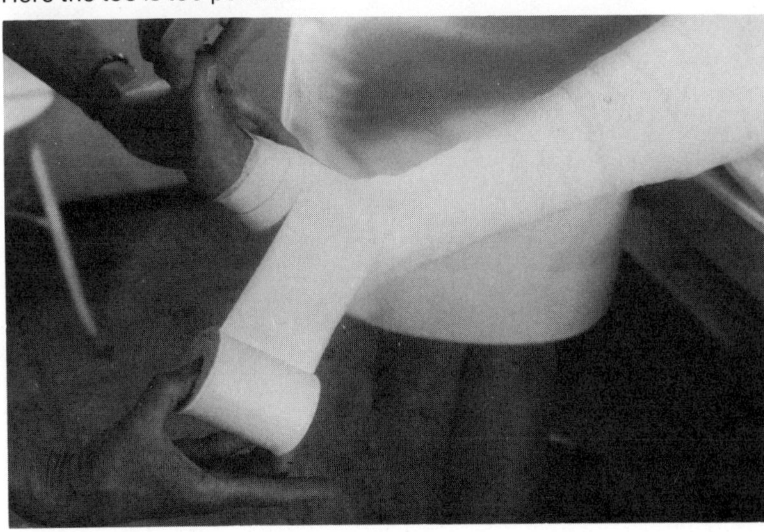

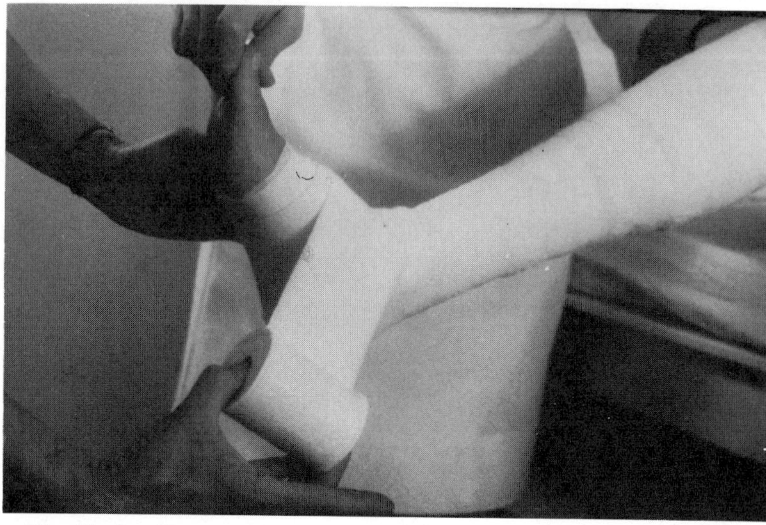

Fig 24–4.—Elastoplast is applied with the ankle at a right angle. A pressure pad of sponge rubber may be incorporated.

Fig 24–5.—Elastoplast wrapped around the corner of the heel.

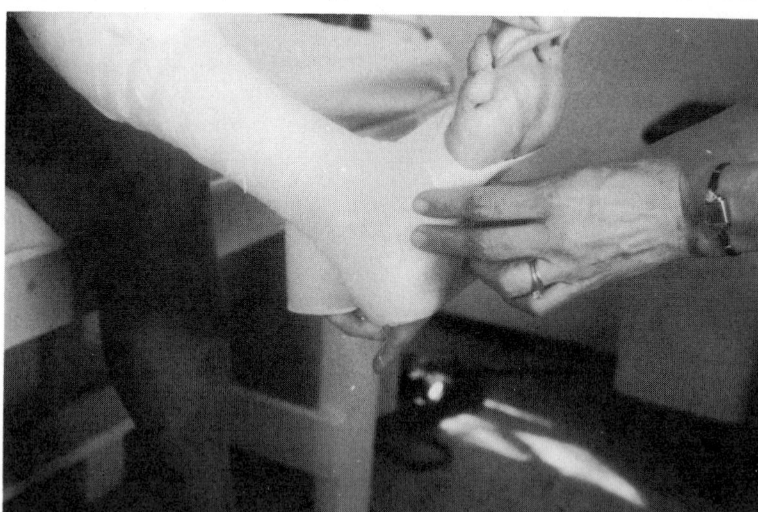

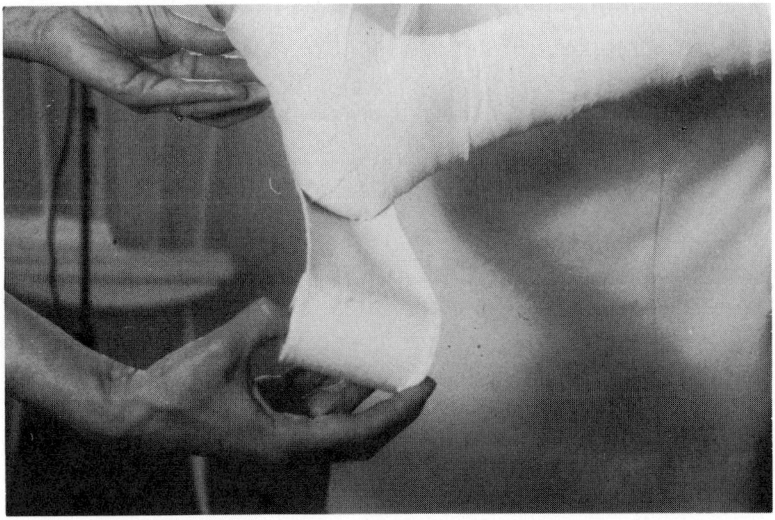

Fig 24–6.—Elastoplast wrapped over the tip of the heel.

Fig 24–7.—Elastoplast wrapped with moderate pressure starting up the leg.

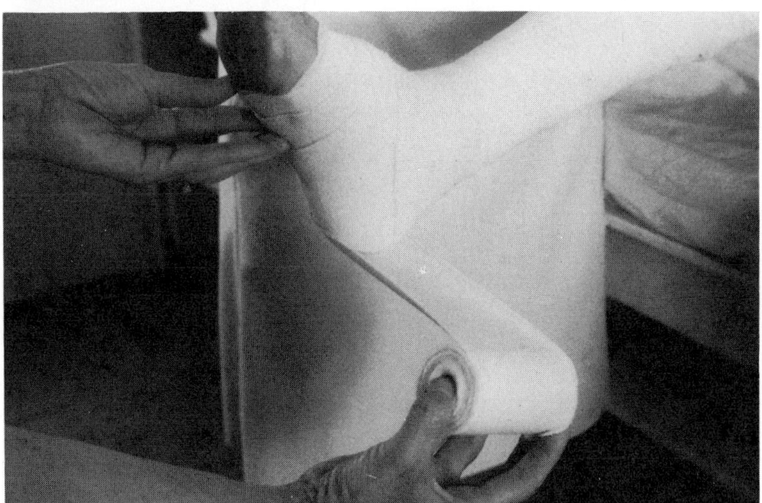

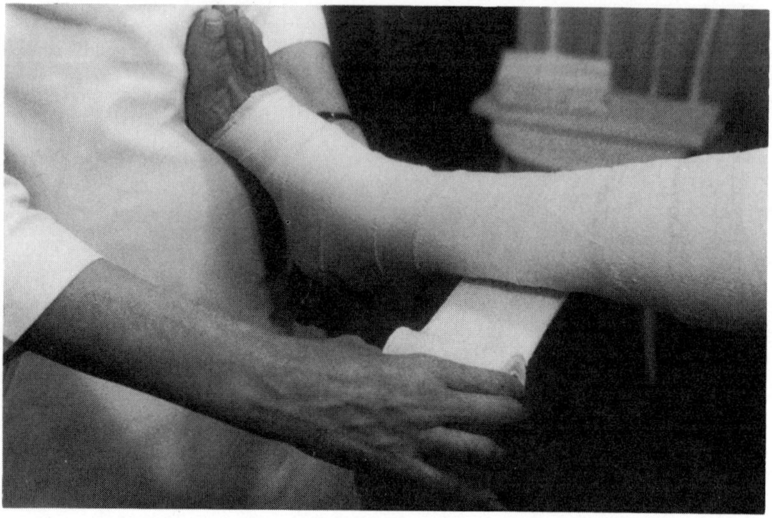

Fig 24–8. – Elastoplast wrapped around the leg.

and superficial phlebitis may occur, or nutritional deprivation may cause the skin to break down, and necrosis and ulceration may occur. Inability of the valves to meet in a dilated vein prohibits the return of venous blood up the leg (venous pressure is about 4 mm water) with the resultant difficulties. Surgical treatment of varicose veins, with ligation of the saphenous and communicating veins (providing the deep veins are patent) is the method of choice.

Steroid-antibiotic creams for treating varicose eczema, with supportive elastic bandages for the varicose veins, will often suffice to keep a patient mobile. Where there is ulceration, enzymatic ointments with hydrocortisone plus sponge-rubber pressure pads and Tensor bandages or Unna boot, carefully applied, are very effective treatment. On occasion, when the ulcers are infected, bed rest, elevation and compresses are necessary. Pinch grafts have their place in speeding convalescence in large ulcers, though I have resorted to prescribing oral steroids more often lately, with or without oral antibiotics, and have had faster and more comfortable healing invariably. This is true of arteriosclerotic ulcers as well.

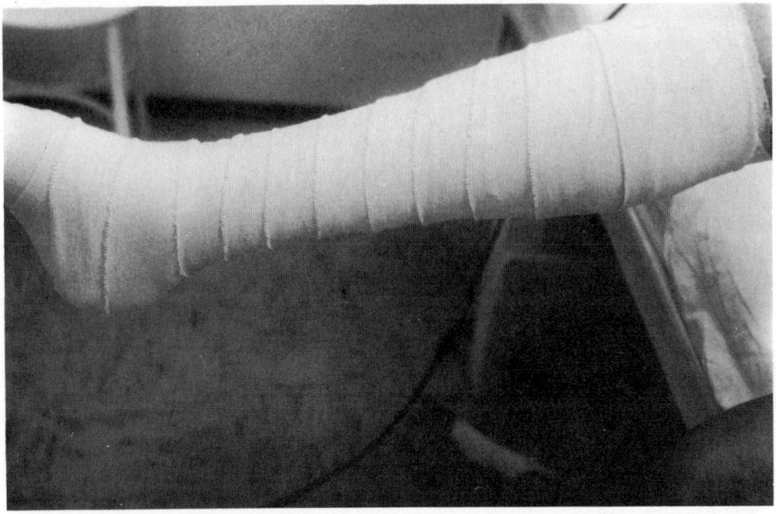

Fig 24–9.—Elastoplast completely wrapped from toes to knee over the zinc paste bandage. This dressing should be checked in three days.

A modified Unna-boot technique is to use Medicopaste (Graham Field), Primer (Edward Taylor, Ltd.) or Dome-Paste (zinc impregnated) bandage applied carefully with no wrinkling from toe to knee, and over this wrap a 3-in. Elastoplast (Figs 24–1 through 24–9).

REFERENCES

1. Winkelmann, R. K., and Ditto, W. B.: Cutaneous and visceral syndromes of necrotizing or "allergic" angiitis: A study of 38 cases, Medicine 43:59, 1964.
2. Sams, W. M., Jr., et al.: Leukocytoclastic vasculitis, Arch. Dermatol. 112:219, 1976.
3. Wishart, J. M.: Wegener's granulomatosis—controlled by azathioprine and corticosteriods, Br. J. Dermatol. 92:461, 1975.
4. Foley, W. J.: The eradication of venous blemishes, Cutis 15:665, 1975.

25 / Erythemas

Localized erythemas resulting from sun, heat or cold (e.g., chilblains or pernio) and other local causes are generally manageable by the exercise of common sense, once the diagnosis has been made.

Exanthematous Erythemas

These can be tantalizingly difficult to categorize correctly. They are almost always of internal origin and very often the result of infection. Toxic erythema occurs in the course of such diseases as typhoid, mononucleosis, brucellosis, rheumatic fever, malaria and meningitis. Generalized erythemas can also occur from fish, berries and drugs (especially belladonna, sulfonamides, barbiturates and chloral hydrate), apart from the ordinary drug rashes that these can cause.

SCARLATINIFORM ERYTHEMAS.—This condition may resemble scarlet fever in everything except the constitutional symptoms, the strawberry tongue and tonsillar exudate. Peeling palms often follow this. (See p. 8, PCAD.)

MORBILLIFORM ERYTHEMA.—This can be distinguished from rubella (German measles) and rubeola (measles) by the Koplik's spots (measles—early) and the occipital nodes. In cases where the diagnosis of German measles is imperative, e.g., in women in early pregnancy, the rubella titer for hemagglutination inhibition can be very helpful.

ROSEOLA INFANTUM (exanthem subitum).—When an infant or very small child is suddenly ill with a high fever for 3 or 4 days and suddenly the fever clears, a reticulated macular erythema on the face and neck may suddenly appear. It rapidly spreads over the body and disappears in 24–48 hours. The palms and soles are not affected.

ERYTHEMA INFECTIOSUM (fifth disease).—This disease is almost asymptomatic except for the erythema. It occurs in spring and summer. Called "slap cheek," it starts on the cheeks and is especially red under the eyes. A general macular erythema develops in 2 days and lasts about 5 days, fading to leave a bluish reticulated network on the skin.

ECHO VIRUS EXANTHEM (Boston 1951—type 16).—This occurs rarely as a slight fever with a morbilliform erythema sparsely scattered over the upper trunk and face. There is no lymphadenopathy.

GIANOTTI-CROSTI SYNDROME.—Also called acrodermatitis papulosa infantum, this condition occurs in young children as an exanthem with an upper respiratory infection, characteristically lichenoid papules on the extensors of the extremities with a copper color and a crusty character. There are hemorrhagic tendencies on the lower extremities, and spontaneous clearing usually occurs in three weeks. This is probably a nonspecific id reaction, though it could be a virus. It is associated with hepatomegaly and splenomegaly.

RAT-BITE FEVER.—whether from *Spirillum minus* (sodoku) or from *Streptobacillus moniliformis* (Haverhill fever) following the bite of a rat or laboratory animal, rat-bite fever starts as erysipelas at the site of the bite, with arthralgia, fever and a morbilliform or scarlatiniform eruption often involving the palms. Penicillin treatment clears it.

Treatment

Recurrent scarlatiniform erythemas as the result of recurrent sore throats, with peeling palms in children, suggest that a tonsillectomy is in order. This recurrent syndrome is akin to guttate psoriasis recurring with sore throat, and yet it is often difficult to persuade the ear, nose and throat surgeon to perform a tonsillectomy. Most of the other erythemas require no treatment beyond explanation and reassurance, though a diagnosis of mononucleosis often has to be ruled out if no easy explanation is forthcoming. A 10-day course of oral antibiotic is often quickly effective.

Erythema Annulare Centrifugum

This rare recurrent polycyclic eruption consists of raised rings that appear, grow, break up and disappear and are replaced by new ones that repeat the same course. It is probably identical with erythema gyratum perstans (Wende). It can be associated with internal malignancy, which should always be looked for. Though the cause is unknown, it is similar to dermatitis herpetiformis in some respects. It is usually asymptomatic, however, and appears on the covered areas of the trunk. A short course of steroids may occasionally abolish it successfully.

Erythema Elevatum Diutinum

Persistent plaques over the joints of the fingers, wrist, knee or Achilles tendon may resemble granuloma annulare. Purplish, smooth and often painful, the disease may last for years. Occasionally steroid treatment seems to be helpful, though recently several articles have appeared showing remarkable remission with dapsone treatment.[1] Extracellular cholesterosis is probably a variant in which lipids are deposited extracellularly in the skin.

Erythema Multiforme

The classic Hebra type of erythema multiforme with recurrent attacks of polymorphous erythema in the spring, involving the hands, feet and face, is probably an infection of the herpes virus. The course of the disease is 3–6 weeks, and there are no scars. The symptomatic type may occur after poison ivy as a sort of "eczematization" or may precede or usher in a serious illness, such as pneumonia or arthritis. It can appear after x-ray therapy of tumors, or after vaccination. The "triggers" can be varied and numerous, e.g., viral, fungal, bacterial, drug, food, malignancy, etc.

Treatment

If itching is a problem, antihistamines help. Local treatment with steroid creams and lotions also helps, though possibly the best control measure is steroid given either orally or by injection in combination with one of the tetracyclines. If the mouth is severely inflamed, treatment with Kenalog in Orabase, mouthwashes with antihistamines in them, or viscous Xylocaine may enable the patient to eat. Mucous membrane lesions in the anus, vagina or penis require lubricating steroid-antibiotic ointments at first, and later powders. Avoidance of potentially allergenic substances, such as exotic foods and not absolutely necessary drugs, is wise. Unless the attack is mild, the hospital is usually the best place for these people.

Granuloma Annulare

An idiopathic and often asymptomatic condition, these granulomas are seen often on the dorsa of hands and feet in children and sometimes in adults, too. They can be treated effectively. Intralesional Kenalog, diluting 10 mg/cc 50–50 with Xylocaine, saline or sterile water, and injecting small quantities at multiple sites (or using the Dermajet) intracutaneously, flattens the raised rings. Pretibial myxedema and necrobiosis lipoidica diabeticorum also can be effectively treated in this manner, although the injections must be more dispersed to avoid necrosis.[2, 3]

REFERENCES

1. Fort, S. L., and Rodman, O. G.: Erythema elevatum diutinum response to dapsone, Arch. Dermatol. 113:819, 1977.
2. Sparrow, G., and Abell, E.: Granuloma annulare and necrobiosis lipoidica treated by jet injector, Br. J. Dermatol. 93:85, 1975.
3. Lang, P. G., Sisson, J. C., and Lynch, P. J.: Intralesional triamcinolone therapy for pretibial myxedema, Arch. Dermatol. 111:197, 1975.

26 / Parasites

Scabies (Sarcoptes scabiei)

This is probably one of the most common parasitic infections, usually spread by bodily contact, though other contaminated objects can also infect. There is severe itching, usually worse at night, with lesions (mostly excoriated burrows) on the fingerwebs, volar wrists, buttocks, penis, axillary folds and around the nipples in women.

Treatment

Treatments such as Kwell lotion given twice daily for 3 days, then repeated weekly for 3 weeks, Eurax cream or lotion (Geigy) twice a day, and the old-fashioned remedy of 10% sulfur ointment applied at night for four nights in a row and washing it off in the morning are effective. The best treatment is benzyl benzoate (Lannette, Inc., Philadelphia) or Zylate (isopropyl alcohol is the base). Benzyl benzoate 25% emulsion applied from the neck down after a hot bath while the skin is still damp, and then left on, is effective if repeated nightly for three nights when the bedding is changed and fresh clothing is worn in the morning. Treatment should be repeated once, a week later. Particular attention should be paid to body folds. If hands are washed, the emulsion should be reapplied for 24-hour contact. (See Formulary, no. 30.) Hernandez-Perez, using 10% Thiobendazole applied once or twice topically, cleared 80% of scabies cases so treated.[1]

Fleas (Siphonaptera)

Plague, rickettsiae and murine typhus are probably transmitted by rodent fleas. Most flea bites seen in this country are from dog and cat fleas, who lay their eggs in floor cracks, rugs or in dust or other debris. Fleas can go without seeking food for long periods of time, and larvae in a rug can take up to a year to reach the adult stage, so infestations can be stubborn. Diagnosis is made by seeing three or four bites in a straight line, evenly spaced, or wheals with a pinpoint central hemorrhagic puncta on the ankles or legs. Another way to detect the presence of fleas in a house is to wear white socks, sit in the dark, then turn on the light suddenly and see the fleas on the socks.

Treatment

Flea powders dusted on the animal or a flea collar, plus spraying the rugs and animals' sleeping places with Raid are necessary. Occasionally naphtha crystals are needed to deinfest a rug. Better yet, all the rugs should be sent out to be cleaned, and repellants should be worn on the ankles. Shuffling across a floor with flypaper leggings will catch many leaping fleas. Black Flag is a good killer spray.

Sand Fleas (Tunga penetrans)

Sand fleas are burrowing insects indigenous to South America, the West Indies and Africa producing shallow lesions usually around the great toenail but in general on the lower extremities. The fleas gradually engorge themselves with blood as they burrow and should be removed carefully with a flat needle. The lesions are referred to as chigo itch (no relation to chiggers). Good solid shoes usually prevent this.

Pediculosis (Lice, Anoplura)

Pediculosis Corporis

The lice live in clothing; the nits hatch in 9 days and must feed within 24 hours. The adult lives about 30 days and is a vector for relapsing fever and typhus. Diagnosis is made by seeing parallel linear scratch marks on the shoulders, back, buttocks and thighs, sparing the face and hands, with small red puncta and an urticarial eruption. In long-standing cases (vagabonds' disease), enlarged regional lymph nodes and a peculiar melanoderma not unlike Addison's disease are features.

Treatment

Historically in large populations, 10% DDT in talc blown into the clothing was used to deinfest; otherwise hot soap-and-water baths and sterilization of the clothing, including bedding, in an autoclave or oven (hotter than 160 F) is satisfactory.

Pediculosis Capitis

Blacks are immune to this infestation of the scalp hair. Characteristically the nape of the neck is excoriated, itchy and may be impetiginized and crusted with a bad odor. The nits can be seen attached to the hair, *firmly*. They have a characteristic fluorescence when tested with Wood's light (white). This pediculosis is more common in children than in adults.

Treatment

Benzyl benzoate emulsion, or Kwell, is effective. A steel fine comb (Derbac Company, Cereal Soap Co. Inc.) facilitates the cure. These fine combs are made of steel and are very good. It is advisable to repeat the treatment several times and *ensure* cure. Sources of infestation must be removed, and family, school mates and other acquaintances should be checked. Soaking the combs in ammonia water for 2 hours allows the nits to be easily removed. Hats are best discarded. Nits hatch in a week, so weekly examination must be done. Vinegar has some dissolving effect on the nit cement as does kerosene (used 50% in mineral oil). Benzyl benzoate is most reliable. (See Formulary, no. 30.)

Pediculosis Pubis

Ordinarily the crab louse is confined to the pubic and anal hair, but in hirsute or heavily infested patients, the chest hair, arm and leg hair, as well as the axilla, beard and eyelashes can be infested. These areas should be examined thoroughly on each visit. The nits attach themselves to the hair and probably are nourished by apocrine secretion. This disease is seen in all classes of society, as opposed to the other varieties of lice which favor the poorer sections of the population. One hairy patient who periodically has to make a 6-week swing through some small towns with inferior hotels, shaves himself from head to foot before and during his trip. Once bitten, twice shy. Undoubtedly some people are more susceptible than others.

Treatment

Often these lice can be exasperatingly difficult to eradicate in a clean person; I continue the treatment for 3 weeks as a rule and treat the marital partner at the same time. Treatment with Kwell shampoo daily and Kwell lotion, or benzyl benzoate applied twice a week from navel to knees and elsewhere as needed, with occasional steel combing, has been necessary despite optimistic one-shot treatments recommended elsewhere. For eyelid infestation, yellow oxide of mercury ophthalmic ointment 1% is very helpful, pulling the nits off with forceps. Maculae caeruleae (taches bleuatres), slate-gray bluish macules 4–10 mm in diameter, are occasionally encountered on the chest, thighs or abdomen of heavily infested patients, and they can in general be disregarded as a vasomotor phenomenon secondary to the material injected into the skin while the louse is dining.

Bedbugs (Cimicidae)

This cosmopolitan disease is caused by a flat, hard 4-mm-long and 3-mm-wide insect that could survive a year in a test tube with no food, generally lives in cracks and wooden beds or furniture or under baseboards, wallpaper or mattress tufts, lays eggs over a long period and has three or four generations per year. It comes out at night to attack the sleeper and takes 10–15 minutes to gorge. For diagnosis, the occurrence of two to five grouped and evenly spaced lesions, usually urticarial papules at the exposed areas, e.g., the wrist, ankle, waist and neck, with new lesions occurring nightly either in a segment of a circle or in a straight line, is strongly suggestive. Often others in the room will be affected, too.

Treatment

The beds should be taken apart and all the joints sprayed with an effective spray, as well as baseboards, mattress tufts, floors and walls. The sprays linger for 3 to 4 months, so perhaps spraying every few months for a year is the best way to deal with this problem. Heating the house to 130 F with the windows closed will also destroy the bedbugs.

Larva Migrans (Creeping Eruption)

This disease consists of irregular wandering tunnels because of the invasion of the skin by a larval form of certain roundworms (usually cat and dog hookworms) in the sands of the southern United States. Cases have been contracted on New England beaches too. Larva currens (cutaneous *Strongyloides*) can mimic larva migrans, though the invasion usually is on the buttocks.[2]

Treatment

Thiabendazole, 50 mg/kg body weight, given either all in one dose or over 2 days, is curative. Ethyl chloride spray refrigeration at the "head" for more than 60 seconds used to be the treatment. The thiabendazole suspension (10%) rubbed in locally either with or without occlusion is effective.[3]

Pinworms (Oxyuriasis)

This usually involves children, though parents can also be infested. The disease manifests itself by anal itching. A flashlight at night will occasionally demonstrate the worms, and anal smears, if done first thing in the morning will catch ova. A small piece of Scotch tape can be used for this purpose, stuck on a glass slide and mailed to the provincial or state laboratory.

Treatment

Any good antibiotic will slow up the worm either internally or externally, since it hatches its eggs outside the anus. Povan (Parke-Davis) pyrvinium pamoate, 5–10 mg/kg body weight, given once and repeated in a week, gives excellent results. The tablets are superior to the liquid, which has an unpleasant oily clinging flavor. Entacyl (piperazine adipate), one teaspoon given three times a day for a week, and Antepar, given according to weight, are alternate treatments. Since the infestation is continued by the fingernails transmitting eggs from anus to mouth, obvious precautions include a nail brush, tight shorts worn in bed at night and frequent changes of bed linen.

Mosquitoes (Culicinae)

Mosquitoes carry malaria, yellow fever, filariasis and other diseases. Aedes aegypti may carry the spirochete of yaws. I suspect that in the United States it carries the virus of molluscum contagiosum. The itching of the bite is severe considering the minuteness of the quantity of saliva the mosquito injects. The mosquito appears to prefer some individuals to others.[4, 5] Reactivity to mosquito extracts is not much inhibited by antihistamine treatment.

Treatment

Netting and repellants such as 612 and Off (or Deet) are very helpful, and there is probably truth in the allegation that thiamine, 100 mg given three times a day, reduces susceptibility to bites.[6] It is said that each purple martin eats 2,000 mosquitoes per day, hence their specially arranged birdhouse apartments sell well. Drainage of swamps is a public health problem. Three generations ago in Canada malaria was common; now it is no longer seen. Excellent public health administration has decreased the prevalence of malaria in the Caribbean.

Stinging Insects

These include ants, bees, wasps and hornets (Hymenoptera). Stings are inflicted only by the females. Prolonged urticaria and even fatalities have occurred following stings. The venom is toxic, as well as sensitizing. As Sutton says, clad in black one is more likely to be stung than when wearing white.[7] Bumblebees do not lose their stings, but can use them repeatedly, whereas when a honeybee stings, the whole stinger separates and is torn off the abdomen. It should be scraped out rather than grasped with forceps to pull it out, since this may force more venom into the wound.

Some ants bite with their jaws and spray poison from the tip of their abdomen into the wound. Most North American ants lack stingers, while stinging ants are common in the tropics. A black species with a scarlet band found on the beach sands of

Lake Erie occasionally stings babies. South American ants are particularly unpleasant.

Granulomas occasionally result from stings, but generally feared is the severe acute anaphylactic reaction or severe generalized urticaria with prostration.

Treatment

For anaphylaxis, epinephrine immediately, intravenous steroids and oxygen, and if possible a tourniquet around the extremity with the sting should be prescribed. The stinger should be removed gently. For less severe reactions, local steroids and antihistamines either by injection, i.e., intravenous Benadryl 2 cc or Chlor-Trimeton intramuscularly 4 mg, or orally, and Decadron spray (Merck) are effective. Desensitization takes 3 years, and it is by no means certain that it is truly effective. The Isuprel inhaler sometimes is good insurance to carry. There are kits (Hollister-Stier) for campers who are very allergic.

Biting Flies (Diptera)

Horse flies, deerflies and gadflies are big sturdy flies that lay their eggs in water plants and marshy ground and produce painful bites on man, occasionally leading to infection. Prevention by wearing protective clothing is about all that can be done. Antibiotic ointments, either with or without steroids, e.g., bacitracin plus systemic antihistamines, assist comfort. Biting midges, gnats, black flies, May flies and "no-see-ums" are attracted to hair spray, and it is not uncommon to see women with bites on the nape of the neck. Decadron spray and Off lead to control, as much as can be obtained. A small piece of a dog's flea collar pinned in the hair works well.

Sand Flies

These should not be confused with *Tunga penetrans* or sand fleas. They are actually small gnats, like mosquitoes, are probably phlebotomi and produce very painful bites around the ankles in visitors to the Caribbean or to Brazilian beaches.

These can develop quite a papular eruption with excoriations and may simulate scabies.

Treatment

Generally treatment should include local creams or combinations of antibiotics and steroids. Rarely, a chronic granuloma will develop that leads to recurrent phlebitis or edema of the ankle, rarely too with ulceration. This should of course be treated symptomatically. Wearing stockings or long trousers helps prevent bites.

Cutaneous Myiasis

Larvae of some Diptera can parasitize man, either via the natural cavities or by burrowing into the skin. Those that burrow into the skin move around leaving a small track, then stop; a tender spot forms and the larva departs, with a furuncular lesion. Cases of this sort have been reported from Ireland, Scotland, Norway and Brittany. Other Diptera deposit eggs in a wound. The eggs may hatch in a few hours and penetrate, and later appear as maggots on the surface of the wound. Maggots do an excellent inexpensive job of wound debridement, though they are rather unesthetic. Urea is probably the principle. They can be washed or flushed off with water and picked out with forceps. Irrigation of chloroform or benzine is reported to be efficacious.[7]

Caterpillars (Lepidoptera)

Fifty different caterpillar species have venomous spines. The brown-tail moth caterpillar creeps around clothing, leaving its hairs behind, which produce a nettling urticaria in the wearer. This occurs in early May in New England. It is almost impossible to eradicate the hairs from the clothing, and the persistence of the condition usually leads to the clothing being cast aside.

Treatment

Local treatment with steroid creams or sprays helps a little, but the condition can be a lasting discomfort. Sutton recommends painting the spots with collodion, which probably prevents the spiny hairs from being moved.[7]

In the Rio Grande valley, "puss caterpillars" have a severe sting that is helped by calcium gluconate taken intravenously.

Spiders

The black widow *(Latrodectus mactans)* is the spider of consequence in Canada, the United States and the Western Hemisphere. It is black with red or orange markings on the underside of a dome-shaped abdomen. There is a red hourglass-shaped spot on the ventral surface. The black widow spins webs in trash heaps and around old lumber. Its bite is painful and leads to a swollen red or purpuric area accompanied by general intoxication with twitching, dizziness, weakness, cramps and even death.

Treatment

Calcium gluconate given intravenously with epinephrine and steroids and specific antivenin (a horse serum product made by Merck, Sharp & Dohme) are the methods of choice. However, 2 cc of 1:2,000 neostigmine methylsulfate with 1/150 grain of atropine relieves the symptoms promptly, according to various sources. For ordinary spider bites, steroid creams are efficacious. Occasionally necrosis poses a therapeutic challenge.

Scorpions

Scorpions are found mostly in the southern United States and Mexico and are decidedly dangerous, especially to children. They are nocturnal and photophobic and sting by a quick stab of the tail. There is *no* inflammation at the site of the sting, but rapidly a numbness spreads up the affected limb and a feeling of tightness develops in the throat. Jitters or twitching may develop later with convulsions, difficulty in breathing and even death.

Treatment

A proximal tourniquet should be applied with an ice bag locally for 2 hours, releasing the tourniquet every 10 minutes or so. Demerol is contraindicated. Oxygen is good; as are steroids intramuscularly injected.

Ticks

Ticks carry rickettsiae and can leave a pruritic nodule at the site of the bite. Wood ticks carry Rocky Mountain spotted fever and Q fever. They are seen in the western United States and Canada, in grass and bushes. In recent years they have been more common along the East Coast as well. Soft ticks carry the spirochete of relapsing fever in central and western United States and Canada. In 24 hours a soft tick bite leads to a rash and relapsing episodes of fever.

Tick bite paralysis from the venom of the tick has been reported; it clears up within 48 hours of removal of the tick. It is seen mainly in children.

Ticks can be removed by touching them with a lit cigarette butt, a hot nail, kerosene, tobacco juice or an essential oil, inducing it to remove itself. Repellents are useful. Toothed forceps grip well. Try not to leave bits of the jaws behind.

Mites (Tyroglyphus)

Grain itch mites, grocer's itch mites and other mites afflict persons in contact with straw, wheat, oats and cheese, producing an itch similar to scabies, with vesicular urticarial papules.

Dermanyssus gallinae

Rat mites transmit rickettsial pox, and bird mites will bite humans when the pigeons abandon their nests. Canaries can be infected. Humans handling chicken coops suffer, and occasionally an air-conditioner will suck in mites and thus infest the human occupant of a room. Bites occur on a person's upper trunk and scalp, although they will occur on any exposed area. They are itchy and urticarial and may be mistaken for delusions of parasitosis.

Treatment

The source must be removed. One should spray along the paths of the migration and use Kwell or 25% benzyl benzoate on the patient.

Trombidiodea

Chigger mites or harvest mites are found in grass and bushes. The reddish mites are 0.3 – 0.5 mm long. They bite the legs and thighs, producing a papular eruption with surrounding urticaria and itching and scratching. The mites drop off when engorged. They are commonly seen in July and August.

Treatment

Treatment is by repellents, for example, 612, Off, Deet and Kwell, or dipping clothing in a solution of 5% dimethylphthalate. Two percent soap assists this repellent action. Spraying the ground with dieldrin (2¼ lb per acre) destroys these mites. It also destroys ticks. The Army impregnates its uniform clothing with "M. 1960" to repel these little mites and chiggers. Twenty-five percent benzyl benzoate or Kwell lotion helps. If a toxic eruption develops, steroids are required.

Beetles (Celeoptera)

Blistering is the result of crushing beetles on the skin; they do not bite. Benzine application followed by soap and water will remove most of the vesicant chemical.

Cercariae

Swimmer's Itch

Ducks, birds, rodents and snails are hosts for the schistosome which is found in calm water, usually at the mouth of a muddy river on a hot day. The schistosome burrows into the skin and dies, producing an itching wheal. Clam digger's itch is the same (seen on Long Island Sound).

Treatment

Brisk rubbing with a towel periodically will wipe off the cercariae before they penetrate the skin. Once the eruption is ensconced, soothing lotions or steroid creams and antihistamines comfort the patient for the short time required to wait for spontaneous cure.

Sea-bather's Eruption

This is similar to the schistosome disease, but probably is caused by jellyfish larvae under the bathing suit. In Honolulu, marine algae give a similar dermatitis, referred to as seaweed dermatitis.

Treatment

Treatment is as for swimmer's itch.

Other Metazoans

Portuguese Man-of-War

These stings can be fatal and always are painful, resulting from contact with the man-of-war's invisible tentacles hanging down from its floating bladder. Stripes of urticarial erythema are the usual sign. Steroids by injection intravenously or intramuscularly, antihistamines orally and steroid creams locally are the treatments of choice. Aromatic spirits of ammonia stop pain promptly.[8] Henrici's meat tenderizer, one teaspoon to ¼-cup water, does the same thing.[8]

Coral Dermatitis

"Dogger-bank itch" is an occupational hazard of fishermen who work in this area. It results in coral cuts leading to a chronic dermatitis of the exposed parts. Many veterans of war in the Pacific can testify to the chronicity of small wounds produced by coral cuts on the ankles. Treatment is with antibiotic-steroid combinations plus protection.

Jellyfish Stings

Jellyfish stings received in tropical waters can cause spasm of the respiratory muscles, nausea, anxiety, abdominal pain and severe toxemia as well as urticaria and burning pain at the site of contact. Treatment is with calcium gluconate given intravenously, as in spider bites, and steroids locally and systemically.

Sting Ray

Effects of bites are similar and treatment is similar to those of the jellyfish.

Worms and Leeches

Trichiniasis

The adult worm inhabits the intestine and the larvae emigrate to the muscles, where they become encysted. This usually results from eating insufficiently cooked pork. Acute urticaria, edema of the eyelids, photophobia, subconjunctival petechiae and splinter hemorrhages under the nails are the common symptoms. Diagnosis is by biopsy of the muscle and, after the second week, a *Trichinella* skin test (which has a 10% false positive reaction rate). Treatment is by thiabendazole.

Hookworm

Human larva migrans is the dog hookworm *(Ancylostoma braziliense)* but human hookworm *(Ancylostoma duodonale)* is common in Europe and the Mediterranean and produces an itchy dermatitis, usually between the toes and progressing over the dorsa of the foot (ground itch, miner's itch or water itch) with vesicles or blisters, pustules, erythematous plaques and macules. Later, via the bloodstream, the organism enters the lungs and travels via the trachea and esophagus to the intestines, where the worm passes its adult life producing eggs excreted in the stool. Loeffler's syndrome and severe eosinophilia are seen. Treatment is by thiabendazole. Another treatment is tetrachloroethylene, 0.1 ml/kg body weight (maximum dose 5 ml in capsules to be given fasting once). This is not to be used if the patient is pregnant, has a cardiac disorder or has an alcoholic history or renal disease.

Ascaris

Ascaris lumbricoides is a 10-in. roundworm found in the intestine. Treatment is with piperazine salts, 75 mg/kg body weight for 2 days; the maximum daily dose is 3–5 gm. *Ascaris* produces erythema nodosum or urticaria.

Oxyuris (pinworms)

These have been previously discussed.

Filariasis

Filiform worms live in the tissues or the body cavity of the host, which in the case of *Wuchereria bancrofti* (a 2-cm-long slim worm) is the human lymphatic system. These worms use mosquitoes as intermediate hosts and multiply in the human bloodstream at night. Photographs of natives in the Congo with their giant scrotums (elephantiasis) perhaps would be adequate refutation to the "silent spring" variety of insect lovers. Treatment is with diethylcarbamazine, a piperazine derivative (Hetrazan—Lederle), 2 mg/kg body weight given three times a day for one to two weeks.

Onchocerciasis

Microfilariae accumulate beneath the horny epidermis as a result of the bite of a black gnat in Mexico and Guatemala. They occasionally cause blindness by entering the cornea. Early lesions suggest erysipelas and later suggest chronic eczema, hyperpigmentation and especially swelling of the ears. The skin nodules range from 1 to 3 cm in diameter, generally on the head in Americans, whereas in Africa the nodules are more generalized. Treatment is with arsphenamine. There is a variety of nonspecific dermatitis connected with filarial infestation which is occasionally similar to dermatitis herpetiformis, polymorphous, urticarial and occurring in repeated attacks. This is referred to as "filarial itch."

Cestodes

TAENEA SOLIUM (tapeworm).—If the larvae stay in man, they cause small round, firm, subcutaneous tumors—cysticercosis; these small tumors can occur anywhere. The adult worms can be cured with Atabrine. Niclosamide (Yomesan) or Atabrine is the treatment of choice.

ECHINOCOCCUS.—These tapeworms cause walnut- to apple-sized translucent tumors under the skin, in about 8% of the cases, or in the liver. Urticaria fever, pruritus, erythema and hyperhidrosis are among the cutaneous symptoms.

SPARGANOSIS.—Long ivory-white ribbons lead to edema, pain and itching, probably because of using contaminated meat as a poultice for wounds or drinking unclean water. Surgical excision cures them.

Leeches

An anticoagulant is introduced by the leech to encourage the flow of blood (hirudin); often the flow of blood from the wound leads to discovery of the leech, since the bite is painless. After the leech is removed, the wound is slow to heal. To hasten its release, strong brine, vinegar, alcohol, a hot match tip or cocaine should be applied. If a leech must be removed from the nasal passage, the patient should be placed head down so the leech will not fall into the trachea! Impregnating clothing with dimethylphthalate helps prevent leeches.

Protozoa

Amebiasis

Skin ulcers occur one to three weeks after surgery in a visceral abscess and begin as erythema with later black necrotic or furuncular anthrax-like lesions. Ragged irregular or round ulcerations also occur around the anus or the genitalia and spread peripherally with scarring. The diagnosis is by organism identification—rosacea, urticaria and pruritus, which can occur from intestinal infestation. Diodoquin and carbarsone are effective treatments, as are Terramycin, Aureomycin and perhaps emetine.

In treating amebic ulcers, local cleansing using antiseptic solution plus systemic treatment with emetine, 1 mg/kg body weight given intramuscularly daily for 6–10 days, is effective. Daily dose should not exceed 60 mg, and repeated treatment should be delayed at least 2 weeks. Pain at the injection site, nausea and occasionally tachycardia plus electrocardiographic change in the T waves are side effects. Oral amebicides for treating intestinal infection include Mebinol, Falmotox and Quixalin, none of which is available in the United States. Furamide, which *is* available (Furentomin—"Entamide Furoate"), should be given 20 mg/kg body weight daily for 10 days (500-mg tablets three times a day usually); this produces the side effect of flatulence. Chloroquine in 250-mg tablets, usually four tablets given the first day and two tablets every day for 20 days, can be used concomitantly. A complete cure is mandatory. Three stools proved normal by trained examiners and a sigmoidoscope are needed to demonstrate cure.

Trichomonas Vaginitis

Flagellate protozoa produce a foamy pruritic discharge from the vagina in women. Cure can be difficult, and the sexual partner should be treated simultaneously. Flagyl (metronidazole) is effective, as are Vioform inserts, 250 mg given three times a day for 10 days, plus one 500-mg vaginal tablet of

Flagyl given every day for 10 days. This leads to total success. The male should be treated three times a day for 10 days also. Allantoin improved vaginal cream (AVC improved) (National Drug Co.) is an additional help.

Leishmaniasis

Oriental Sore (Alleppo button)

Specific ulcers develop on the face, usually from the bite of the sand fly, which carries the flagellate principle. (See p. 65, PCAD.) It takes a number of months to evolute and heal. It can take up to a year to pass through this cycle, and a characteristic stellate scar remains. Treatment is with stibosan or potassium antimony tartrate, but spontaneous cure is the rule.

American Leishmaniasis (Brazil, Peru, Bolivia)

This form differs in that it fails to produce immunity in adults.

Uta

A benign self-limiting form occurs in children in the Andes (where verruga peruana is endemic—*Bartonella*). This is a sort of wart.

Espundia

This leishmaniasis occurs in adults in forest regions and affects mucous membranes. The treatment is with 2-hydroxystilbamadine.

Rattlesnake Bites

Treatment is with antivenin, 1 vial per 250 cc, 5% glucose given intravenously over 90 minutes, or locally infiltrated 0.02 M calcium disodium editate.[9]

REFERENCES

1. Hernandez-Perez, E.: Topically applied thiabendazole in the treatment of scabies, Arch. Dermatol. 112:1400, 1976.
2. Smith, J. D., Goette, D. K., and Odom, R. B.: Larva currens: Cutaneous strongyloidiasis, Arch. Dermatol. 112:1161, 1976.
3. Stone, O. J.: Systemic and topical thiabendazole for creeping eruption, Tex. Rep. Biol. Med. 27:659, 1962.
4. Editorial: The mosquito and its prey, Br. Med. J. 1:1131, 1951.

5. Muirhead-Thomson, R. C.: The distribution of anopholine mosquito bites among different age groups, Br. Med. J. 1:1114, 1951.
6. Shannon, W. R.: Thiamin chloride: An aid in the solution of the mosquito problem, Minn. Med. 26:799, 1943.
7. Sutton, R. L., Jr.: *Diseases of the Skin* (11th ed.; St. Louis: C. V. Mosby Co., 1956), p. 300.
8. Frohman, I. G.: Treatment of physalia stings (Portuguese man-of-war), J.A.M.A. 197:733, 1966.
9. Russell, F. E.: Treatment of rattlesnake bite, J.A.M.A. 207:159, 1969.

27 / Pruritus

The sensation of itching varies widely in intensity in various locations and at various times. It can come in waves, or continue as a persistent debilitating torture affording the victim no rest. It is in general intensified by heat and humidity, rough wool clothing, sweating, sudden changes in temperature (from stove to refrigerator to sink), excessive washing, and often attempts to seek peace and quiet and rest. It is generally relieved by cool compresses, soothing local lubricants, concentration on something else, light loose soft clothing, an airy atmosphere and, finally, scratching!

Itching is a symptom and requires relief, since the reflex scratching produced frequently aggravates the condition and leads to further complications in many instances, such as infection, autoeczematization and lichenification.

Systemic Causes of Itching

Metabolic diseases such as diabetes, uremia, thyroid dysfunction and hepatobiliary disease (with or without jaundice) can be the source of unexplainable itching. Lymphomas, such as mycosis fungoides, Hodgkin's disease or leukemia, and lymphosarcomas, will often be ushered in with generalized pruritus. (See pp. 161–163, PCAD.) Hidden malignancies, intestinal parasites, polycythemia vera, drug eruptions with scant objective evidence and dermographism can also produce itching. Orchiectomy, pregnancy, carcinoid and various neurologic and psychogenic conditions, as well as occasionally habit, can produce itching.

The itching of uremia can be relieved quickly by treatment with oral cholestyramine, 5 mg given twice a day, though it comes back when the medication is stopped.[1] Itching also can be alleviated by giving twice-weekly erythema-producing doses of ultraviolet light, using the sunburn spectrum, and whole-body irradiation. Nine of 10 patients have been helped in this manner.[2]

Unapparent External Causes of Itching

These include prickly heat, fiber glass particles in clothing, strong detergent or bleach in clothing (especially in sweaty people), long, hot frequent baths with strong defatting soaps, senility, maculae ceruleae in pediculosis pubis and delusions of parasitosis. Exposure to insecticide sprays, chafing from tight clothing, deodorants and disinfectants all can give irritation on the inner thighs, axillae and neck folds. Itching scalp can be from mere dryness, irritant hair creams or mild seborrhea; occasionally a scant pediculosis in a very clean person may be difficult to diagnose. Too much shampooing occasionally explains itching of the scalp; the temporary relief afforded leads to greater and greater frequency of shampooing. Occasionally a brain tumor will cause itching of the nose.

General Philosophy of the Symptomatic Treatment of Itching

There are times in the life of every dermatologist when, due to an unfortunate combination of circumstances, he is either unable to get an adequate history or unable to make an adequate examination of the patient's skin. This can be due to nocturnal poor light, an insensible patient, a language barrier or many other reasons. At such times relief of the itching includes doing things that will not obscure the diagnosis or run any risk of injuring a sick patient. Generally at such times antihistamines are safe and moderately effective. Pyribenzamine 50 mg, Chlor-Trimeton 4 mg, Perazil 25 or 50 mg, Polaramine 2 mg, Dimetane 4 mg, Periactin 4 mg, Benadryl 50 mg, Phenergan 12.5 or 25 mg, and sometimes Tacaryl, which is also a phenothiazine, are effective antihistamines. Some are less sedative than others. Temaril, 2.5 or 5.0 mg, is another phenothiazine derivative that is helpful in treating itching, although it is not classified with the antihistamines. Bear in mind that phenothiazone derivatives can have side effects producing muscle spasms or extrapyramidal reactions as well as jaundice or allergic skin reaction.

Local applications of soothing, cooling and drying lotions (shake lotions with or without camphor, menthol and phenol) will give relief when the skin is acutely inflamed with vesicles and perhaps with serous oozing. Steroid emulsions, or lotions or creams, used in treating the less inflamed perhaps slightly drier and lichenified eruptions will often give adequate symptomatic relief. Cooling soothing baths with starch or oatmeal and cool boric acid or Burow's solution or saline compresses will give symptomatic relief.

Holding the itching member under the hot-water tap is a form of self-treatment to be condemned.

Removal of the cause is the ideal treatment. Only too often this is not possible. In most instances an educated balance of avoiding causative or aggravating factors compatible with the patient's occupational survival in his environment is the modus vivendi.

In some specific regions the itching is so all-pervasive as to make symptomatic relief imperative and in fact essential to cure. A judgment can be developed as to when to use which remedies, although the present choice of steroids has made management easier. For example, calcium gluconate given intravenously and slowly is very helpful, as is calcium strontium bromide 10% given intravenously similarly. Anticholinergic drugs such as Syntropan or atropine sulfate grains 1/150, Pro-Banthine 15 mg, Prantal 100 mg, and on occasion Pathobamate, which is a combination of meprobamate and Pro-Banthine, can be helpful. Antiserotonin agents, especially Periactin, are very helpful, and occasionally icebag compresses or an intracutaneous injection of steroid by needle or Dermajector is also helpful treatment.

Any change in the patient's routine, such as drastic change in diet, avoidance of stimulating spicy foods, such as coffee, tea, hot soup, sharp cheese, port, chocolate, carbonated cola drinks, berries and tomatoes, may be helpful.

Local Treatment of Itching

Dry Conditions

LARGE AREAS.—Emulsion bases, such as lipid-free Cetaphil lotion, which does not take antibiotics or Burow's solution (Texas Pharmacal), is an excellent remedy for treating atopic persons. They can have menthol 0.25%, camphor 0.25–0.50%, or phenol 0.5–1.0% and/or steroids suspended easily, e.g.:

Kenalog suspension—parenteral 50 mg (1 vial)
Cetaphil lotion—q.s. ad 240

Calamine liniment, a water-in-oil emulsion, will take antibiotics, and phenol can be added:

Calamine	8%
Zinc oxide	8%
Olive oil	50%
Calcium hydroxide solution q.s. ad	100

Schamberg's lotion is as follows:

Menthol	0.25%
Phenol	1.0%
Peanut oil	45%
Calcium hydroxide solution	45%
Zinc oxide powder	8%

Burow's emulsion (George Andrews) is given below:

Zinc oxide	30 gm
Talc	30 gm
Lanolin anhydrous	30 gm
Olive oil	130 gm
Burow's solution	6 gm
Lime water q.s. ad	300 gm

Antipruritic agents to add include coal tar solution USP in 2–8% strength and benzocaine 1–10% strength, usually 2% (which is quite sensitizing). Solarcaine cream for sunburn gives quick relief. Lidocaine (Xylocaine) is less sensitizing, as is perhaps Quotane. Their anesthetic action is considerable, but they should be used only in emergencies because of their power to sensitize. Pontocaine and Nupercainal are similar anesthetic agents. Tincture of benzoin, chloral and resorcin also have antipruritic properties, although milder.

SMALL AREAS.—Pastes or lotions can be used; a good antipruritic ointment is:

Menthol	0.15%
Phenol	0.3%
Ichthamol	1.8% (or it can be left out)
Zinc oxide ointment	60.0%

or

Menthol	0.15%
Phenol	0.3%
Crude coal tar	1.2%
Zinc oxide ointment	
q.s. ad	60.0

Moist Oozing Conditions

LARGE AREAS.—Shake lotions can be used; good antipruritics are calamine and bentonite:

Menthol	0.25%
Camphor	1.0%
Calamine	10.0%
Zinc oxide	10.0%
Glycerin	2.5%
Bentonite magna	45.0%
Lime water	
q.d. ad	120.0

Make a lotion and label *Apply as needed.*

Other antipruritic lotions for treating large moist areas are 1% hydrocortisone in Allercreme skin lotion; 0.25% hydrocortisone lotions, e.g., Cort-Dome and Cetaphil; triamcinolone lotions, such as Kenalog 50 mg and Cetaphil q.s. ad 240; and Wise's shake lotion:

Aluminum acetate	12.5%
Glycerin	20.0
Talcum powder	25.0
Zinc oxide	25.0
Lime water	17.5%

Compresses should be used to cleanse the skin twice a day.

SMALL AREAS.—Plain Lassar's paste is often very helpful, using oil to cleanse. (See Formulary, nos. 2, 3, 5, 22, 39, 40, 43.)

Pruritus Ani

Sweating, obesity, friction and long periods of sitting, such as taxi drivers are subjected to, in tight unabsorbent clothes, often produce this disorder. Scratching the area leads to small excoriations which rapidly crust or get infected and intensify the itching. Further scratching or rubbing may lead to lichenification of the anal skin with edema and fecal material in folds, which rapidly produces a red, hot, sore anal region. If home treatment with anesthetic ointments (e.g., benzocaine, Americaine, Surfacaine, Nupercainal) supervenes, a severe contact dermatitis may develop so that the patient may not be able to walk. This same chain of events can occur as a result of overcleansing the anal skin with strong soaps, inappropriate or overtreatment of psoriasis, seborrheic dermatitis or atopic eczema. Often moniliasis following antibiotic therapy for an unrelated infection will initiate this chain of events, especially in diabetics. Oral treatment with Mycostatin, as well as 1% hydrocortisone in Mycostatin cream, will promptly relieve such cases. Usually 2 or 3 months of taking oral B-complex vitamins subsequently heads off relapses. This same cream is useful in treating cases caused by simple intertrigo, though Caldesene dusting powder (Maltbie Company) is effective. Occasional cases of pinworm infestation can be uncovered by anal swabs taken first thing in the morning before the victim gets out of bed.

Tinea produces a marginated erythema that is easily recognized in most instances, but occasionally in a clean patient, culture for fungus or microscopic examination for mycelia is the only way the diagnosis can be made. There is almost always coincidentally tinea pedis, and the organism is usually *Trichophyton purpureum.* Castellani's paint used daily for 3 weeks is a satisfactory cure, though Tinactin is less colorful. Other useful remedies include Halotex (Westwood) and Lotrimin (Delbay).

Other causes of pruritus ani include scabies, condyloma acuminatum (occasionally high up in the rectum), rectal carcinoma, hemorrhoids, cryptitis, and anal fissures or fistulae. These last usually produce *pain* rather than *itching.* If, after excluding the above causes, itching persists or recurs, then *idiopathic* pruritus ani is most likely involved. This can challenge the therapeutic ingenuity of the most gifted physician. Excessive use of mineral oil, codeine, coffee, tea, alcohol, emotional strain, intestinal parasites, drugs such as Diodoquin, excessive looseness of the bowels and constipation all play a part.

Management of Idiopathic Pruritus Ani

Since many patients admit that many flare-ups of their itching appear to be related to periods of anxiety or high emotional stress, it is probable that active enzymes passed with the feces may coat the anal skin and initiate a mild "digestion" of the surface epithelium. Hence, gentle but thorough cleansing after defecation is essential, using cotton or Kleenex tissue and warm water, and then blotting dry. On occasion Phisoderm for normal skin assists in reestablishing a normal pH, and this should be used in preference to soap, which should be prohibited in the acute phase. Another good cleanser is Balneol (Westwood). Glycerin-impregnated cotton swabs or wipes can be obtained. (Tucks – Fuller Pharmaceutical Co.).

Treatment with a mild evening sedation, using Phenobarb or meprobamate, plus long-acting antihistamines taken at night (e.g., Teldrin spansules, 12 mg hour of sleep) will allow the patient to rest, as well as possibly act within the intestinal tract to lessen the irritative powers of the fecal contents. Sitz baths, 15 minutes in Aveeno or Bur-veen soaks, every evening or even more often, will soothe. Spicy foods, especially coffee and alcohol, should be avoided, and underpants should be seamless and not tight. The patient should use one of the well-made steroid creams, e.g., Aristocort, Kenalog, Cordran, Synalar or Vioform hydrocortisone lotion 1%, or an emulsion, and should be instructed in applying it with the fingertips, rubbing in gently until it more or less disappears, at least four times a day. The patient must understand that he is not to wash it off prior to each application. Occasionally a patient will say that even though he cleanses scrupulously after defecation, within a half hour he feels sticky, and on wiping his anal area again, he is surprised to find more fecal staining. The inflamed anal skin may conceal folds and crypts in which fecal material can remain unnoticed, only to ooze as it becomes more liquid with a rise in temperature. Such a patient should be advised to recleanse the anal area one-half hour after defecation, or syringe out the rectal ampulla with a small 2 oz enema of plain tap water after defecation, reapplying the steroid cream immediately. In treating stubborn cases, treatment with grenz rays or x-rays may be necessary, although this should be only a last resort. For very loose stools, Metamucil, 1 level tablespoon taken every night, will give a drier bulkier stool and avoid postevacuation mucus discharge. Instructions to the patients to avoid loose stools, wear light loose clothing, use Kleenex or Tucks instead of harsh toilet paper, keep the area clean but avoid strong soaps, and not sit or lie on the back for long periods of time are helpful. The diet should be bland, and rest should be adequate. Occasionally, lactic acid bacillus orally can be very helpful.

Pruritus Vulvae

Since orifices are usually warm, moist and loaded with sensory nerve endings, itching at such sites tends to be more intense and calls for more complaining than appears to be justified by the amount of visible changes. All of the causes listed for pruritus ani (such as seborrheic dermatitis, atopic eczema, psoriasis, moniliasis, contact dermatitis, intertrigo, pinworms, tinea, scabies and warts) can be factors here. In addition are irritations produced by douches, contraceptive jells or jellies, tampons, sanitary napkins and vaginal discharges secondary to either *Trichomonas* or *Monilia*, often both. Occasionally a sugary urine alone will cause pruritus vulvae. Senile vaginal changes, vulvar dysfunction and dyspareunia have been successfully treated with progesterone made up in an ointment using 200 mg of the injectable material in 2 oz of hydrophilic ointment USP and given twice daily. Improvement occurs within 2–4 weeks.[3]

Monilial Vaginitis

Patchy white spots on a reddish mucous membrane appear with a diagnostic culture. Treatment is by Mycostatin tablets to be inserted vaginally, or A.V.C. improved gel every night with douching in the morning. This is to be repeated nightly for 7 days and then tapered gradually, or pre- or post-menstrually for two periods. Gyne-Lotrimin inserted nightly for a week also cures, although it has to be repeated.

Trichomonas Vaginalis

This disease, causing a foamy discharge, is diagnosed by the hanging drop showing motile organisms. Flagyl metronidazole (250 mg given three times daily for 10–20 days, but not during pregnancy) with a 500-mg vaginal tablet inserted nightly is very often curative. Tetracycline treatment also helps. Another suppository is called Milibis.

Lichen Simplex Chronicus

Itchy plaques produce unreasonably intense desires to scratch, perpetuating the thickening which leads to itching from relatively minor stimuli such as mild overheating. Intracutaneous steroid using Kenalog suspension 50–50 is probably the best treatment, or grenz rays or steroid creams, perhaps Aristocort 0.5%.

Presenile Atrophy

Atrophic changes in women after the menopause occasionally lead to itching of the vulva, which usually can be relieved by steroid-estrogen combinations applied locally. Replacement therapy with oral estrogens also helps.

Lichen Sclerosus et Atrophicus

This is often confused with kraurosis (leukoplakia) vulvae. It consists of pearly white, flat papules that coalesce to produce patches around the vaginal orifices and on the labia. There is usually extension to the anal area, and other spots can be seen, sometimes on the back, chest and volar wrists. Treatment with vitamin A orally is helpful, as is steroid applied under occlusion using Aristocort 0.5%. Es-A-Cort cream (Dome) is useful. Some West Coast dermatologists like to use dextrorotary alpha-tocopherol given three times a day. Patients treated with 2% methyltestosterone in a water-soluble base are reputed to show improvement in 4–6 weeks. A report of improvement in patients with balanitis xerotica obliterans (which is similar to lichen sclerosus et atrophicus) who used 2.5% testosterone propionate ointment makes this certainly worth a trial.[4]

Lichen Planus

Purplish flat-topped polygonal papules respond to grenz ray treatment and the usual treatment for lichen planus. I favor 80 mg Kenalog IM for this disease.

Incontinence

Incontinence can cause irritation in elderly females, especially if they are bedridden and have a flaccid bladder. Keri hand cream or Silicote protective creams are helpful, and if the irritation gets out of hand, Biozyme hydrocortisone ointment (Armour) is occasionally helpful. Lidex ointment is effective.

In general, the management of idiopathic pruritus vulvae is to:

1. Avoid obesity, heat, sweat and friction.
2. Avoid tight clothing.
3. Avoid soap.
4. Avoid long car rides.
5. Avoid local irritants, especially contact irritation from douches.
6. Apply triamcinolone creams locally and take sitz baths in oatmeal or compress with Bur-Veen, Burow's or boric acid solution.
7. Take antihistamines or Atarax for sedation.
8. Use gentle attempts to ventilate psychological hangups (e.g., death of an only child, wandering husband).

Pruritus of Overbathing

Asteatosis, xerosis, pruritus hiemalis, senile pruritus and "eczema crackilee" usually can be recognized by the early localization of itching over the extensors, hips, shoulders and calves, with dry flaky skin present. The history of fondness for long, hot, frequent baths or showers with Dial, Zest, Lifebuoy, Safeguard, or other strong shriveling soaps, is usually the case. Patients will often readily admit that they are addicted to hot baths, and often they will not be too willing to desist. The condition is usually worse in the winter, and in certain parts of the world where the water contains large numbers of alkaline salts, which tend to dry the skin, it can occur in summer *or* winter. Old people are much more susceptible since their skin contains much less sebum. Wearing rough tweeds and confinement to bed in a hospital, where the linens are washed in sodium triphosphate or other strong alkaline detergents, will aggravate the condition. The treatment, of course is to make the baths short, cool and few and use a superfatted soap, a bath oil and plenty of lubrication. Mild soothing steroid emulsions are a very effective remedy. (See Formulary, nos. 5, 43.)

Pruritus of the External Ear

The orifice of the ear canal is often the site of mild scaling erythema which may be due to improper cleansing, with accumulation of ear wax and bacterial growth in it. Other irritations may result from the tickling of vibrissae while a person is chewing or after swimming or bathing. Occasionally occlusion of the canal by swollen wet wax will induce a person to dig in the ear canal with a fingernail or a hairpin, leading to infection with *Pseudomonas*, which probably is the most common cause of otitis externa. The discharge occasionally will drop onto the neck, producing the classic *infectious eczematoid dermatitis* with rapidly appearing widespread dirty crusting lesions; more often an underlying seborrheic dermatitis, psoriasis or atopy is to blame. These conditions can be recognized by involvement of the other usual areas of the face and body. Occasionally lichen simplex will involve the area immediately in front of the ear. Contact dermatitis of the ear lobe from nickel earrings, of the whole ear from medications, and of the upper ear from hair dyes can usually be recognized, too.

Treatment with wet compresses, with boric acid or Burow's solution for the acute oozing ears initially and wicks in the canal inserted every 5 minutes for 40 minutes three times daily will soothe the average acute attack. Very severe swelling may require wicks to be inserted by a physician and nurse. The ear canal is almost completely surrounded by cartilage, so edema can cause severe pain. Systemic antibiotics may be needed.

Syringing of the ear with small rubber-tipped syringes, using 1:10,000 aqueous Metaphen, will remove much debris and dead skin and permit medication to be inserted. Two percent hydrocortisone in aerosporin otic solution, and later hydrocortisone-Terramycin powder insufflated with a small spray or Coly-Mycin otic, are excellent.

Essential management involves convincing the patient of the danger of putting *anything* in his ear once the ear is quieted down and more or less normal. The dog-leg bend in the canal makes retention of infection a problem best dealt with by a healthy intact epidermis. Scratching or wiping with cotton tips can easily remove the skin, leading to oozing serum and acute flare-ups.

For dry scaling external ears, treatment measures suitable for seborrheic dermatitis or psoriasis elsewhere are appropriate. For example, Mycolog cream (watch for ethylene diamine sensitivity), 1% hydrocortisone in bacitracin ointment at night, or triamcinolone cream with 3% liquor carbonis detergens in it usually work well. Lidex ointment is excellent.

Diving should be avoided temporarily.

Picker's Warts

Many patients will present small lichenified thickened nodules on the occiput, neck or dorsa of the hand, wrist, knuckle or ankle. These are too small to be called lichen simplex, and yet not profuse enough to be prurigo nodularis. They are often warty, and the patient will complain that they itch. Patients often admit to picking them, especially when perplexed or thinking, and several will call a nodule their "think button." Electrosurgical removal is the only hope of cure, with a good hot electrodesiccating spark to curette it right off. Recurrences occur about 25% of the time. In my hands, intralesional triamcinolone has been disappointing.

Lichen Simplex Chronicus

Lichenification is the term used to describe a cobblestone-like cross-hatched thickening of the skin caused by incessant rubbing. The patch is usually fairly sharply defined and in an area accessible to the fingers, such as the ankle, wrist or neck. The surface is dry and sometimes scaly, with persistent and severe itching. The alternate term for the condition, "circumscribed neurodermatitis," implies a nervous patient, but such is not always the case. Persons with obsessive compulsive personalities, whose parents did not chastise them for scratching when they were little, are apt to develop this following whatever mild initial lesion occurs, such as a mosquito bite, sweat or rash. Patients start rubbing the area to relieve a superficial transient itching sensation, which may be provoked by wearing rough fabric against their skin or perhaps by 2 cups of coffee awakening their "nerve endings." This rubbing further stimulates the "nerve endings" (perhaps to a little hypertrophy?), so that when the next stimulus occurs, the threshold is a little lower for the initiation of the itching sensation. Each day the frequency of the rubbing increases, as does the intensity of the itching sensation, until finally we arrive at the diseased state of pruritic lichenified patch.

Treatment involves covering the patch with an occlusive coating of collodion or Elastoplast, with or without the application of crude coal tar first; this was an effective remedy in the presteroid era. At present, the therapy of choice involves steroid creams or ointments applied locally many times a day, and perhaps with occlusion overnight, or any variation on this theme depending on the location. In some areas intracutaneous injection of Kenalog suspension 50–50 is extremely effective, dilution being required to lessen subcutaneous atrophy. Generally 30% steroid and 70% water will not produce subcutaneous atrophy; 50% steroid and 50% water seldom does; 30% water and 70% steroid often does; and 100% steroid usually produces atrophy.

Triamcinolone suspension should be well diluted and well shaken before injection to disperse the micronized particles. Blindness following scalp injection—though very rare—has occurred, possibly from crystallized particles entering an artery.[6] X-ray therapy has a place here, too: 75 rad repeated at weekly intervals for 4 or 6 weeks almost always will stop the rubbing. Sutton believes that many of the patients he sees have low serum protein levels or other blood abnormalities, e.g., the mild anemia which when corrected leads to prompt recovery.[5] Mild sedation late in the day helps when fatigue and frustration tend to take their toll (e.g., Meprobamate 200 mg or Phenobarb 0.25 grain). Antihistamines taken at bedtime will often allow a mildly restless patient to stop scratching (Teldrin, Benadryl or Periactin). The patient should be given a *definite* follow-up date and encouraged to apply the cream regularly; he should continue to apply it four or five times a day *after* he stops itching, for several weeks.

I remember one patient, a nurse, whose patellar areas of the knees were so lichenified and so itchy that when all else failed, substitution of a pliable scar following electrodesiccation and curettage was followed by grateful relief. Dry ice can also be used. However, the reaction is *always* exaggerated in patients with lichen simplex.

Exudative Discoid and Lichenoid Dermatitis
(Sulzberger-Garbe, "oid-oid")

The onset is sudden, with severely itching disks on the penis or bridge of the nose. Intractable and uncontrollable itching with nocturnal exacerbations leads to widespread dermatitis which can be unresponsive to treatment. The diagnosis is difficult, and the treatment more so. The condition seems to occur in aggressive men who take gamblers' risks for high stakes in business or other activities involving "nerve." Removal from the environment to sunny seashore or desert climes offers the most lasting benefit.

Cutaneous Neuroses

Hallucinations of sensation, e.g., the smell of burning milk, which is seen in patients with certain varieties of brain tumor, can point to organic disease and should never be casually disregarded or cavalierly dismissed, exasperating though these cases may be.

Hyperalgesia, anesthesia and paresthesia, especially around the nose or mouth, may be manifestations of central nervous system disease, and the patient should have a good and complete neurologic examination. Queer sensations at the tips of the extremities occur in women during the menopause and may be relieved by estrogen treatment. Many of us are familiar with the wave of sensory change occurring at about 10:30 A.M. associated with hypoglycemia, and some of us have experienced the unpleasant pounding in the ears referred to as the "Chinese restaurant syndrome" (monosodium glutamate). Gustatory sweating and prickling of the skin serve to point up the relation that cutaneous sensory changes have with internal physiologic function. Similarly deranged function can lead to exaggerated cutaneous sensations, which may range from painful to anesthetic.

Dermatalgia, pains in or under the skin, occur often in localized areas, especially the scalp. It is often based on a psychoneurosis. There is no effective treatment for erythromelalgia, which is usually characterized by periodic attacks of deep dusky erythema, with or without pain, involving a group of toes or the whole foot or hand, made worse by dependency and blanching on elevation.

Meralgia paresthetica, or "pinched nerve syndrome," often seen in pregnant women toward the end of their pregnancy, is probably due to an abnormal leaning-back posture, producing pain and hyperesthesia in areas in the chest and abdomen. This can also occur in persons with spinal arthritis, or disk or other disorders. Trichotillomania and trichokryptomania are neurotic manifestations, characterized by continually plucking or breaking scalp or eyelid hair. It is an obsessive-compulsive manifestation perhaps best helped by referral to a psychiatrist skilled in hypnosis, or at least in the instruction of autohypnosis.

Phobias

ACAROPHOBIA.—An obsession with digging out small parasites from the skin is a pitiful condition for which there appears to be no hope. Such patients bring in bits of skin (and occasionally insects!) in jars and bottles and sometimes taped to slides for the physician to look at in the hope that he will confirm the righteousness of their belief. Again hypnosis offers some help.

SYPHILOPHOBIA.—This fear of having syphilis can lead to suicide and should be treated with batteries of blood tests, argument, persuasion and reaffirmation periodically.

BROMIDROSIPHOBIA.—A patient's belief that his sweat has a repulsive odor is most difficult to treat and may be an inner manifestation of dementia praecox. Obsession with scalp odor is another example of this.

Neurotic Excoriation

Digging and picking at the accessible areas of the skin produce a myriad of dug-out, scabbed-over small excoriations. Often these marks are produced by the patient's attempt to dig out a persistently difficult hair (real or imagined) with forceps and a magnifying glass. Anyone who has chased an evasive splinter can realize the mechanism. Occlusion by Gelocast or

Elastoplast dressing heals the lesions, but it is seldom that the patient can be induced to permanently desist. Again hypnosis and Atarax treatment help.

Factitial Dermatitis

This condition produces bizarre destructive lesions, *consciously* inflicted by the patient in a desire to avoid duty or elicit sympathy or other compensation. A weird variety of this condition is when the patient tries to induce others to produce the mutilation, as in a patient I had once who imitated the symptoms of acute abdomen disorder so thoroughly that she had had 16 laparotomies over a period of a few years!

Trophic Skin Changes

Occasionally the dermatologist will be consulted to assist in the treatment of such changes after section of the gasserian ganglion for tic douloureux. The trigeminal nerve-supplied area, when unilaterally deprived of its sensory protection, becomes extremely susceptible to cold, heat, wind, soap and water, and sun, and may suffer repeated attacks of inflammation and dry desquamation. Steroid protective creams for the skin and protective glasses for the eyes, if needed, serve to inhibit the severity of these changes.

Mal Perforans

Degenerative changes in the dorsal column of the spinal cord leading to absence of pain sensation on the sole of the foot produce a deeply invading ulcer of the sole of the foot, usually at the ball, due to the whacking of the head of the metatarsal bones against the ground on walking. The skin destruction is severe and painless. (See p. 198, PCAD.) It is seen in persons with tabes, diabetic neuropathy, leprosy and arteriosclerosis as well. Padding and hygiene are essential.

Causalgia

Peripheral nerve injury can produce periodic attacks of burning pain and intense sensitivity to cold with or without trophic changes in the joints and skin of an individual extremity. There is no specific treatment, the object being to protect the area involved from injury and to increase blood flow perhaps by administering vasodilating drugs occasionally, such as Priscoline (Ciba) 1 Lontab (80 mg) twice a day. Side effects such as flushing usually disappear after continuance of the treatment.

REFERENCES

1. Silverberg, P. S., et al.: Cholestyramine in uraemic pruritus, Br. Med. J. 1:752, 1977.
2. Gilchrest, B. A., Rowe, J. W., Brown, R. S., Steinman, T. I., and Arndt, K. A.: Relief of uremic pruritus with ultraviolet phototherapy, N. Engl. J. Med. 297:136, 1977.
3. Jasionowski, E. A., and Jasionowski, P.: Topical progesterone in treatment of vulvar dystrophy, Am. J. Obstet. Gynecol. 127:667, 1977.
4. Pasieczny, J. A. H.: The treatment of balanitis xerotica obliterans with testosterone propionate ointment, Acta Derm. Venereol. 57: 275, 1977.
5. Sutton, R. L., Jr.: *Diseases of the Skin* (11th ed.; St. Louis: C. V. Mosby Co., 1956), p. 872.
6. Salmanowitz, V. J., and Orentreich, H.: Cutaneous corticosteroid injection and amaurosis, Arch. Dermatol. 110:729, 1974.

SUGGESTED READINGS

British Journal of Dermatology
International Journal of Dermatology
Journal of the American Medical Association
Lancet

Formulary

1. Lotio alba, for acne and rosacea; strength can be varied

Rx. (A)	Zinc sulfate	4.0	(8.0) (12.0) (16.0)
	Rose water q.s. ad	60.0	
(B)	Potassium sulfuretta	4.0	(8.0) (12.0) (16.0)
	Rose water q.s. ad	60.0	

Mix A and B after filtering B.
M. Ft. Lotio. Shake well and keep tightly closed.
Sig: Apply at night. Beware chapping.

2. Calamine lotion USP; soothing, cooling, absorptive

Rx.	Calamine	8.0
	Zinc oxide	8.0
	Glycerin	2.0
	Bentonite magma	25.0
	Lime water q.s. ad	100.0

Sig: Daub on p.r.n.

3. Menthol-camphor antipruritic lotion

Rx.	Menthol	0.25
	Camphor	1.0
	Calamine	
	Zinc oxide $\overline{aa}$	10.0
	Glycerin	2.5
	Bentonite magma	45.0
	Lime water q.s. ad	120.0

M. Ft. Lotio
Sig: Daub on p.r.n.

Rx.	Menthol	2.5
	Spirit of camphor	
	Alcohol $\overline{aa}$ q.s. ad	120.0

Sig: Daub on p.r.n.

4. "Prickly heat" lotion

Rx.	Resorcin	2.0
	Sulfur precipitate	5.0
	Zinc oxide	20.0
	Talc	20.0
	Glycerin	10.0

(balance of formula on next page)

Lime water	35.0
70% Alcohol q.s. ad	120.0

M. Ft. Lotio

Sig: Daub on p.r.n.

5. Modified calamine liniment (Sulzberger's variant of Pusey's lotion)

		Thin	Thick
Rx.	Tragacanth powder	4.0	1.25
	Phenol	0.66	0.8
	Glycerin	0.66	0.75
	Prepared calamine	30.0	30.0
	Zinc oxide	30.0	30.0
	Olive oil	120.0	120.0
	Distilled water q.s. ad	240.0	240.0

6. Cold cream, USP XVII

Rx.	Spermaceti	12.5
	White wax	12.0
	Mineral oil	56.0
	Sodium borate	0.5
	Purified water q.s. ad	100.0

7. Vleminckx solution, can be supplied as Vlem-Dome packets (Dome Co.) which contain about 60% calcium polysulfate, 5% sulfur and 3% calcium thiosulfate. One packet per pint of warm water makes the solution. Sig: Compress 15 minutes with cloths (tarnishes silver). Useful in treating cystic acne. The local skilled pharmacist can compound it as follows:

Rx.	Vleminckx solution	60.0
	Saturated solution of zinc sulfate	40.0
	Glycerin	10.0

Add 40 gm zinc sulfate to 50 cc water, and stir with a little heat so you can get a saturated solution. Then decant 40 cc into a mortar, and add Vleminckx solution gradually and stir. Glycerin will assist this.

Dispense in wide-mouth jar and label one tablespoon in three-fourths glass hot water as a compress. Avoid silver spoons.

8. Magma alba

Rx.	Saturated solution of sulfurated potash	30.0
	Saturated solution of zinc sulfate	20.0
	Glycerin	5.0
	Odor q.s., e.g., 10 drops	

Though tricky to make, the resultant paste is effective in treating all types of acne.

Sig: Apply at night.

9. Two-bottle lotio alba

Rx. Bottle 1 – Saturated solution sulfurated potash
Bottle 2 – Saturated solution zinc sulfate

Mix equal parts (eyedropper measuring tops) in third container, allowing the gas to escape. Then apply at once.

Lascoff's Apothecary (New York City) supplies a finely made two-bottle lotio alba as a kit, which they will mail to patients. A prescription has to be written out for 25% two-bottle lotio alba and then mailed to them.

10. Tars

Rx. A. Coal tar ointment USP = 1% Coal tar in zinc oxide paste (with polysorbate 80, 0.5%)

B. Eczema paste = 5% cade oil in zinc oxide paste

C. Psoriasis starter

Rx.	Salicylic acid	0.6
	Phenol	0.6
	Liquid carbonis detergens	3.0 to 6.0
	USP Hydrophilic ointment q.s. ad	60.0
	Sig: Rub in b.i.d.	

D. Tar paste (Doak) = about 1% tar extract in Lassar's paste, useful in treating eczema

11. Scalp night ointment (psoriasis)

Rx. A.	Salicylic acid	1.0
	Hydrarg. amm.	15.0
	Aquaphor q.s. ad	60.0

Sig: Rub in scalp overnight. Shampoo in morning.

B. An oil:

Salicylic acid	1.0
Ammoniated mercury	7.5
Castor oil	10.0

Olive oil q.s. ad 100.0
M. Ft. Lotio
Sig: Rub in overnight and cover with shower cap. Shampoo in the morning.

When shampooing an oily or greasy head, put shampoo in dry *first*, emulsify the oil, and *then* add water *last* before rinsing.

12. Psoriasis (for nonhairy areas)
Rx. Salicylic acid 0.6
Hydrarg. amm. 3.0
Liquid carbonis detergens 3.0
USP Hydrophilic ointment ad 60.0
13. "Freckle peeler," for bleaching, light peeling, helpful in flat warts
Rx. Camphor 1.0
Salicylic acid 2.0
Bichloride of mercury 0.06
Alcohol q.s. ad 50.0
Sig: Paint on t.i.d. until peeling occurs, then stop and later resume.
14. Ophthalmic mercury ointments
A. Yellow oxide of mercury 1%, for sties and blepharitis. Sig: Insert inner lower lid o.n. and p.r.n.
B. Ammoniated mercury ointment 3%, useful for nits on lashes. Sig: Rub in o.n.
C. Hydrarg. bichlor. ophthalmic ointment 0.03%, as above.
15. Chrysarobin ointment
Rx. Chrysarobin 0.1 to 0.5 to 5% in petrolatum q.s. ad 60.
Sig: Rub in once or twice daily. Use fresh chrysarobin; stains, useful in treating psoriasis.
16. Anthralin ointment
Dermik made this 0.1, 0.25, 0.5 and 1%; supplies are still available.
17. Vioform (Ciba), can be used in powder form for extemporaneous Rx. Also, 3% cream and 3% ointment with or without hydrocortisone in 1% or 0.5% concentration.
18. Castellani's paint
Rx. Basic fuchsin solution (5% alcoholic) 10.0

Boric acid	1.0
Acetone	5.0
Resorcinol	10.0
Phenol 5% aqueous to make	100.0

Add the fuchsin to phenol and filter; add boric acid and let the substance stand for 2 hours. Add acetone and wait 2 hours. Add resorcinol. It stains.

19. Soft corns—a good substitute for Quatrasol is as follows:

Rx.	Urea crystals	7.5
	Aqueous Zephiran (1:750)	7.5
	Cordran lotion (Lilly)	15.0

Sig: Paint t.i.d. for soft corns.

20. Hairy brown tongue

Rx. Podophyllin 2–20% in alcohol and acetone.

Sig: Paint daily.

21. Wart paint

Rx.	A.	Podophyllin resin	7.5
		Acetone	
		Tincture benzoin aa q.s. ad	15.0

This will dissolve if warmed a little and allowed to sit overnight.

B.	Salicylic acid	1.5
	Lactic acid	1.5
	Glacial acetic acid	1.5
	Collodion flex q.s. ad	15.0

Make a paint. Sig: Apply daily until irritation occurs. Then rest and later resume. Clean up with nail polish remover periodically.

C. Cantharone (Ingram Pharm. Co., San Francisco); 0.7 cantharidin in collodion, useful but sometimes tricky, consult manufacturer's instructions, e.g., in the Physicians Desk Reference.

D. Glutaraldehyde wart paint

Bottle 1, 25% glutaraldehyde solution (aqueous)

Bottle 2,	sodium bicarbonate	2.3
	Tween 80	0.2
	Water q.s. ad	100.0

Mix bottles 1 and 2 equal parts with an eye dropper in a small container (shelf life less than 2 weeks) and use this to rub and tattoo into the plantar warts daily.

22. Steroid preparations—stable with a long shelf life
    A. Hydrocortisone—less expensive and can be easily compounded using the hydrocortisone powder in the USP hydrophilic ointment, or aquaphor, or can be extemporized in other ways. Numerous manufacturers make 1% cream and ointment in all suitable sizes.
    B. Fluorinated preparations
        1. Betamethasone or Valisone (Schering) comes as a cream in 0.1%, 5, 15 and 60 gm tubes; ointment 0.1%, 5, 15 and 60 gm tubes; lotion 0.1%, 20 and 60 cc plastic bottles; spray 0.15%, 80 gm; reduced strength 0.01%, 15 and 60 gm tubes.
        2. Betamethasone dipropionate (Schering) Diprosone, cream and ointment 0.05%; lotion 15 and 45 gm tubes.

           Flurobate (Texas Pharmacal) comes as a cream, 0.025%, 15 and 60 gm tubes; gel, 0.025%, 15 and 60 gm tubes.

           Benisone (Warner Chilcott) comes as a cream, 0.025%, 15 and 60 gm tubes; gel, 0.025%, 15 and 60 gm tubes.
        3. Dexa Methasone (Merck) Decadron cream, spray 90 gm; ophthalmic preparations 0.1%. The spray is especially useful for nickel-sensitive women who want to wear earrings. A spray on the earlobes and earrings protects for about 4 hours.
        4. Fluocinolone or Synalar (Syntex) or Neo-Synalar cream, 15 and 60 gm tubes only; ointment or cream 0.025%, 15 and 60 gm tubes, 120 gm and 425 gm jars; cream 0.01%, 5, 45 and 60 gm tubes; lotion 0.01%, 20 cc and 60 cc plastic bottles; emollient cream 0.025%, 15 and 60 gm tubes; High potency cream 0.25%, 5 and 12 gm tubes.

           Fluonid (Derm Arts) cream and ointment 0.01%, 0.025%, 15 and 60 gm tubes and 425 gm jars; solution 0.01%, 20 and 60 gm plastic bottles.

5. Fluocinonide—Lidex (Syntex) 0.05% cream, ointment and gel (Topsyn), 15, 30 and 60 gm tubes. Very effective in treating psoriasis, especially the ointment.
6. Fluorandrenolide, Cordran (Lilly) cream and ointment, 0.05%, 7½, 15 and 60 gm tubes, 225 gm jars; cream and ointment, 0.025%, 30 and 60 gm tubes, 225 gm jars; lotion, 0.05%, 20 and 60 gm plastic bottles; tape, 0.05% in small and large sizes.
7. Halcinonide Halog (Squibb) cream 0.1%, 15 and 60 gm tubes, 240 gm jars.
8. Triamcinolone—Aristocort (Lederle) 0.1% topical; cream and ointment (A is more lubricating) (acetate) supplied in 15 and 75 gm tubes, ½ lb and 5 lb jars; and 0.5% topical cream and ointment, 15 gm tubes, ½ lb jars; 0.025% topical cream, 15 and 75 gm tubes, ½ lb and 5 lb jars.

   Kenalog (Squibb) (Acetonide), 0.1% cream and ointment in 15, 60 and 80 gm jars, 240 gm, 5¼ lb jars; 0.1% cream and ointment in 15, 60 and 80 gm tubes, 240 gm jars; 0.5% cream and ointment, 20 gm tubes; 0.025% cream and ointment, 15 and 80 gm tubes, 240 gm jars; 0.1% lotion, 15 and 60 cc squeeze bottles; 0.025% lotion, 60 cc squeeze bottle; spray in 50 or 150 gm spray can. Kenalog 0.1% in Orabase for treating canker sores, 5 gm tube.
9. Locorten (Ciba) cream 0.03% fluoromethasone, 5, 15 and 60 gm tubes.

   Oxylone (Upjohn) cream 0.025% fluoromethalone, 15, 60 and 120 gm tubes.

C. Other preparations

Medrol and Neo-Medrol (methylprednisolone) creams (Upjohn); Neo-Medrol and Medrol cream 0.25% and 1.0% with or without neomycin 7.5, 30 gm, 1.5 oz tubes.

Tridesilon (Dome Co.) cream and ointment 0.05%, 5, 15 and 60 gm tubes, 5 lb jars, cream only.

Note: Continued long-term use of topical steroids, particularly the fluorinated steroid creams, can produce atrophy, telangiectasia and perioral dermatitis resembling acne with seborrhea. If occlusive techniques are used, spreading folliculitis or aggravation of any preexisting minor infection can occur.

D. Steroids combined with antibiotics and antimonilial agents

Mycolog cream (Squibb)—Nystatin, neomycin, gramicidin and Kenalog especially mentioned because of occasionally markedly superior effects in treating seborrheic dermatitis and nummular eczema.

23. Topical antibiotic preparations

A. Polysporin ointment (Burroughs & Wellcome) hits gram-negative bacteria except *Proteus*, polymyxin, bacitracin (no neomycin).

B. Neosporin ointment (B & W), polymyxin, bacitracin, and neomycin.

C. Neosporin G cream (B & W), polymyxin, gramicidin and neomycin.

D. Neosporin aerosol (B & W), polymyxin, bacitracin and neomycin. Neomycin hits gram-negative organisms.

E. Neosporin powder (B & W), polymyxin, bacitracin and neomycin.

F. Neopolycin (Pitman Moore), polymyxin, bacitracin and neomycin in a carbowax base.

G. Aerosporin otic solution (B & W), polymyxin and bacitracin (no neomycin).

H. Chloromycetin cream 1% (Parke-Davis), vanishing base, 1 oz tubes only.

I. Garamycin cream or ointment 0.1% (Schering), gentamicin hits *Pseudomonas, Proteus, E. coli* and some gram-positive cocci.

J. Spectrocin cream and ointment (Squibb), also lotion, gramicidin and neomycin.

K. Terramycin ointment and powder (Pfizer), 3% terramycin, 1% hydrocortisone.

L. Colymycin S. Otic (Warner Chilcott), colistin, hydrocortisone, neomycin, effective in treating external otitis, hits *Pseudomonas, Aerobacter*, and *E. coli.*

M. Bacitracin ointment, plain (various manufacturers) hits gram-positive cocci, tetanus, diphtheria.
N. Ilotycin cream 0.5% (Dista division of Lilly), useful in treating coral red-fluorescing erythrasma.

24. Antibacterial cleansers and antiseptics
A. Betadine shampoo and skin cleanser (Purdue Fredericks), 1 oz and 4 oz, povidone-iodine preparations reported to kill bacteria, fungi, viruses, protozoa and yeasts.
B. Prepodyne scrub (West Co.), poloxamer iodine in lathering base, also on swabs. Available in 1 pint and 1 gallon bottles, action similar to above.
C. Phisohex (Winthrop) should not be used on skins through which it can be absorbed, e.g., premature infants or burned skin, since cerebral injury can occur. It is a bacteriostatic cleansing agent, but requires continued use for true effectiveness.
D. Zephiran chloride (Winthrop) (1:750 aqueous) (1:750 tinted tincture) (spray tinted tincture 1:750) Benzalkonium chloride USP, an excellent antiseptic, see manufacturer's data in Physicians Desk Reference. Can be used as preoperative preparation or aftercare to daub on small wounds and to store instruments.
E. Mercurial preparation, e.g., tincture of merthiolate 1:1,000, mercurochrome 2%, mercury bichloride aqueous 1:1,000, useful for treating small cuts and infections.
F. Hibiclens (Stuart), excellent antibacterial effect.

25. Antifungal preparations
A. Antimonilial, vulvovaginitis, Propion Gel (Wyeth); Mycostatin suppositories (Squibb), also cream, ointment, powder and oral tabs; AVC Improved (National Drug) contains allantoin and sulfa; Sporostacin cream and ointment (Ortho), benzalkonium and hydantoin; Candeptin (Schmid Labs.), candicidin, vaginal tabs, ointment or vaginal capsules; Fungizone (Squibb), amphotericin B, cream, lotion, ointment, not recommended, Gyne-lotrimin vaginal tabs (Delban), excellent.
B. Paronychia, Sopronol solution (Wyeth), sodium pro-

pionate and caprylate; 20% sodium caprylate (Rx by any good pharmacist) solution; 3% thymol iodide in chloroform (again Rx), 3% chrysarobin in chloroform (black, again Rx), 1% gentian violet aqueous—stains; Fungizone solution (Squibb), not recommended; Romanol (light iodine) (Jamol Labs) Lotrimin lotion (Delbay), excellent.

C. Tinea versicolor, Akrinol ointment (Schering), akrisorcin, 50 gm, has to be used for 6 weeks at least twice daily; Photographer's hypo, or 20% sodium thiosulfate aqueous twice daily for months; Fostex or any other sulfur soap, wash daily; Selsun (3% selenium sulfide suspension) (Abbott) overnight, two or three nights a week, washing off in morning; Tinver lotion (Barnes Hind), 25% sodium thiosulfate solution has to be used twice daily for a long time, 5-oz bottles.

D. Dermatophytes, 3% salicylic 3% sulfur in USP hydrophilic ointment or petrolatum; 3% salicylic acid and 6% benzoic acid in USP hydrophilic ointment (½ Whitfield's); Desenex (5% undecylenic acid, 20% zinc undecylenate) (Pharmacraft) powder in morning and ointment at night; Tinactin (Schering) tolnaftate, powder, solution, cream and aerosol 1%, can sensitize, but often strikingly effective; Halotex (Westwood), Haloprogin 1%, cream and solution, often very effective; Micatin (J & J), miconazole cream; Verdefam liquid and cream combination (Texas Pharm.), helpful; Castellani's paint, excellent in treating tinea cruris; Onycho-phytex (Unimed) borotannic complex, excellent for nails.

E. Griseofulvin preparations, Fulvicin (Schering) tablets, 125 ultrafine, 250 and 500 mg; Grifulvin V (McNeil), tablets 125, 250 and 500 mg, and suspension 125/tsp; Grisactin (Ayerst), capsules and tablets, 125, 250 and 500 mg, Gris-Peg (Dorsey), 125 mg ultramicronized tablets.

26. Antihistamines

Allerest tablets (Pharmacraft), primarily for pollen and

inhalant allergies, one three times a day after meals (contains two antihistamines, chlorpheniramine maleate and methapyrilene fumurate, and a decongestant phenylpropanolamine HCl).

Actidil (B & W), triprolidine HCl tablets, 2.5 mg. syrup, 1.25 mg/tsp, usually given two or three times daily.

Benadryl (Parke Davis), diphenhydramine HCl capsules, 25, 50 and elixir 12.5 mg/tsp, usual dose three times a day after meals, also as injection 50 mg/ampule.

Dimetane (Robins), brompheniramine maleate tablets 4 mg, extentabs 8 gm and 12 mg, elixir 2 mg/tsp, also injectable 10 mg/cc or 100 mg/cc; has anticholinergic effects.

Chlor-Trimeton (Schering), chlorpheniramine maleate tablets 4 mg, repetabs 8 mg and 12 mg, also Teldrin (Smith, Kline & French) 8 mg and 12 mg, long-acting; also syrup Chlor-Trimeton, 2 mg/tsp and injection 10 mg/cc ampule.

Atarax (Roerig), hydroxyzine HCl tablets 10 mg, 25 mg, 50 mg and 100 mg, syrup 10 mg/tsp, antihistamine, anticholinergic and sedative.

Vistaril (Pfizer), hydroxyzine pamoate, oral suspension 25 mg/tsp, capsules 25, 50 and 100 mg, intramuscular; solution supplied as 25 mg/cc or 50 mg/cc.

Periactin (Merck, Sharp & Dohme), cyproheptadine HCl tablets 4 mg and syrup 2 mg/tsp; often makes people very drowsy.

Phenergan (Wyeth), promethazine HCl tablets 12.5, 25 and 50 mg, also syrup 6.25 mg/tsp or 25 mg/tsp; it is a phenothiazine and occasionally strange muscle spasms can occur.

Temaril (S.K.F.), trimeprazine tablets 2.5 mg, spansule 5.0 mg, and syrup 2.5 mg/tsp; in addition to antihistamines and antiseritonin activity, it has a central effect in suppressing itching; it is a phenothiazine.

Pyribenzamine (Ciba), tripelennamine, tablets 25 and 50 mg, lontabs, 50 mg and 100 mg, syrup 25 mg/tsp.

Forhistal (Ciba), dimethindene maleate, tablets 1 mg, syrup 1 mg/tsp.

Polaramine (Schering), dexchlorpheniramine maleate, repetabs 6 mg, 2 mg tablets, syrup 2 mg/tsp.

Tacaryl (Westwood), methdilazine HCl (a phenothiazine), tablets 8 mg, syrup 4 mg/tsp.

The main side effects of antihistamines are drowsiness or dryness of the mouth, and occasionally dizziness.

27. Acne preparations (proprietary)

A. Cleansers

Acne-Aid detergent soap (Stiefel), 6.3% sulfated surfactants.

Acnaveen soap (Cooper), oatmeal, 2% sulfur, 2% salicylic acid in soap-free surfactant; excellent for treating comedones.

Fostex cake and cream (Westwood), sulfur 2%, salicylic acid 2%, wetting agents and surfactants.

Proseca—"dry wash" (Westwood), sulfur 4%, polyoxyethylene lauryl ether in combination of cleansers and wetting agents.

Acne-Dome cleanser (Dome), soybean paste with supplied sponge; this is the mildest cleansing paste; good for sensitive skins.

Brasivol 1 and 2 (fine, medium, coarse) (Stiefel), abrasive cleanser with aluminum oxide scrubbing particles.

Ionax scrub (Owen) and foam, benzalkonium chloride 0.2% in blend of polyoxyethylene ethers and the scrub polyoxyethylene granules, quite effective in treating comedone acne.

Pernox scrub (Westwood), similar to above but without the benzalkonium and with 2% sulfur and 1.5% salicylic acid; it is sometimes irritating, but effective; 60 seconds of scrubbing with lots of water is enough.

Plain sulfur soaps are manufactured by many different companies, but they tend to chap the skin.

Neko soap (Parke-Davis), a very strong, almost caustic soap.

Polybrade (Texas Pharmacal), sodium lauryl sulfate polyoxyethylene granules with fatty acid also.

Fat solvents, such as Sebanil solution (Texas Pharmacal), Therapads (Fuller), Tyroderm packets (Summers) are useful for very hot weather or where washing facilities are few.

B. Nighttime cream or paste

Sulfo-lac (Kelgy), mild vanishing polysulfide cream.

Vleminckx and magma alba (see no. 8) and lotio alba (no. 1).

C. Anytime, clear

Benzoyl peroxide lotions, e.g., Benoxyl 5% or 10% (Stiefel); Persadox (Texas); Panoxyl gel, 5% or 10% (Stiefel); Benzagel 5% or 10% (Dermik); Desquam-X 5% or 10% (Westwood); Persadox gel (Texas); Vanoxide (Dermik); Benzoyl peroxide with chlorhydroxyquinilone 0.25% = Benoxide (Dermik) 5% and 10% benzoyl peroxide lotion (Dermik); Xerac 5-BP (Person & Covey), slightly less irritation.

Sulfur-resorcin preparations can be extemporized in alcohol or ordered, such as Contrablem (Texas) 5% sulfur, 2% resorcin, or Transact (Westwood), 6% polyoxyethylene lauryl ether and 2% micropulverized sulfur in an alcohol gel.

Retin-A lotion and cream, while clear, are occasionally extremely irritating, the cream less so, and the gel even less than that, 0.025% recently introduced; patients have to be warned to not wash for an hour before applying it and to avoid sun while using it (e.g., do not use in June, July and August in northern climes) and when redness, burning, chapping or dryness occurs, rest at once for 5 or 6 days.

D. Anytime, tinted

Liquimat (Texas), comes in many shades, cosmetically elegant, a 5% sulfur lotion with alcohol.

Acne-Aid lotion (Stiefel), 10% sulfur, 10% alcohol, well made and effective.

Fostril (Westwood), same as Transact, but tinted, with sulfur, quite effective.

Acnomel (S.K.F.), sulfur and resorcin.

Dermik products: Sulfacet R, with sodium sulfacetamide 10%; sulfur 5%; Rezamid, resorcinol 2%, sulfur 5%, parachlorometaxylenol 0.5%, alcohol 28.5%; Postacne, sulfur 2%, alcohol 25%. There are many others such as Resulin (Almay), Sulforcin Base, (Texas), Microsyn (Syntex), Clearasil (Vick) and Komed (Barnes-Hind).

28. Antiseborrheic preparations

3% sulfur 3% salicylic acid in USP hydrophilic ointment.

Pragmatar (S.K.F.), as above, but with the addition of a small amount of tar distillate 4%.

Sulforcin lotion 5% sulfur, 2% resorcin (Texas).

Mycolog cream (Squibb), Kenalog, gramicidin, neomycin and Mycostatin (preserved with ethylene diamine and thimerosal), beware.

Rx. 0.5% salicylic acid, 2% ammoniated mercury, 10% zinc oxide in aquaphor, every night to the face.

Sodium salumyd ophthalmic ointment (Schering), sulfacetamide 10% for blepharitis; also Metimyd ophthalmic ointment and solution, similar but with prednisone added, very helpful; yellow oxide of mercury 1%.

Selsun (Abbott) for seborrhea capitis, three times a week to start, then gradually less often over a 6–8 week period. This is the best antiseborrheic preparation available; if used alone, the hair becomes oily rather quickly, so using Dara shampoo (Owen) before and afterward helps this.

Capitrol shampoo (Westwood) is a good anti-seborrheic shampoo, although it can yellow gray hair.

A. Also, for otherwise intractable seborrhea capitis, Ol. Sulf., a useful overnight preparation, consists of

Rx.	Salicylic acid	1.0
	Sulfur ppt.	7.5
	Castor oil	10.0
	Olive oil q.s. ad	100.0

Sig: Make a lotion and rub in scalp overnight and wash out in the morning, putting the shampoo in before wetting the hair. Wear a shower cap to bed.

B. Diasporal cream (Doak), 3% sulfur and 3% salicylic acid in a washable base. Rub in overnight, shampoo in the morning.

C. Scalp lotion for blondes:

Rx.	Thymol	0.1
	Mercury bichloride	0.1
	Salicylic acid	2.0
	Tincture of capsicum	5.0
	essential oil q.s. for odor	
	50% alcohol q.s. ad	100.0

M. Ft. Lotio, Sig: Rub small amounts into scalp daily.

Sebucare (Westwood) is also suitable for white hair, imparting a sheen.

D. Scalp lotion for brunettes

Resorcitate (Almay), with or without oil, contains salicylic acid and resorcin monoacetate.

E. A similar formula using bay rum:

Rx.	Salicylic acid	1.2
	Resorcin monoacetate	4.0
	Mercury bichloride	3.0
	Bay rum q.s. ad	120.0

M. Ft. Lotio, Sig: Rub into scalp with fingers.

F. Other good antiseborrheic shampoos are Meted (Texas Pharmacal), Sebulex (Westwood), Metasep (Summers), Zincon (Lederle) and Ionil (Owen), all sometimes very effective.

For seborrheic dermatitis of the groin and axilla: Vioform lotion 1% (Ciba) is excellent, as is Mycolog cream occasionally.

29. Sabouraud's (Stoke's modifier of Sabouraud's ointment)

Rx.	Oleum Cadine (Merck)	12.0
	Sulfur ppt.	6.0
	Salicylic acid	3.0
	USP hydrophilic ointment q.s. ad	60.0

Sig.: Rub in scalp overnight. Shampoo in morning, putting shampoo in *first*, adding water last.

30. Antiparasitic preparations

Pediculocides: Kwell lotion and shampoo, also cream (Reed and Carnrick), gamma isomer of benzene hexachloride 1%; manufacturers recommend one application, leaving it on 24 hours and then rinsing and repeating in 4 days. It takes more than this to be effective; mildly drying. A-200 Pyrrinate (Norcliff), reputed to be effective. Topicide (Lilly) and Cuprex unfortunately are no longer available, nor is DDT, which as a 1% powder was helpful. Ten percent kerosene in mineral oil is fairly effective if nits are difficult to remove, but easier and safer is water and white vinegar equal parts left in 15 minutes and then showered off.

Scabicides: Kwell, as above, but must be used over a week at least. Benzyl benzoate emulsion, the best. Supplied as an emulsion 50%, e.g., the Burroughs & Wellcome preparation, but obtainable from the Lannet Co. It is used diluted 50-50, about a cupful covers the body and rubbed in from the neck down every night for 3 nights, changing clothes and bedding on the morning of the fourth day, repeating once a week. Eurax cream (Geigy), "crotamiton," antipruritic and sensitizing, occasionally very useful for treating stubborn resistant nodules in scabies.

31. Soaps and shampoos

Mild soaps, Basis (Beiersdorf), Oilatum (Stiefel), Kauma (Stiefel), Neutragenia, Alpha-Keri (Westwood). Phisoderm (normal, oily and dry skin types), Soy-Dome cleanser, Lowila cake and Acidolate are all "soapless" cleansers. Aveenobar (Cooper) and Emulave (Cooper) are mild oatmeal cleansers.

Antibacterial soaps, Dial, Zest, Lifebuoy, Safeguard, Palmolive Gold, Irish Spring, Coast, Gamophen, Hibiclens.

Mild shampoos, Daragen (so-called hair-repair shampoo), Ionil shampoo contain benzalkonium chloride;polypeptides and coconut fatty acids, soapless (Owen); Purpose (Johnson & Johnson), similar to their baby shampoo; DHS shampoo (Person & Covey); Pernox

(Westwood), reported to help oily hair; Drysum (Summers) has acetone, helps oily hair; Panoxyl (Stiefel) also helps dry oily hair. Dara is a good shampoo.

Tar shampoos, 10% L.C.D. (coal tar solution USP) in tincture of green soap is an old standby; Iocon Gel (Owen); Zetar (Dermik); Sebutone (Westwood); Ionil T. (Owen); Polytar (Stiefel); Pentrax (Texas Pharmacal); Tersatar (Doak).

32. Peeler for oily acne (Dr. McKee's)

Rx.	Resorcin	4.0
	Sodium hyposulfite	15.0
	Alcohol USP	30.0
	Witch hazel q.s. ad	120.0
	Sig: Apply to face t.i.d.	

33. Efudex (Roche), 5-fluouracil as solution 2% or 5%, 10 cc or 5% 25 gm tube, cream; used in clearing actinic keratoses via inflammatory reaction.

Fluoroplex (G.S. Herbert), 1% solution, 30 cc bottle, or 1% topical cream 30 gm; used as clearing agent in keratoses via the inflammatory reaction. Strong triamcinolone cream used with it may, if fluorinated, cause erythema to persist.

34. Depigmenting agents, with sunblock: Eldopaque Forte (Elder), 4% and 2%; without sunblock: Eldoquin 2% or 4%, lotion or ointment.

35. Repigmentation, 0.5% Oxsoralen alcoholic solution (usually start with 0.1% and short black light exposures, increasing the time) is locally applied (Cambridge Chemists).

36. Cream for fissured hands (D.E.H. Cleveland)

Rx.	Salicylic acid	0.6
	Balsam of peru	1.0
	Oleum ricini (castor oil)	4.0
	Hydrous lanolin	10.0
	Petrolatum alba q.s. ad	30.0

37. Eczema cream (Dr. Harry Katz)

Rx.	Menthol	0.2
	Phenol	0.5
	L. C. D.	3.0

Petrolatum
Neobase q.s. ad 60.0

38. Birch tar tincture

Rx.	Rectified oil of birch tar	5.0
	Alcohol (96%)	50.0
	Ether ad	100.0

M. Ft. Pigmentum
Sig: Paint scalp as directed.

39. Ichthyosis (U. Wile's old formula)

Rx.	Salicylic acid	1.0
	Cocoa butter	10.0
	Unguentum aquae rosae USP ad	100.0

Rx. Glycerin
Camphor water
70% Alcohol
equal parts of each to make 180

40. Patchy nummular eczema (Sulzberger & Wolf's formula)

Rx.	Resorcin	2.4
	L. C. D.	12.0
	Red sulfide of mercury	1.0
	Zinc oxide	20.0
	Talc	20.0
	Glycerin	10.0
	Water	
	Alcohol q.s. ad	120.0

41. Creams for bleaching hair
"Jolen" (proprietary)

Rx.	Superoxal (Merck)	5.0
	Unibase (Parke-Davis)	10.0

42. Makeup base

Rx. Zinc oxide
Talc
Calamine
Glycerin $\overline{aa}$ 10.0
Alcohol 95%
Water $\overline{aa}$ 40.0

Neutracolor 1.0 to 3.0 (usually 2.0) to the required shade.

43. Nummular eczema (additional formula)

Rx. 2% Hydrocortisone in Terramycin ointment (turns dark with time)

SUGGESTED READING

Physicians' Desk Reference
AMA Drug Evaluations, 3d ed.

List of Product Sources*

Balloon cushion (ROHO)
ROHO Research & Development Co., P.O. Box 658, Belleville, IL 62222 (p. 160)

Bismuth subsalicylate
Barclay Pharmacy, 18th & Spruce Streets, Philadelphia, PA 19103 (p. 134)

Comb, steel fine
Cereal Soap Co., Inc., P.O. Box 329, Boonton, NJ 07005 (p. 327)

Creams, protective
The West Co., 42-16 West Street, Long Island City, NY 11101 (p. 296)

DNCB – dinitrochlorobenzene
Aldrich Chemical Co., 940 W. St. Paul Avenue, Milwaukee, WI 53233 (p. 59)

Dressing, spray (Aeroplast)
Medical-Surgical Products Div., Parke, Davis & Co., GPO Box 118, Joseph Campau Ave. At the River, Detroit, MI 48232 (p. 226)

Ferric subsulfate solution (Monsell's solution)
J. T. Baker Chemical Co., Phillipsburg, NJ 08865 (p. 257)

Gloves, surgical
B. F. Goodrich Industrial Engineered Systems Div., Sun-

*Numbers in parentheses refer to pages where products are described.

dries Sales Dept., 500 S. Main St., Akron, OH 44318 (p. 280)

Pioneer Rubber Co., Div. of Sherwood Medical Industries, 1831 Olive St., St. Louis, MO 63103 (p. 280)

V. K. Gloves, P.O. Box 490083, Atlanta, GA 30349 (p. 280)

Herpes vaccine (Lupidon-G)

Bergedorfer Apotheke, Walter Mester D., 2050 Hamburg 80, Vierandenstrabe 15, West Germany (p. 47)

Hermal-Chemie Co., 2057 Reinbeck b. Hamburg, Danziger Strasse 5, West Germany (Kurt Herman) (p. 47)

Media, culture

GIBCO Diagnostics, 421 Merrimack St., Lawrence, MA 01843

Microbiologic Associates, Bldg. 100, Biggs Ford Road, Walkersville, MD 21793 (p. 123)

Nitrogen, liquid, method of applying (Foster Froster)

Medical Specialties, 3214 Howard Avenue, New Orleans, LA 70113 (p. 236)

Oleoresins, prepared

Hollister-Stier Labs., 550 Industrial Park Drive, Yeadon, PA 19050 (p. 272)

Port wine stain (Covermark)

Lydia O'Leary, 41 E. 57th Street, New York, NY 10022 (p. 246)

Shoes

Alden Shoe Co., Middleborough, MA 02346

G. H. Bass, Wilton, ME 04294 (p. 277)

Musebeck-Foot-So-Port Shoe Co., Forest & Westover, Oconomowoc, WI 53066 (p. 278)

Sandak, 1004 E. Orangefair Lane, Anaheim, CA 92803 (p. 278)

Shoes, arch supports for

H & W Orthopedic Arch Supports, Inc., 66-07 Myrtle Avenue, Brooklyn, NY 11227 (p. 299)

Shoes, box-toe (Celastic)

Celastic Box Toe Co., 609 Schuyler Avenue, Kearny, NJ 07032 (p. 277)

Shoes, pads for (Morton's)

Hersco Arch Products Corp., 137 E. 25th Street, New York, NY 10010 (p. 299)

Tars (Naftex Lascoff)

Lascoff's Pharmacy, 82d Street & Lexington Avenue, New York, NY 10016 (p. 23)

Tarpaste

Doak Pharmacol Company, 700 Shames Dr., Westbury, L.I., N.Y. 11590 (p. 24)

Index

C

T

U